POSTGRADUATE MEDICINE

Postgraduate Medicine

I. J. T. DAVIES

FRCP, FRCPE

Consultant Physician (Highland Health Board)
Raigmore Hospital, Inverness;
Regional Director of Postgraduate Medical Education
for Northern Scotland (Highlands & Western Isles);
Clinical Senior Lecturer in Medicine,
University of Aberdeen

Fourth edition

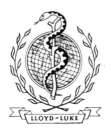

LLOYD-LUKE (MEDICAL BOOKS) LTD
49 NEWMAN STREET
LONDON
1983

FIRST EDITION 1969
Spanish translation 1971
SECOND EDITION 1972
Reprinted 1972
Italian translation 1974
THIRD EDITION 1977
FOURTH EDITION 1983

PRINTED AND BOUND IN ENGLAND BY
HAZELL WATSON AND VINEY LTD
AYLESBURY, BUCKS

ISBN: 0 85324 163 5

For

JOYCE, EDWIN, BENJAMIN AND ELEANOR

PREFACE TO FOURTH EDITION

I have revised the whole book, continuing to try and cater for those who require a reasonably concise, albeit personal, overview of general medicine. Basic medical knowledge is assumed, but where I know that biochemical or physiological principles are often misunderstood I have sometimes gone back to first principles. It might be questioned these days whether there is still a place for a single-author review of general medicine. However, it is known that consultant physicians with a special interest spend at least 80 per cent of their time doing general medicine; candidates for the MRCP diploma are still required to cover the whole span of general medicine—it does not therefore seem unreasonable that some of their examiners should be expected to do the same. The popularity among general physicians of the annual Royal College of Physicians Advanced Medicine Symposia, at which the range of topics is complete, signifies that general physicians still feel an obligation to have a working knowledge of each of the major specialties which make up internal medicine. The success of previous editions both in the UK and abroad testifies that the book fulfills a need.

I take heart from a quotation from Sir Geoffrey Vickers' *The Art of Judgement*:

"Even the dogs may eat the crumbs which fall from the rich man's table; and in these days, when the rich in knowledge eat such specialized food at such separate tables, only the dogs have a chance of a balanced diet."

In the United States, with medical relicensure mandatory and recertification so frequent, a book which provides a balanced die. of internal medicine should be especially valuable.

The eponyms are a personal quirk; they either intrigue or antagonise, and I hope the reader will comment. The bane of a book is the Index; I am most grateful to Mr Frank Wallis of Stratford-upon-Avon, who, in return for a donation to charity, has taken the burden from me.

IEUAN DAVIES

Lentran House
Lentran
By Inverness   IV3 6RL
September, 1982

PREFACE TO FIRST EDITION

Medical textbooks fall into two main groups: those intended for medical students and those which are large, comprehensive and intended mainly for reference purposes. It seemed to me that there was need for a book intended to be read from cover to cover which served the needs of those engaged in general medicine and which attempted to bridge the gap between the theoretical knowledge of the final year medical student and the practice of sound, safe and orthodox medicine.

Medical education has now achieved the status of a distinct discipline with the increasing recognition that the haphazard, do-it-yourself system of undergraduate and postgraduate medical education should be replaced by co-ordinated, well-taught and applicable courses of instruction. These courses require a great deal of enlightened thought, clear analysis of the problems, energy and expertise in their construction and delivery. I am grateful for the countless fruitful discussions I have had with friends and colleagues experienced in the problems of medical examination who have given considerable thought to the difficulties in overcoming the knowledge, experience and interest gaps.

Concepts, facts and ideas which I know are often ill-understood by those working for the membership diploma of one of the Royal Colleges of Physicians have been explained and amplified. I hope I have given some guidance to the important practical considerations in general medicine as well as crystallising some of the current problems.

Into one compact and convenient volume I have tried to distil the basic requirements of current postgraduate medicine which will be useful not only to general and specialist physicians but also to final-year medical students, to interested general practitioners, and to those working for surgical, anaesthetic and obstetrical postgraduate degrees.

In order to make the book as viable and useful as possible I would be pleased to hear from any reader who has views about other information that might have been included and grateful for guidance which would clarify any of the explanations.

I wish to express my sincere thanks to those who have given me so much encouragement; to the medical secretaries who have typed the manuscript and to the staff of the photographic department of Llandough Hospital who prepared the illustrations.

My thanks are due to the Editor of the *British Journal of Hospital Medicine* for permission to use the section on Shock which has been revised but appeared originally in that journal.

I am grateful for the assistance of Doctors Jeremy Cobb, Sam

Davies and Neville Hodges who helped in the preparation of the index. Mr. Douglas Luke, the publisher, has been most helpful, courteous and understanding and it is a joy to express my gratitude to him.

Finally, I have received from my kind and patient wife, Dr Joyce Davies, M.R.C.P., such help and encouragement that without her I would never have contemplated, let alone complete, the work.

IEUAN DAVIES

Llandough Hospital,
Penarth,
Glam. CF6 1XX
October, 1968

CONTENTS

CARDIOLOGY

Complicated new investigations have not replaced the need for careful clinical assessment of the heart. Most of the specialised techniques are based on simple physiological principles; knowledge of their application and limitations is of value in the full assessment of a patient.

DYSPNOEA

The grading of dyspnoea is helpful in recording the progress of symptoms and in briefly communicating the degree of disability. The accepted convention is:

Grade 1. Dyspnoea on severe exertion such as running up two flights of stairs.

Grade 2*A*. Dyspnoea on moderate exertion such as walking normally up two flights of stairs.

Grade 2*B*. Dyspnoea on mild exertion such as walking slowly up one flight of stairs.

Grade 3. Dyspnoea on minimal exertion such as walking from room to room.

Grade 4. Dyspnoea at rest.

It is of value to record the extent of interference with the patient's way of life, for example, dyspnoea which prevents a housewife from doing the family shopping or a husband from driving the family car is usually severe. It is helpful to record the exact disability which breathlessness imposes on a patient. For example can a housewife make one, two or three beds "on the trot" without having to rest in between each, can she sweep out one room without resting, can she carry the week's shopping home or can she run downstairs to answer the door? The number of flights of stairs that can be climbed at a normal pace is a useful guide; or if the patient has only tried one flight—does he think he *could* climb a second flight if there was one?

Dyspnoea is a subjective, uncomfortable awareness of breathing. It is mainly due to excessive use and fatigue of the respiratory muscles. The pulmonary venous congestion which occurs with left-sided heart failure results in congestion of the interstitial lung tissue and airways diminishing the elastic properties of the lungs and increasing the ventilatory effort needed to transfer air through the airways. Normal expiration is probably triggered by a number of reflexes of which the best known is the Hering[1]-Breuer[2] reflex, in which stretch receptors in the alveolar walls are stimulated during inspiration, and impulses pass via the vagus to the respiratory centre which initiates relaxation of the inspiratory muscles. Expiration is a passive process due to the inherent elastic properties of the lungs. The normal rate and depth of breathing at rest are probably mainly due to the inherent rhythmicity of the respiratory centre secondarily modified by afferent reflexes from the lungs and, during exercise, by alterations of the gas tensions in the blood. Congestion of the alveolar walls will accelerate the afferent reflexes (increasing the rate of breathing). Later, breathing becomes further accelerated because of hypoxia of the respiratory centre, due to alveolar-wall oedema interfering with the diffusion of oxygen from the alveoli into the blood. Early cardiac failure is accompanied by dyspnoea before there is any alteration in pH, oxygen or carbon dioxide content of arterial blood perfusing the respiratory centre. The rapid relief of cardiac dyspnoea by morphia is probably due to a decrease in awareness of breathing as well as depression of the respiratory centre and inhibition of the vagus, slowing the rate of breathing and thereby reducing fatigue of the respiratory muscles.

Paroxysmal nocturnal dyspnoea when lying flat at night, and orthopnoea (*Gk.* orthos: straight) are due to reduced mechanical advantage of the diaphragm, redistribution of oedema fluid from dependent parts, and reduced sensitivity of the respiratory centre during sleep, leading to failure of early compensatory mechanisms and increase in cardiac output and venous return in the recumbent position.

Occasionally, patients who are dyspnoeic due to a pulmonary embolus *prefer* to lie flat; the reason for this is that they feel faint if they sit upright because they have a low cardiac output.

Breathlessness when the patient lies in a particular position is seen in the uncommon occurrence of a pedunculated tracheal or bronchial polyp.

CARDIAC PAIN

Ischaemic cardiac pain arises from pain receptors in the myocardium, and is transmitted via the sympathetic nerves to the upper thoracic sympathetic ganglia and thence to the upper five thoracic spinal nerves. This explains the radiation of cardiac pain in the distribution of T 1–5 and the relief of pain by division of these sympathetic ganglia. These nerves supply the upper oesophagus, accounting for the frequent similarity of oesophageal pain and angina; they also supply some of the muscles and ligaments surrounding the shoulder joints, accounting for the reflex spasm and disuse of the left shoulder which may occur following cardiac infarction. Disuse of the joint may be accompanied by a periarthritis and calcification. The left joint is much more frequently involved than the right but the converse is true when periarthritis is due to excessive use, because most people are right-handed. The first thoracic nerve supplies sensation to the inner side of the upper arm and occasionally to the lower arm and little finger accounting for the radiation of cardiac pain down the arm. Distinction between oesophageal and cardiac pain may sometimes be made by infusing dilute hydrochloric acid or dilute sodium bicarbonate through an oesophageal tube, and noting whether this induces the patient's pain. Following a large meal, T-wave changes may occur in the ECG in the absence of ischaemic heart disease, and are due to slight alteration in the position of the heart. Occasionally, pain due to reflux oesophagitis, motor inco-ordination of the oesophagus and hiatus hernia may induce ischaemic ECG changes, and may be relieved by trinitrin.

The pain of pericarditis is occasionally confused with angina. The lower part of the parietal pericardium alone is pain-sensitive and is supplied by the phrenic nerve (C 4–5). Gross distension of the pericardium with fluid gives rise to a dull ache in the front of the chest which may be referred to the back of the neck and shoulder in the distribution of C 4–5. Usually the occurrence of a pericardial effusion in acute pericarditis leads to a lessening of pain because of separation of the inflamed visceral and parietal pericardium. The characteristic pain of pericarditis is usually sudden in onset and frequently pleuritic in nature, due to involvement of contiguous diaphragmatic parietal pleura. Acute pericarditis is accompanied by superficial inflammation and necrosis of the myocardium, which is responsible for the accompanying ST elevation in the ECG and for any similarity between the pain of pericarditis and myocardial ischaemia. However, no pathological Q waves occur in the ECG in pericarditis.

Dissection of the aorta may be similar to myocardial infarction, as shock is a common accompaniment in both. The pain of dissection is unlike that of myocardial infarction in that it is usually "tearing" and it is maximal at its onset and gradually wanes, whereas the pain of myocardial infarction is frequently preceded by premonitory pain. The pain of dissection usually radiates to the back and abdomen; following aortic dissection, occlusion of peripheral arterial pulses is less common than is generally believed. Dissection involving the aortic valve leads to severe aortic incompetence. The dissection may continue over several days and if the abdominal aorta is involved abdominal pain is usually severe and continuous; bleeding into the peritoneum gives rise to paralytic ileus and signs of peritonitis. The clue may be the presence of a pathological arterial bruit. Occasionally, bleeding is into the gut. An unexplained and puzzling feature of dissection of the thoracic aorta is a gap of several days between the onset of the tearing pain of dissection and enlargement of the aortic knuckle on the chest x-ray.

Other causes of chest pain which may simulate the pain of myocardial ischaemia include pain of musculo-skeletal origin, Tietze[3] syndrome (tenderness and swelling of upper costochondral junctions), pleuritic pain, and bronchial carcinoma, especially if it causes rib erosion.

THE PULSE

It is traditional for doctors to feel the radial pulse; however, the character and rhythm of the pulse are best assessed in the more proximal pulses—the carotids and brachials are the most convenient. Occasionally the radial pulses are most suitable for detecting pulsus paradoxus and the femorals for detecting a collapsing pulse.

The normal peripheral arterial pulse is made up of three components. The first, known as the percussion wave, is due to a forward moving column of blood expanding the peripheral arteries as a result of the relatively high resistances it meets in the arterioles as compared with the main arteries. The second is the tidal wave and is probably caused by two separate mechanisms—one is reflection of a pressure wave from the high-resistance arterioles back up the column of blood, and the other is transmission of a wave along the wall of the arteries, beginning at the aorta with the ejection of blood from the left ventricle. The third wave—the dicrotic wave—is due to transmission down the column of blood of a wave resulting from bulging downwards, into the ventricle, of the cusps of the closed aortic valve (Fig. 1).

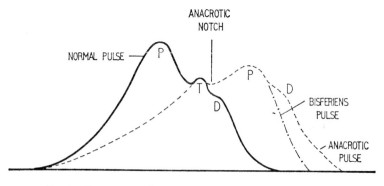

FIG. 1.—Components of the normal and abnormal peripheral pulse.
P—Percussion wave. T—Tidal wave. D—Dicrotic wave.

In aortic stenosis the ejection of blood from the ventricle is prolonged and there is delay in arrival of the full percussion wave at the periphery. The tidal wave is less affected. If the stenosis is severe, the percussion wave is delayed beyond the tidal wave which is felt as a notch on the upstroke of the pulse tracing—the anacrotic notch (*Gk.* ana—up; krotos—stroke). The tighter the stenosis, the more delayed will be the percussion wave and the lower on the upstroke will be the anacrotic notch.

The collapsing pulse of aortic incompetence or arteriovenous shunting is due to disappearance of the dicrotic wave, since leaking valves will not abruptly stop retrograde flow and will not reflect a pressure wave towards the periphery. The bisferiens pulse (*L.* to beat twice) of combined stenosis and incompetence has two easily palpable impulses, the first due to the tidal wave, as in the anacrotic pulse, and the second to an apparently forcible percussion wave due to disappearance of the dicrotic wave. The dicrotic pulse of widespread peripheral arteriolar dilatation, usually due to fever, is a combination of a rapid upstroke due to early run-off into the arterioles, and an easily palpable dicrotic notch on the downstroke (*Gk.* dictrotos—twofold beating). The characteristic pulses of hypertension and atherosclerosis of the major vessels are similar in that there is a rapid and strong upstroke due in the one case to a high arteriolar resistance, and in the other to loss of elasticity of the aorta.

Other abnormal pulses are:

Pulsus alternans, in which *regular* alternate beats are diminished in volume. It is specially easy to appreciate this by palpating the radial pulse while deflating a sphygmomanometer cuff around the upper arm—as the pressure falls there will be a sudden doubling of the pulse rate.

Pulsus bigeminus (or coupling), in which every alternate beat is an extrasystole and therefore of diminished volume, *but* following this extrasystole there is a long compensatory pause; unlike pulsus alternans every beat is not equidistant (*L.* geminus—a twin).

Pulsus paradoxus occurs in constriction of the heart, whether by thickened pericardium, pericardial effusion or, rarely, in severe asthma when there is a gross trapping of air within the chest. During inspiration there is a fall in pulse volume. It is important to note that this is not paradoxical but is an exaggeration of the normal. During inspiration the pulmonary vascular bed increases in size due to traction on the vessels by the expanding lung. If the heart is constricted, the volume of the right ventricle is fixed during inspiration and expiration, therefore, the increased volume of the pulmonary vascular bed cannot be accommodated by increased output from the right ventricle. The left ventricle is underfilled and the pulse volume falls. Also, if the pericardium is tethered to the diaphragm by adhesions, as the diaphragm descends the heart elongates and decreases in volume, reducing the filling of both ventricles. Additional mechanisms suggested for pulsus paradoxus are that the large intrathoracic pressure-swings in asthma and emphysema result in direct compression of the thoracic aorta, and in constrictive pericarditis the volume of the pulse falls with inspiration because the increased volume of blood in the right ventricle causes bulging of the interventricular septum into the left ventricle (reversed Bernheim effect).

Peripheral Arterial Insufficiency

Relative ischaemia of a limb is suggested on inspection by:

Atrophic shiny skin with loss of hair
Brittle deformed nails
Persistent skin infections
Skin which looks permanently red, or cyanosed, due to chronic anoxia, causing the superficial vessels to become permanently dilated.

The skin of the ischaemic limb is cooler than the normal side; before deciding for certain about differences in temperature between the two sides make sure that the limbs are in the same position and that they have been exposed for the same length of time. The peripheral pulses should be carefully palpated at rest, and if there is a suspicion of arterial insufficiency and the pulses appear equal in volume at rest, it is most important to exercise the limbs and palpate the pulses again. Occasionally peripheral pulses appear equal at rest, but after exercise the pulse on one side may disappear due to blood being diverted by the exertion to the leg with the most patent arteries.

Simple Confirmatory Tests of Arterial Insufficiency

1. With the limbs horizontal press the skin of both limbs in corresponding positions. After removing the pressure blanching will be seen; the blanched area should normally begin to flush in 5 seconds. If the circulation is completely obstructed and the skin permanently cyanosed, blanching will not occur. This situation exists in early gangrene.

2. Elevation of both limbs to 45 degrees normally does not result in much change of colour of the limbs. If part of the limb becomes pale, the arterial supply is impaired. With the limbs in this position the skin compression test can be carried out as above; flushing of the blanched area should occur within 10 seconds.

3. If elevation of the limbs to 45 degrees results in pallor, the patient should be asked to hang the legs over the couch so that they are below the level of the body. In this position the pink colour should return to

the skin within 10 seconds. At 10 seconds the veins on the dorsum of the feet should also have filled when the legs are in a dependent position.

Reactive hyperaemia test.—A blood pressure cuff is inflated to the systolic pressure around the limb when it is elevated. The limb then rests in the horizontal position for 5 minutes and the cuff deflated. Flushing gradually extends down from the level of the deflated cuff to the foot; this is followed by progressive fading. If the arterial supply is good the whole process—flushing plus fading—should be complete in 2 minutes. The cuff occludes the arteries and temporarily paralyses the sympathetic supply to the cutaneous vessels, which become maximally dilated, so that when the cuff is removed, blood immediately enters the dilated cutaneous vessels—if it reaches them.

THE JUGULAR VENOUS PULSE (JVP)

The internal jugular vein runs in a straight line from the angle of the jaw to the medial end of the clavicle. It lies *deep* to the sternomastoid and platysma; when the internal jugular vein is examined it is mandatory that the patient's head be resting comfortably on the back-rest, and the head be slightly flexed so that the platysma and sternomastoid are relaxed. The *vertical* height of the top of the venous pulse above the sternal angle (the angle of Louis)[4] should be measured by placing a rule on the sternal angle. If the venous pulse cannot be seen, pressure on the abdomen may cause it to be visible above the clavicle for one or two heart beats; if the level remains more than 4 cm above the sternal angle for more than two beats, the filling of the right atrium is impaired and mild heart failure is present.

The simplest way of appreciating the mechanism of the jugular venous pulse is to consider it in relation to ventricular contraction (Fig. 2). The two main waves of the JVP are a and v. The a wave is due to atrial contraction ejecting the last portion of blood from the atrium into the ventricle at the end of the diastole. As well as forcing blood into the ventricle, atrial contraction causes reflux into the superior vena cava and jugular veins. The x descent, following the a wave is due to the atrium expanding (atrial diastole) and accommodating the blood which has refluxed up into the veins. As the ventricle begins to contract the tricuspid valve closes, blood returning to the right atrium gradually fills it, and once it is full, further blood is accommodated in the veins, causing the v wave. As the ventricle relaxes the intraventricular pressure falls, and as soon as the hydrostatic pressure of blood in right atrium and veins exceeds the intraventricular pressure, the tricuspid valve opens and blood enters the ventricle. Any blood entering the heart during diastole can flow direct into the ventricle.

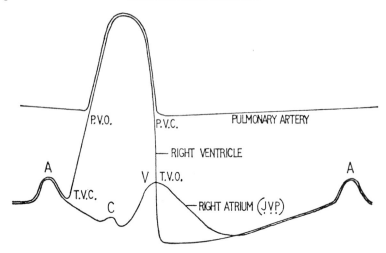

FIG. 2.—Pressure in pulmonary artery, right ventricle and right atrium during systole and diastole. A—A wave. C—C wave. V—V wave. T.V.C.—Tricuspid valve closes. P.V.O.—Pulmonary valve opens. P.V.C.—Pulmonary valve closes. T.V.O.—Tricuspid valve opens.

The *a* wave will be elevated (giant *a* wave) in conditions which prevent normal filling of the ventricle, e.g. tricuspid stenosis and right ventricular failure, the latter being most commonly due to pulmonary hypertension and pulmonary stenosis. If the right atrium contracts while the ventricle is also contracting and the tricuspid valve is closed, all the blood in the atrium will reflux up the veins, causing a big *a* wave. In complete heart block, the atria and ventricles are beating independently; atrial systole will sometimes occur during ventricular systole and sometimes during diastole. This results in irregular big *a* waves of varying height, called cannon waves.

In tricuspid incompetence, part of the force of right ventricular contraction is transmitted to the atrium—this occurs during ventricular systole and causes the giant *v* wave. Atrial fibrillation will abolish the *a* waves but may be associated with some elevation of the *v* wave even in the absence of heart failure—the fibrillating atrium is unable to accommodate as much blood as the normal atrium. In constrictive pericarditis, the walls of the ventricle are held apart by the adherent pericardium so that when the ventricle is filling there will be an initial rapid flow, this is reflected in the JVP as a rapid *y* descent (Friedreich's[5] sign). A rapid *x* descent also occurs because the walls of the atrium are similarly held apart; this rapid *x* descent occurring during ventricular systole is responsible for the so-called "systolic collapse of the JVP" in constrictive pericarditis. Conditions which obstruct venous filling of the heart (congestive failure and constrictive pericarditis) will cause an elevation of the JVP during inspiration (Kussmaul's[6] sign).

THE BLOOD PRESSURE

The blood pressure in the legs is best measured by an occluding cuff around the thigh and palpation or auscultation of the popliteal artery, or foot pulses; if the foot pulses are used, the patient can remain in the supine position and the ordinary arm band can be used around the lower leg. By this method the systolic pressure is usually 20 mm higher than in the arm; in coarctation, the systolic pressure in the femoral artery is less than 20 mm higher than in the brachial. The circumference of the arm has an effect on the blood pressure. If the circumference is more than 25 cm the ordinary sphygmomanometer will register a diastolic pressure above the true value.

The diastolic pressure is often taken as the point at which the sound becomes muffled (4th Korotkoff[7] sound). Ideally, band width should be about 20 per cent more than arm diameter. Indirect blood pressure measurements tend to underestimate systolic and overestimate diastolic blood pressure when 4th sound is taken. The WHO expert committee recommends recording the 4th and 5th Korotkoff sounds. The casual BP in hypertensives is higher than that in normotensives.

THE APEX BEAT

The apex beat is normally defined as the lowest, outermost point at which the cardiac impulse is palpable. Some people prefer the point of maximum impulse (PMI) as the best method of detecting displacement or enlargement of the heart. The outward displacement of the chest wall during systole at a time when the heart itself is getting smaller is due to the fact that the base of the heart is anchored by the great vessels but the apex is mobile. The outward movement during ventricular contraction occurs because of partial rotation of the heart. In constrictive pericarditis there is retraction of the apex during systole because the pericardium is adherent to the chest wall, so that decrease in size of the ventricle will be transmitted to the chest wall and the thickened pericardium will not allow forward movement of the apex. The apical impulse may be double if atrial contraction is forcible, as in hypertrophic obstructive cardiomyopathy (palpable 4th sound).

Hypertrophy of either ventricle may often be assessed by the character of the precordial impulse. Left ventricular hypertrophy characteristically causes a sustained apical impulse, palpable over a small area if only hypertrophy is present; if dilatation of the left ventricle is present as well as hypertrophy, the heaving sustained impulse is felt over a wider area. Right ventricular enlargement causes a tapping apical impulse which is short and poorly sustained. Right ventricular hypertrophy may also cause a palpable impulse at the left sternal edge—the parasternal heave. Mitral stenosis may cause a tapping apex beat even though the right ventricle is *not* hypertrophied; this tapping apex beat of uncomplicated mitral stenosis is due to rapid and forceful closing of the mitral valve and is, therefore, a palpable first heart sound. If the apex beat is not palpable, the patient should be asked to turn on the left side and a further attempt made to locate it. It is often not palpable in obesity, emphysema, pericardial effusion, pleural effusion and pneumothorax. The apex beat will be found on the right side in dextrocardia, whether congenital or acquired (from fibrosis of the lower lobe of the right lung).

The various types of apical impulse are:

Normal
Left ventricular
Right ventricular (usually with a parasternal heave)
Displaced
Retractile (i.e. moving *inwards* during systole) as in constrictive pericarditis
Paradoxical—outward movement of some part of the precordium other than over the apex of the heart during systole. This occurs when there is a ventricular aneurysm which fills and expands during systolic contraction of the ventricle.

Percussion of the heart does not accurately delineate its borders but the cardiac dullness is abnormally extensive with a pericardial effusion or large aortic aneurysm. Dullness occurs to the right of the midline in dextrocardia.

HEART SOUNDS AND MURMURS

The mechanism of the production of the heart sounds and heart murmurs was first established by James Hope[8], who was also the first physician to codify the process of clinical examination—inspection, palpation, percussion and auscultation. Sounds and murmurs are caused by turbulence of the blood and vibration of the vessels and valves.

Turbulence of the blood. This occurs when there is rapid flow through narrowed tubes or when there is a sudden change in size of a tube. At high flow rates turbulence produces high-pitched sounds and at low rates, low-pitched sounds.

Vibration of vessels and valves. Rapid distension of the chambers of the heart causes vibration of their walls. Vibration of valves occurs when blood is flowing rapidly over them, or when they open or close forcefully.

HEART SOUNDS

The first sound is due to a combination of mitral and tricuspid valve closure. In mitral stenosis the first sound is loud because prolonged flow of blood through the narrowed valve means that the valve is wide open at the beginning of ventricular systole, resulting in more forceful closure when the ventricle contracts. In the normal the cusps of the mitral valve have time to "float" into the closed position before the onset of ventricular systole. The first sound will vary in intensity if the valve is sometimes fully open and sometimes nearly closed when ventricular systole starts. This is the situation in complete heart block (when atria and ventricles are beating completely independently) and in ventricular tachycardia which is always slightly irregular so that the cusps of the mitral valve are in a slightly different position at each ventricular systole. The second heart sound consists of two components, the first is due to closure of the aortic valve and the second to closure of the pulmonary valve. During inspiration, blood is drawn into the chest increasing the load on the right ventricle. The increased volume of blood takes longer to expel, resulting in prolongation of right ventricular systole during inspiration, and closure of the pulmonary valve occurs after the aortic valve.

Conditions prolonging systole of one ventricle will result in delaying the component of the second sound produced by that ventricle. Right bundle-branch block, pulmonary stenosis and atrial septal defect will delay the pulmonary component of the second sound resulting in audible aortic and pulmonary components widely separated; furthermore, the splitting may already be maximum in expiration so that increasing the volume of blood entering the right ventricle by inspiration will not result in any further splitting (fixed splitting). Conditions which increase the pressure in the pulmonary artery result in a narrowed split but a loud pulmonary second sound because of the rapidity with which the valve shuts. Pulmonary stenosis, in which there is a lowered pressure in the pulmonary arteries, results in a quiet pulmonary second sound, as the lowered pulmonary artery pressure does not shut the valve so abruptly, and it causes a delay in the sound because of prolongation of right ventricular systole. In the case of the aortic valve, left ventricular systole is prolonged in aortic stenosis and in late activation of the left ventricle (left bundle-branch block). The aortic component may be so delayed that it occurs after the pulmonary component; if the pulmonary component is delayed normally during inspiration the two sounds may be superimposed so that only one sound is audible. This means that during inspiration only one sound is heard but in expiration two components are heard; this is the reverse of normal and is, therefore, called reversed or paradoxical splitting. Reversed splitting may occur in the absence of left bundle-branch block; it is then a sign of left ventricular dysfunction, and occurs commonly following myocardial infarction. High systemic pressure or reduced elasticity of the aorta will result in forceful closure of the aortic valve and a loud aortic component to the second sound.

The third heart sound occurs during the period of rapid filling of the ventricles (at least 0·12 sec after the second sound); it is caused partly by sudden distension of the ventricular walls—mainly the wall of the left ventricle—and partly by turbulent flow at the mitral valve. Conditions which cause early rapid filling of the ventricles will produce a pathological third sound; these are heart failure (in which venous pressure is elevated causing rapid flow into the ventricle), mitral incompetence, ventricular septal defect, and constrictive pericarditis (by holding the ventricular walls apart and thus allowing a sudden influx of blood). A third sound is physiological in youth (up to the age of 40).

The fourth sound is due to contraction of the atria—this occurs at the end of the diastole and is responsible for ejecting the remaining small volume of blood into the ventricles (the ventricles fill mainly due to hydrostatic pressure of blood in atria and great veins). The occurrence of the fourth sound at the end of the diastole is the reason for its alternative name—presystolic triple rhythm (the rhythm that occurs with a third sound is sometimes called protodiastolic). The fourth sound will be heard in conditions which hinder the filling of the ventricles at the end of diastole, the most usual causes are left ventricle failure and myocardial infarction or ischaemia in which the fibrotic or necrotic myocardium is more resistant to distension than normal. In tachycardia, the third and fourth sounds cannot be identified separately and are heard as one sound—summation gallop.

The opening snap is a high pitched sound, best heard at the left sternal edge; it occurs in mitral stenosis. The sound is due to sudden rapid opening of the mitral valve because of the elevated left atrial pressure—the higher the atrial pressure the quicker the valve will open. The height of the left atrial pressure is related to the severity of the valve stenosis. Hence, the earlier the opening snap occurs in diastole the more severe the stenosis. If the valve is heavily calcified it is unable to open as quickly as when supple, therefore an opening snap is unusual in calcific mitral stenosis (this is not an absolute rule—there are exceptions). The opening snap does not usually occur if here is associated mitral incompetence.

At the beginning of ventricular contraction the aortic and pulmonary valves open and blood is ejected into the aorta and pulmonary arteries. Dilatation or rigidity of these vessels will result in turbulence of blood or in excessive vibration of their walls leading to a high pitched sound called an "ejection click." Hypertension, atherosclerosis and post-stenotic dilatation may cause early systolic ejection clicks. Clicks also occur in pulmonary and aortic valve stenosis (without post-stenotic dilatation) and are due to vibration of valve cusps resulting from the high rate of flow (because of the narrowing) across them. The importance of clicks is that they do not occur in stenosis other than at the valve. Occasionally pulmonary and aortic "stenosis" is due to narrowing below the valve, this may be muscular narrowing (hypertrophic obstructive cardiomyopathy) or more rarely fibrous narrowing. Narrowing above the valves is exceptionally rare.

MURMURS

The loudness of murmurs depends on the quantity of blood flowing past the lesion which causes them. During ventricular systole blood is pumped into a high-pressure system (the aorta)—the speed of flow increases as ventricular pressure increases and then decreases as the high pressure system becomes full. If outflow from the ventricle is narrowed a murmur is produced whose loudness increases to a maximum and then declines; because they occur during ejection of blood such murmurs are called "ejection" murmurs (*synonyms:* "diamond shaped" murmurs and crescendo-decrescendo murmurs). If the flow of blood from the ventricle is into a low-pressure chamber of large volume, blood will begin to flow at the beginning of ventricular contraction and will continue to the end of systole unabated, such murmurs are, therefore, called pansystolic (holosystolic) and occur in incompetence of the atrioventricular valves (separating high pressure ventricles from low pressure atria). The definition of an ejection murmur is, therefore, one whose maximum intensity is near mid-systole and a pansystolic murmur is one more or less equally loud throughout systole.

Diastolic murmurs occur when blood is flowing into a ventricle during diastole, either from the aorta or pulmonary artery because of incompetence of their valves, or from the atria through a narrowed atrioventricular valve. Like systolic murmurs their loudness will depend on the volume of blood flowing. In the case of aortic incompetence the pressure is higher in the aorta at the beginning than at the end of diastole (the pressure falls off as blood is distributed to the arterioles). In the case of mitral stenosis the murmur will be loudest during the period of maximum ventricular filling, which is towards mid-diastole, and during the ejection of the last portion of blood from the atria (i.e., during atrial systole). The murmur of aortic (and pulmonary) incompetence begins early in diastole and then gradually wanes, whereas the murmur of mitral stenosis begins towards mid-diastole (after the opening snap), wanes and then rises again as the atrium contracts. The longer blood takes to enter the ventricle from the left atrium the tighter is the stenosis, hence, the severity of the stenosis can be judged by the length of the murmur. The auscultatory methods of assessing the severity of uncomplicated mitral stenosis are:

Length of the mid-diastolic murmur
Closeness of the opening snap to the second sound
Loudness of the first heart sound.

The site and radiation of a murmur is often as important as its character in deciding its origin. Sounds arising from the cardiovascular system seem to be better conducted to the surface through blood than through tissues; murmurs from the aortic valve will, therefore, be heard best when blood in contact with the valve is nearest the surface, i.e., over the ascending aorta (second right intercostal space), and over the left ventricle (i.e., apex). Murmurs originating from the mitral valve will be heard over the left ventricle but the left atrium is too deep to conduct sound to the surface. This phenomenon gives rise to one of the most useful rules in cardiology, namely, murmurs arising from the base of the heart (aortic and pulmonary valves) are often heard at the apex, but murmurs arising from the apex (mitral and tricuspid valves) are never heard at the base. The main use of this rule is in distinguishing a long aortic ejection systolic murmur (which sounds like a pansystolic murmur) from a true pansystolic murmur arising from the mitral valve or a ventricular septal defect. Murmurs arising from the right side of the heart will generally be louder during inspiration, due to increased blood entering the right side of the heart.

The effect of various drugs on murmurs is of little value in practice. Amyl nitrate causes vasodilatation and increases venous return, leading to an increase in the murmur of pulmonary stenosis. After a few more seconds the murmur of aortic stenosis will increase (when the increased venous return reaches the left side of the heart). Vasopressor drugs such as phenylephrine, which increase peripheral resistance and hence left ventricular pressure, increase the intensity of murmurs arising from mitral incompetence and left-to-right shunt, such as ventricular septal defect. In practice these drugs may also affect the pulmonary vascular resistance and so are not used widely.

Grading of murmurs.—In order to communicate in a shorthand way the intensity and duration of murmurs, their loudness and length can be graded. There are two conventions of grading: one has six grades of loudness and length and the other four grades. It is good practice always to record *graphically* the auscultatory findings.

Innocent and Functional Murmurs

Functional murmurs are murmurs which arise in the absence of organic disease at their site of origin, e.g. the ejection systolic murmur at the pulmonary area in an ASD or the diastolic murmur at the mitral valve in a VSD. The aortic and/or pulmonary systolic murmurs which are present in anaemia, thyrotoxicosis and pyrexias are also examples of functional murmurs.

Innocent murmurs are a common source of confusion and considerable experience is sometimes required in deciding whether a murmur indicates underlying heart disease or not and whether further cardiac investigation is indicated. As a rule all innocent murmurs are systolic in timing; they are heard only over a small area and do not radiate widely; they are *not* loud and often vary with the patient's posture. It is axiomatic that the ECG and chest x-ray should be within normal limits and the patient be free of cardiac symptoms if a murmur is assumed to be innocent. A previous history of rheumatic fever or a rheumatic fever type of illness (pain in the joints or confinement to bed with an undiagnosed illness during childhood) should make one very wary of diagnosing an innocent murmur.

Examples of Innocent Murmurs

Cardiorespiratory murmur.—Most of these are due to obstruction of blood flow to a small part of the left lung overlying the heart. Some are possibly due to distortion of the pulmonary valve cusps from traction on the pulmonary artery by surrounding lung. These murmurs are nearly always systolic and are loudest in inspiration.

Venous hums.—These are often loudest in diastole or may be continuous. They are common in childhood, pregnancy and thyrotoxicosis. They are usually best heard at the base of the heart and at the root of the neck. They are loudest in inspiration and in the upright posture because of increased venous return with these manoeuvres; the murmur may become louder when the head is turned away from the side being auscultated, because of stretching and narrowing of the jugular veins on the side being examined. Venous hums can usually be abolished by the Valsalva manoeuvre, lying down, and manual compression of the jugular veins. The most difficult differential diagnosis is usually a patent ductus arteriosus.

Pericardial sounds.—These are due to pleuro-pericardial adhesions and are often very variable in their site, timing and variation with respiration. They can sometimes be increased by firm pressure of the diaphragm of the stethoscope on the precordium.

Carotid and arterial bruits are fairly common in normal people.

Chest deformity may cause a short systolic murmur.

Still's murmur is any high-pitched, innocent, systolic, apical murmur occurring during childhood.

Mammary souffle.—This is due to dilated arteries and veins in the breast during pregnancy.

ELECTROCARDIOGRAPHY

Muscular contraction of the myocardium is associated with a change in the surface charge on individual muscle cells (depolarisation). The electrocardiogram measures the summation of the surface charges of all muscle cells in the myocardium. It is convenient to place the electrical contacts for recording these changes at a number of sites on the body which have been found empirically to reflect either electrical activity of a known part of the heart or flow of electricity in a known direction. The limb leads reflect the amount of electricity flowing in their direction and the chest leads (V leads) show the electrical activity in the part of the heart which they overlie.

It is conventional to describe the flow of electricity during ventricular contraction in terms of the predominant direction of flow (a system which describes both direction and strength of flow is known as a vector system). The Einthoven[9] triangle is a convenient mnemonic for remembering which ECG leads are attached where, and in what direction electricity is flowing when one limb lead shows a bigger deflection than another (Fig. 3a).

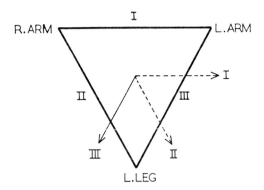

FIG. 3(a).—Einthoven triangle showing the direction of the three limb leads parallel to the sides of the triangle.

Example: if the biggest QRS deflection of any of the limb leads is in lead II then the QRS vector is said to be +60°. This is the direction of flow of the largest amount of electricity when viewed from the front; it is, therefore, the mean frontal QRS vector.

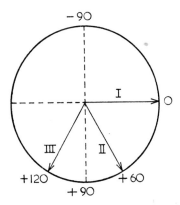

Fig. 3(*b*).—Direction of limb leads viewed from the front.

The direction of flow of electricity could be viewed from other sites, e.g., from the side or from above, however, these other sites are not as useful as considering the flow of electricity from in front. From Fig. 3*b* it will be observed that the three main limb leads record electricity flowing in the lower half of the circle; in order to improve the "pick up field" leads which record electricity in other directions are introduced—these are known as the augmented limb leads (aVR, aVL, and aVF) and they record flow in the directions shown (Fig. 4).

The chest or V leads record electrical activity as follows:

V1+V2—from right ventricle
V3+V4—from interventricular septum
V5+V6—from left ventricle.

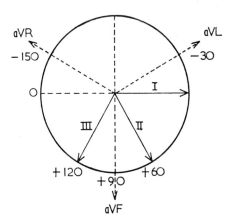

Fig. 4.—Direction of standard and augmented limb leads viewed from the front.

The normal waves of the ECG are P Q R S and T
The P wave is due to atrial depolarisation
The Q wave is due to depolarisation of the interventricular septum
The R and S waves are due to depolarisation of the ventricles
The T wave is due to repolarisation of the ventricles.

The size of these waves depends on the leads in which they are recorded. Under certain circumstances the P and T waves may be inverted, but when the QRS complex is considered, Q and S waves are always downward deflections and R waves always upward deflections. It is the convention to call upward deflections positive and downward deflections negative.

(Note that this may give rise to confusion, because in the frontal plane vector reference circle directions below the horizontal are positive and above the horizontal are negative.)

The Normal Direction of the QRS Vector

The lead in which the positive deflection is greatest is taken as the direction of the QRS vector. Usually it is accurate enough to note the height of the R wave, but strictly speaking the depth of any negative deflection (Q or S) should be subtracted from the height of the R wave to determine the lead in which the true positive deflection is the greatest.

Noting the lead in which the negative deflection is maximum is a useful method of checking the vector (which will be in a direction diametrically opposite the lead with the greatest negative deflection). The lead in which the sum of the positive and negative deflections is zero is the lead at right angles to the vector.

In normal adults the mean frontal QRS vector should be between 0° and +110°. Vectors of 0° to −90° are known as left axis deviation and vectors more than +100° as right axis deviation. Conditions which alter the mechanical position of the heart may also alter the direction of the vector. For example left axis deviation may be caused by a high diaphragm due to ascites or pregnancy, as well as hypertrophy of the left ventricle. Right axis deviation is normal in young children, and occurs in right ventricular hypertrophy.

Examples of frontal QRS vectors.—(i) Figure 5: the frontal QRS vector is +105°. The leads with the largest positive QRS complexes are leads II, III and aVF, which means that the vector lies between +60° and +120°. The leads in which the total of the QRS complexes most nearly approaches zero are leads I and aVR; these leads are nearly at right angles to the vector. Lead aVF is at right angles to lead I (see Fig. 4). On close inspection it will be seen that the negative deflection in lead I is slightly more prominent than the positive

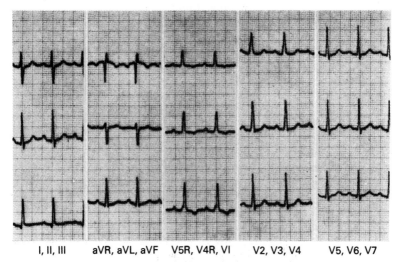

I, II, III   aVR, aVL, aVF   V5R, V4R, VI   V2, V3, V4   V5, V6, V7

FIG. 5.—ECG showing right ventricular hypertrophy. Note frontal plane QRS vector of +105°, tall R waves in V1, small S waves in V5 and 6, and T-wave inversion in V1.

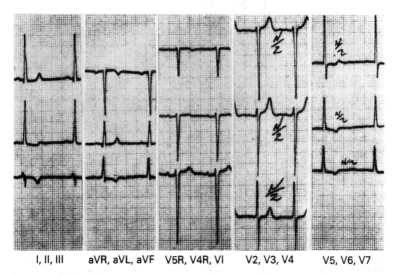

I, II, III   aVR, aVL, aVF   V5R, V4R, VI   V2, V3, V4   V5, V6, V7

FIG. 6.—ECG showing severe left ventricular hypertrophy. Leads V2 to V6 are recorded at half the normal sensitivity. Note QRS frontal plane axis of +25°, deep S wave in V1, tall R and V6, and inverted T waves in leads V6 and V7.

deflection, i.e., the vector is almost at right angles to lead I but is pointing slightly away from the direction of lead I; it lies around + 100°. Applying the same rules to lead aVR (which records electricity at − 150°), again, the negative deflection is slightly more prominent; therefore, the vector is slightly less than + 120° (which is the direction at right angles to aVR), i.e., around + 110°. We have now located the vector between + 100° and + 110°, which for practical purposes we call + 105°.

(ii) Figure 6: the frontal QRS vector is +25°. The leads with the biggest deflection are leads I and II, hence the vector lies between 0° and +60°. The size of the QRS complexes in aVL and aVF are more or less the same (slightly more in aVL). The direction midway between aVL (− 30°) and aVF (+ 90°) is + 30°. In fact the positive deflection is slightly more in aVL than aVF, therefore the direction is nearer aVL, i.e. less than + 30°, say + 25°. This is confirmed by the fact that the sum of the QRS complexes in lead III (+ 120°) is almost zero; in fact the negative deflection is slightly more than the positive, hence the vector is directed slightly away from lead III, more or less at right angles to it, i.e. at + 25°.

The Electrocardiogram and Myocardial Disease

A damaged myocardial cell loses its ability to pump out sodium and becomes persistently negative electrically. At rest this results in the remainder of the myocardium having a slight negative charge. With contraction and depolarisation the remainder of the myocardium becomes electrically negative, but the injured area cannot take part in this depolarisation, so that although it is negatively charged, it is not as much so as the remainder of the myocardium. This positivity as compared with the remainder of the myocardium causes elevation of the ST segments in the leads which face the area of damage. The current of injury is found with damaged muscle, but if the muscle dies, then it is electrically silent and the ST segments revert to normal. If myocardial infarction involves the whole thickness of the wall of the ventricle, it is electrically silent, and any lead overlying the infarcted area will record electricity seen through the "window" of the infarcted area; in practice, the electricity recorded through the window arises from the septum, and is thus seen in the overlying lead as a Q wave. Thus, an area of myocardial ischaemia near the surface (subepicardial) is seen as elevation of ST segments, and an area of complete infarction of the ventricular wall (transmural infarction) is seen as a Q wave in the appropriate leads.

The Anatomy of the Coronary Arteries

The left coronary artery divides into:
Left anterior descending
Left circumflex
Diagonal branches.

The left anterior descending artery descends in the groove between the two ventricles, and sometimes passes around the heart to the groove on the back of the heart, where it is joined by the posterior descending artery, which is a branch of the right coronary artery. The anterior descending artery supplies branches to the anterior part of the interventricular septum and the anterior wall of the left ventricle. The left circumflex artery supplies a branch to the posterior portion of the left ventricle, and in about 10 per cent it supplies the whole of the posterior/inferior part of the left ventricle. The left circumflex artery supplies the sino-atrial node in about 45 per cent of cases. The diagonal branches supply a variable amount of the lateral side of the left ventricle.

The right coronary artery forms the conus artery near its origin (which usually supplies most of the posterior part of the left ventricle) and later it divides into the right circumflex and right anterior descending arteries. In 55 per cent of cases the sino-atrial node is supplied by the right coronary artery.

Blood Supply of Special Sites

Interventricular septum.—Anterior two-thirds supplied by anterior descending (left coronary), and posterior one-third from posterior descending (right coronary). In 10 per cent of cases the whole of the septum is supplied by the left coronary artery.

Papillary muscles.—*Anterior papillary muscle.*—Usually two or three supplies from the branches of the left coronary, i.e., anterior descending, circumflex and diagonal branches.

Posterior papillary muscle.—This usually has two supplies from right and left coronary arteries, but when the right coronary supplies most of the diaphragmatic portion of the heart it also supplies the posterior papillary muscle. The order of frequency of occlusion is: anterior descending (anterior and anteroseptal infarcts), right coronary (true posterior and inferior infarcts), and left circumflex (anterolateral and inferior infarcts).

Patterns of infarction.—Subepicardial infarcts will have elevation of appropriate ST segments and transmural infarcts will have additional Q waves. Subendocardial infarcts can only be appreciated if they involve the anterior surface (they cause symmetrical inversion of the T waves).

Anterior infarcts:
Changes in lead I, aVL and V1, 2 and 3

Anteroseptal infarcts:
Changes in lead I, aVL, and V3, 4 and 5

Anterolateral infarcts:
Changes in lead I, aVL and V4, 5, 6 and 7

Posterior infarcts:
Tall R waves only in leads V1 and 2

(Q waves do not occur because the "window" is at the back of the heart and ST segment changes do not occur because none of the leads lies over the infarcted area.) The reason for the tall R waves in the right ventricular leads is that with loss of the posterior wall of the heart, the leads record straight from the anterior wall without the effect of some neutralisation from electricity arising from the opposite side of the heart.

Inferior infarcts:
Changes in lead II, III and aVF.

All the above changes indicate acute infarction.

As fibrosis and healing occur, the Q waves usually remain, but the ST elevation and T inversion return to normal. These changes start after about seven days; the speed with which they occur is variable, but usually the ST segments are isoelectric in three weeks after an acute infarct. The development of a ventricular aneurysm is suggested by persistent ST elevation.

It is important to note that Q waves are not always pathological; they are caused by normal septal depolarisation and are only abnormal in certain leads or if they are more than a certain size. They are usually normal in lead III but should be considered abnormal if they:

Exceed 0·04 second
Exceed a quarter of the height of the R wave
Are present in several leads.

Exercise electrocardiogram.—An ECG taken during and after exercise is sometimes helpful in deciding whether atypical chest pain is due to myocardial ischaemia. But it is important to be aware of the limitations of the exercise ECG. The only *certain* sign of myocardial ischaemia on the exercise ECG is ischaemic elevation or depression of the whole of the ST segment of more than 1 mm—this alteration only occurs if the lumen of the coronary arteries is reduced to less than half of normal. A negative exercise ECG does not exclude myocardial ischaemia—approximately 25 per cent of patients with classical *angina*

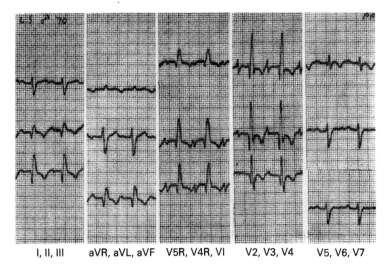

I, II, III   aVR, aVL, aVF   V5R, V4R, VI   V2, V3, V4   V5, V6, V7

FIG. 7.—ECG showing right bundle-branch block. Note widened QRS complexes
beyond 0·12 sec., tall R wave in V1, and deep S wave in V6.

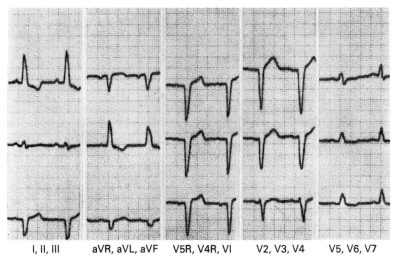

I, II, III   aVR, aVL, aVF   V5R, V4R, VI   V2, V3, V4   V5, V6, V7

FIG. 8.—ECG showing left bundle-branch block. Note widened QRS complexes, but
relatively normal shape and direction.

have a *normal resting* and *exercise* ECG. Other abnormalities are often seen in the exercise ECG and undoubtedly occur more frequently when there is myocardial ischaemia; however, these same abnormalities are also seen commonly in normal people, so that these changes occurring in an individual patient with atypical chest pain must *not* be taken as evidence that the patient's pain is due to myocardial ischaemia. These changes are:

Frequent ectopic beats
Widening of the QRS complexes
T-wave inversion
Depression of the beginning of the ST segment.

Myocardial Ischaemia

The ST elevation and Q waves described above imply actual infarction of myocardium; nevertheless, the myocardium may become transiently ischaemic due to narrowing of the coronary arteries. These are the signs of myocardial ischaemia without infarction:

Divergence of QRS and T vectors of more than 60°. Transient T-wave inversion may occur in the absence of ischaemia in a large number of conditions such as after a heavy meal, hypoglycaemia, head injuries, exercise, smoking and hiatus hernia.
Deep persistent inversion of the T waves is usually pathological
Flat T waves in several leads
Abnormally tall T waves
Inverted U waves
Depression of the ST segment
An abnormally sharp angle between ST segment and T wave
Left bundle-branch block
QRS vector more than $-30°$.

Bundle-branch Block

The bundle of His[10] divides into right and left branches after leaving the atrioventricular node.

Prolongation of the QRS complex more than 0·12 seconds (3 small squares on the ECG paper) implies that there is delay in the spread of depolarisation—this is due to injury to either the right or left branches of the bundle of His. Lead V1 records electrical activity over the right ventricle; however, because the left ventricle is so much thicker than the right, the electricity picked up by V1 is due to left ventricular activity as "seen by" a right ventricular lead. The electricity arising from the right ventricle is swamped by that from the left. In right bundle-branch block, activation of the right ventricle is delayed but left ventricular activity is normal; therefore, in V1 right ventricular

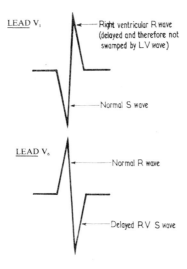

LEAD V₁

Right ventricular R wave (delayed and therefore not swamped by L V wave)

Normal S wave

LEAD V₆

Normal R wave

Delayed R V S wave

FIG. 9.—Right bundle-branch block.

electricity is seen after the normal V1 deflection—it is seen as a positive R wave. Conversely in V6 right ventricular activity is seen after the normal R wave as an S wave.

The characteristic patterns of right bundle-branch block are shown in Fig. 9, while Figure 7 shows these patterns in an ECG.

In the chest leads, left bundle-branch block is seen as prolongation of the QRS complexes, but without alteration of their general shape and direction (Fig. 8).

In the limb leads, right bundle-branch block is frequently accompanied by right axis deviation, and left bundle-branch block by left axis deviation.

Ventricular Hypertrophy

In the limb leads hypertrophy of either ventricle is usually seen as right or left axis deviation. The increase in size of the hypertrophied ventricle causes an increase in the voltage recorded by leads over that ventricle. In the case of left ventricular hypertrophy (Fig. 6) the R wave is taller than normal in V6 (this is accompanied by a deep S in V1—since this is also due to left ventricular electricity). In right ventricular hypertrophy (Fig. 5) the normally hidden right ventricular R wave in the S of V1 may appear and be more powerful than the LV

S wave, so that right ventricular hypertrophy is accompanied by a positive R wave in V1. If right ventricular hypertrophy is severe, there may be delay in activation, i.e. the appearances may be those of right bundle-branch block. In addition there may be T-wave inversion in leads recording the appropriate ventricle (lead I and V6 for the LV, and lead III and V1 for the RV).

Hypertrophy of the atria, the left in mitral stenosis and the right in cor pulmonale, may also be appreciated in the ECG. The best lead is limb lead II; right atrial enlargement causes a tall P wave (P pulmonale) and left atrial enlargement causes a wide bifid P wave (P mitrale).

Other Important ECG Abnormalities

Digitalis effect.—Shortened QRS complex, prolongation of P-R interval, T-wave inversion, and coupling (alternate normal and ectopic beats). It is important to remember that almost every known arrhythmia may be caused by digitalis so that if a patient has been taking digitalis this should be considered as a possible cause. Characteristically digitalis slows the heart rate when given in therapeutic doses; nevertheless, if the dose exceeds the patient's needs a tachycardia may be produced which will aggravate pre-existing heart failure (which may lead to the mistaken conclusion that the patient is underdigitalised).

Hypocalcaemia causes prolongation of the Q-T interval; the normal Q-T interval varies according to the heart rate. The upper limits of normal with different rates are given in tables. The Q-T interval is also prolonged in any condition which delays repolarisation of the ventricles, such as myocardial ischaemia, myocarditis and procainamide.

Hyperkalaemia causes tall, pointed T waves and widening of the QRS complex.

Hypokalaemia causes flattening of the T waves, prominent U waves and prolongation of the P-R interval.

The Effect of Drugs on the Electrocardiogram

The main mechanisms of action of drugs in altering the electrocardiogram are:

Direct effect on myocardial fibres
Direct effect on conducting tissue affecting rate, rhythm and
    conduction
Alterations of general haemodynamics or metabolism
Structural damage to myocardium
Combinations of any of the above.

Digitalis.—The effects of digitalis on ventricular repolarisation cause:

Depression of the ST segments
Decreased amplitude of the T wave often with reversed polarity
Shortening of the Q-T interval
Increase in amplitude of the U wave.

The characteristic sharp downward curve of the ST segment running into the inverted T wave gives rise to the so-called reversed correction mark configuration (i.e. $\vee$ instead of $\sqrt{}$). The effects of digitalis toxicity are often most marked in leads II, III, and aVF and in the right chest leads in contrast to the changes of left ventricular hypertrophy. Occasionally digitalis can produce elevation of the ST segment, and pointed, inverted or upright T waves. It is essential to realise that the effects of digoxin on the ECG may last up to 6 weeks. Effects of digitalis on rhythm and rate include bradycardia, nodal rhythm, ectopic beats, supraventricular tachycardia, coupling, and ventricular tachycardia.

Quinidine and procainamide.—Therapeutic doses usually slow the sinus rate and increase the P-R interval. In atrial fibrillation the rate is slower and atrial flutter may develop with an increase in the ventricular rate, which may then slow if more quinidine is given; eventually sinus rhythm may be restored. These drugs in higher doses increase the duration of the QRS complex and cause lowering and widening of the T waves so that they resemble those seen in hypokalaemia. Toxic doses of these drugs cause gross widening of the QRS complexes, a high degree of A-V block, and bradycardia.

Lignocaine.—Therapeutic doses of lignocaine do not produce any effects on the rate or form of the normal ECG, although they may slow or abolish ventricular ectopic beats.

Phenytoin.—The most common effect of phenytoin is to slow the sinus rate and to produce some A-V block.

Propranolol. The main effect is to prolong A-V conduction and to produce ventricular slowing. There is normally no change in the QRS complexes and T waves.

Suxamethonium.—This may produce hyperkalaemia in the presence of soft-tissue injury or burns.

Phenothiazines.—The main effects are prolongation of the Q-T interval with widening and lowering of the T waves.

Imipramine.—The effects are similar to those of the phenothiazines. Supraventricular and ventricular tachycardia may also occur.

Emetine, chloroquine and antimony compounds.—These may produce non-specific T-wave changes, which are usually transitory and best seen in the right chest leads.

RADIOLOGY OF THE HEART

The heart size and silhouette as well as a number of other diagnostic features may be gleaned from a routine P-A film of the chest. The usual rules for inspection of chest x-rays should be observed (see p. 124). The size of the heart is best expressed as a percentage of the maximum diameter of the chest (the cardiothoracic ratio or CTR); this should normally be below 50 per cent. Care should be taken to exclude conditions which may increase the apparent size of the heart. These include:

Too short a distance between x-ray tube and plate (as in a portable x-ray)
Film exposed with the patient not taking a full inspiration
High diaphragm
Bradycardia
Pericardial effusion
Depressed sternum
Kyphoscoliosis.

Increase in the CTR in the absence of any of the above means enlargement of one or both ventricles. It is usually not possible to say with certainty on a P-A film which ventricle is enlarged, but left ventricular enlargement is said to produce a round apex which encroaches on the diaphragm. Right ventricular enlargement is said to produce a straight left border to the heart. In the lateral views it may be easier to distinguish isolated ventricular enlargement. When the left ventricle enlarges the cardiac silhouette is seen overlapping the spine in the left lateral view, and in right ventricular enlargement the retrosternal translucency is encroached upon. It is generally thought that pure hypertrophy of either ventricle does not cause cardiac enlargement; if the heart is enlarged it implies dilatation as well as hypertrophy.

Left atrial enlargement is seen as an abnormal shadow below the left pulmonary artery in the plain film, and in a barium swallow lateral film the barium-filled oesophagus will be indented. The left main bronchus may be lifted upwards by a giant left atrium so that it comes off from the trachea at an angle of more than 45° from the vertical. Enlargement of the right atrium is seen on the right lower border of the cardiac silhouette.

Descriptions of the cardiac silhouette should begin at the left border of the upper mediastinum, where a left-sided superior vena cava or subclavian artery may be seen. The normal structures seen in the silhouette should be described in order: the aortic knuckle may be enlarged, calcified, double as in coarctation, or small in conditions with a low cardiac output such as mitral stenosis. Next, the left pulmonary artery, left atrium, left border of the heart (left ventricle), right atrium, right pulmonary artery and superior vena cava should be described. An over-penetrated film of the heart may show calcification in one of the valves or coronary arteries; it may also show left atrium, descending aorta or an abnormal shadow behind the heart such as a hiatus hernia, paravertebral abscess or collapsed left lower lobe. Calcification may occur in the coronary arteries (particularly the left), a ventricular aneurysm, or pericardium. It is not possible to say for certain from a P-A film whether calcification is in the mitral or aortic valve; a working rule is to draw a line between the right cardiophrenic angle and the junction of pulmonary artery and left atrium—calcification above this line is probably in the aortic valve and below the line is probably in the mitral valve. Screening of the heart gives a much better idea of the site of the calcification; screening should also demonstrate the degree of pulsation of the cardiac silhouette, which is reduced in the presence of pericardial effusion, and any paradoxical (i.e., expanding during systole) pulsation suggestive of a ventricular aneurysm. Conditions associated with an increased pulmonary blood flow (such as an ASD) cause excessive movement of the pulmonary arteries ("hilar dance") which will be seen on screening.

The proximal pulmonary arteries may be enlarged in pulmonary hypertension, increased pulmonary blood flow or in post-stenotic dilatation due to pulmonary stenosis. The distal pulmonary arteries will be prominent ("pulmonary plethora") if there is increased flow. In pulmonary hypertension there is often an abrupt decrease in size of the pulmonary arteries ("peripheral pruning"). In Eisenmenger's syndrome the dilatation of the proximal pulmonary arteries is often gross. Haziness of outline of enlarged proximal vessels may be due to pulmonary oedema.

The upper-lobe veins are prominent if there is an elevated left atrial pressure as in left ventricular failure or mitral stenosis. Anomalous pulmonary veins may be seen draining into the superior vena cava.

The lung fields should be carefully inspected for evidence of pulmonary oedema which may be manifested by:

Kerley's[11] "B" lines (septal lines) which are small, horizontal, parallel lines 1–2 centimetres in length occurring at the costophrenic angles. They are due to dilated lymphatics within the interlobular septa
Pleural effusions either in the costophrenic angles or in the transverse or oblique fissures
Ill-defined homogeneous opacities radiating out from the hila
Bilateral lower-zone haziness
Haziness over the whole of the lung fields
Dilatation of the upper-lobe veins

Hazy outline to the hilar vessels.

Rarely, pulmonary oedema may occur in one lung only; the explanation for this is not known. Other abnormalities in the lung fields which may occur with heart disease are:

Deposition of haemosiderin which may calcify or ossify
Pulmonary infarcts
Notching of the under-surface of the upper ribs which may occur in coarctation of the aorta.

Occasionally pulmonary oedema occurs when the heart size is not increased. These are the main conditions to think of:

Constrictive pericarditis
Mitral stenosis
Constrictive type of cardiomyopathy
Blocked lung lymphatics (e.g. in pneumoconiosis and silicosis) preventing normal drainage of fluid from the lungs
Viral pneumonias
Inhalation of toxic fumes
Head injury or cerebrovascular accident.

ECHOCARDIOGRAPHY

The frequency of ultrasound waves is about 50 times the audible sound range. The waves travel in straight lines and are reflected back only by the interface between structures of different densities. The transducer, which both transmits and receives the ultrasound, produces 1000 pulses every second. The echocardiogram records the time taken by every pulse to return to the transducer; thus a moving structure will alter the time of return of successive pulses. By sophisticated recording and analysis over a period of time, a visual record of movement of all structures in the path of the ultrasound pulses can be seen on an oscilloscope, and can be recorded photographically; Fig. 10 shows the anatomy of the standard echocardiographic views. Fig. 11 shows diagrammatically the appearances of the various cardiac structures visualised in the standard echocardiographic views.

Interpretation of the Echocardiogram

The normal echocardiographic examination should include, where possible:

Examination of all four valves
Measurement of size of left atrium, and right and left ventricles
Measurement of left ventricle wall thickness.

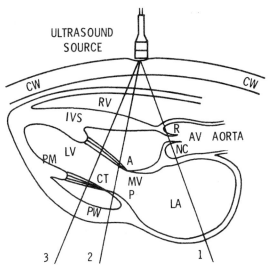

FIG. 10.—Anatomy of the standard echocardiographic views. CW: Chest Wall; RV: Right Ventricle; LV: Left Ventricle; IVS: Interventricular Septum; PW: LV Posterior Wall; LA: Left Atrium; AV: Aortic Valve (Right+non Coronary Cusps); MV: Mitral Valve (Anterior+Posterior Leaflets); PM: Papillary Muscle; CT: Chordae Tendinae.

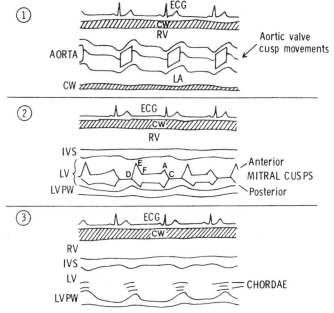

FIG. 11.—Diagrammatic appearance of the various cardiac structures visualised in the standard echocardiographic views.

Normal Structures (Fig. 12)

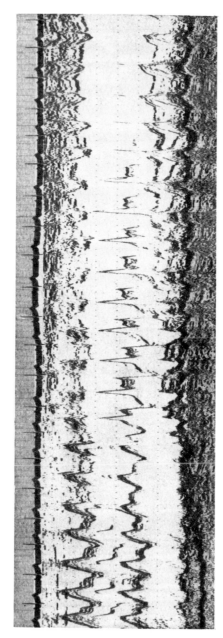

FIG. 12.—The normal appearance when the transducer is "swept" from aorta to left ventricle.

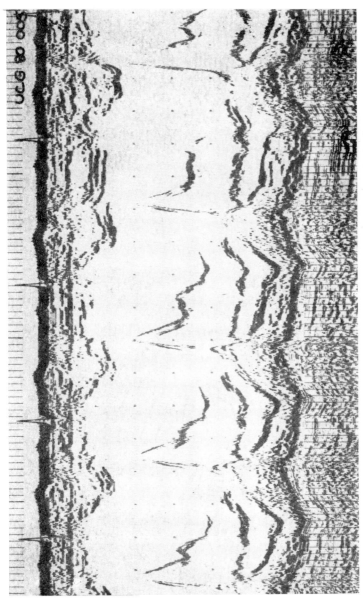

Fig. 13.—Echocardiogram showing the normal appearance of the mitral valve.

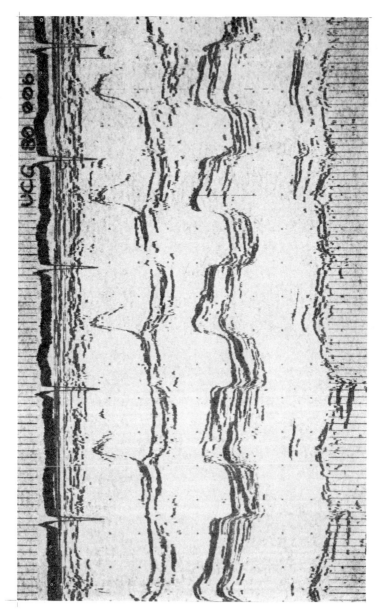

FIG. 14.—Echocardiogram showing mitral stenosis with the thickened valve cusps remaining open during most of diastole. The heavy echoes are due to valve calcification.

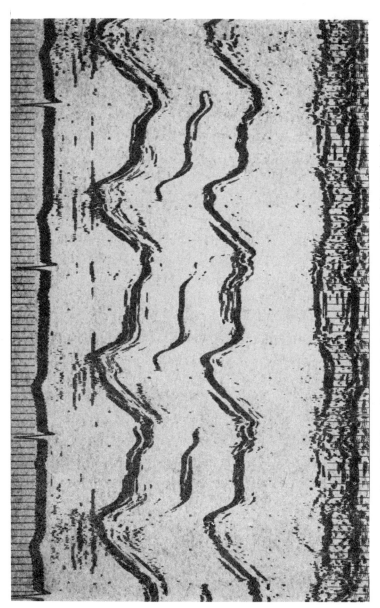

FIG. 15.—Echocardiogram showing the normal appearance of the aortic valve.

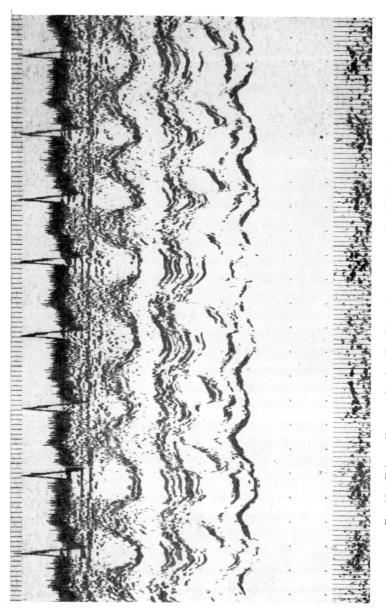

Fig. 16.—Echocardiogram showing the distorted movement of calcified aortic valve cusps.

Mitral valve.—The mitral valve serves as a reference point and is inspected first. The valve opens during diastole, the movements of both cusps are a mirror image of each other. The movement of the valve (Fig. 11 and 13) shows two peaks in diastole: the first (or E point) is due to early rapid filling of the ventricle, the valve then floats back into a partly closed position (F point), only to open again during atrial systole (A point) and close again at the onset of ventricular systole (D point). In mitral stenosis the valve remains completely open during most of diastole; thickening of the valve cusps and calcium deposition may also be seen (Fig. 14). Echocardiography has enabled prolapse of the cusps of the mitral valve to be increasingly recognised. Atrial myxomas can be detected relatively easily, but thrombosis in the left atrium, unfortunately, is difficult to detect.

Aortic valve.—The aortic valve cusps are seen as two echoes, one moving anteriorly in systole and the other posteriorly; the echoes remain more or less parallel to each other (Fig. 15). The cusps should be seen to open completely, and during diastole the single echo should be seen in the middle and not to one side of the aortic root shadow. The echocardiogram is useful in the diagnosis of obstructive cardiomyopathies, which affect mainly the left ventricular outflow tract, although the hypertrophied muscle may interfere with the function of the anterior cusp of the mitral valve, which is seen to move anteriorly during systole.

Echocardiography and the Evaluation of Left Ventricular Function

The echocardiogram has a useful role in evaluating the mechanical performance of the left ventricle by:

Documenting the size of the ventricle and percentage change in ventricular diameter during systole and diastole

Allowing calculation of ventricular volumes and the volume of blood ejected with each beat (ejection fraction)

Showing appropriate or inappropriate movement of the ventricular walls during systole as well as speed of movement

Demonstrating disturbed initial valve closure rates if ventricular compliance is reduced.

Figure 16 is an echocardiogram showing the distorted movement of calcified aortic valve cusps.

APEX CARDIOGRAPHY

Major abnormalities of the apex cardiogram. (Fig. 17).

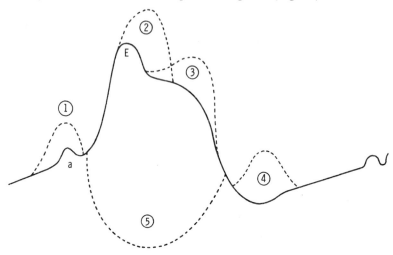

FIG. 17.—Diagram of apex cardiogram showing the main variations from normal.

1. Increased A wave (more than 15 per cent of total displacement), due to left ventricular failure causing raised end diastolic pressure in the left ventricle and increased atrial contraction, to force blood into the ventricle during diastole.
2. Increased amplitude during systole, due to left ventricular hypertrophy.
3. Abnormal shape of systolic impulse, due to left ventricular aneurysm, myocardial infarction, or cardiomyopathy.
4. Increased rapid filling wave, due to increased flow into the left ventricle as in mitral or aortic incompetence.
5. Retraction of apex during systole, due to pericarditis.

SYSTOLIC TIME INTERVALS

By recording simultaneously the phonocardiogram, carotid pulse wave, apex cardiogram, and electrocardiogram it is possible to obtain a measure of ventricular ejection time, pre-ejection time (electromechanical interval), and isovolumic systole. These measurements when related to heart rate and exercise can give useful information about stroke volume, ventricular function and valve function. The ejection time index is a derived measurement which when low indicates a reduced stroke volume and when prolonged indicates the degree of outflow obstruction, such as occurs in hypertension and aortic stenosis.

RADIOISOTOPE IMAGING OF THE HEART

It was noted incidentally that some radioisotopes used for bone scanning would accumulate in areas of acute myocardial infarction. Calcium pyrophosphate accumulates in areas of ischaemia; technetium-labelled phosphate (or similarly behaving compounds) will accumulate within 12–24 hours of a myocardial infarction. At present this technique is expensive and is only used in specialised units.

Thallium, an isotope which behaves like potassium, is rapidly taken up by the heart, depending on the blood supply; areas of reduced perfusion or ischaemia are seen as cold areas. The test can be repeated before and after exercise to establish if there are reduced areas of perfusion during exercise. It may be useful in patients with atypical chest pain or suspected angina which cannot be confirmed by other means.

CARDIAC CATHETERISATION

The purposes of catheterising the heart are to sample blood, to measure pressures and to inject radio-opaque contrast material. The right heart is catheterised via a peripheral vein, usually the saphenous or median basilic in the antecubital fossa. The aorta and left ventricle are catheterised by inserting the catheter into the femoral artery by the Seldinger[12] technique.

The pressures and wave forms of every chamber entered are recorded. The ventricular and atrial pressures are necessary in order to know the extent to which a lesion may be putting a strain on the appropriate chamber. The gradient across the aortic or pulmonary valve during systole is a measure of the narrowing of the valve. Normally the systolic pressure in the left ventricle and aorta is the same, but if the valve is narrowed the pressure in the aorta will be low and in the ventricle high; this difference in pressure is the gradient. The same is true of the pulmonary valve. The site at which the gradient occurs indicates the site of the stenosis; this is important if it is anticipated that the stenosis is below the valve (subvalvar or infundibular) as in hypertrophic obstructive cardiomyopathy. Mitral stenosis causes an elevation of left atrial pressure; this can be indirectly recorded by wedging a catheter into a distal pulmonary artery. The left atrial pressure is transmitted to the pulmonary veins and back to pulmonary arterioles. Thus, it is possible to know left atrial pressure without catheterising the left heart.

If a shunt is suspected, the oxygen saturation of the blood at known sites is estimated; the site at which there is an increase of oxygen saturation in the right heart will indicate the level of a left-to-right shunt. The extent of the step up in oxygen saturation will indicate the size of the shunt. The cardiac output can be calculated if the mixed venous (right atrial) and arterial oxygen saturations and the amount of oxygen consumed in a given time are known (Fick[13] principle). Another method of demonstrating a shunt is by dye-dilution curves. An instrument which can detect the presence of a dye in the blood is attached to the lobe of the ear. Dye is injected in the right side of the heart; if a right-to-left shunt is present, the dye will appear early at the ear ("early appearance time") because it has not had to go through the lungs to enter the left heart. In a left-to-right shunt with the dye injected into the right heart, it traverses the lungs and enters the left heart; some will return to the right heart via the left-to-right shunt and will again pass through the lungs into the left heart. The instrument will, therefore, record a normal peak and a second smaller peak ("recirculation peak").

Angiocardiograms taken during the injection of radio-opaque material will delineate the heart chambers. To demonstrate the extent of leakage of a valve a cine-angiogram is preferable; to demonstrate disordered anatomy of a valve or chamber a series of bi-plane "stills" are better.

RHEUMATIC FEVER

The incidence of rheumatic fever is declining in highly developed countries but it is still common in the underdeveloped countries. The diagnosis of rheumatic fever is facilitated by application of the diagnostic criteria formulated by Ducket Jones[14] and known by his name. The major criteria are the cardinal features of rheumatic fever. The minor criteria are non-specific evidence of a systemic disorder which gives an indication of the progress of the disease or evidence of previous streptococcal infection.

DUCKET JONES CRITERIA FOR THE DIAGNOSIS OF RHEUMATIC FEVER

Major Criteria	*Minor Criteria*
Carditis (unexplained murmurs, congestive heart failure, cardiac enlargement)	Fever
	Raised ESR or leucocytosis
	Previous attack of rheumatic fever
Arthritis	
Rheumatic nodules	Arthralgia

Sydenham's[15] chorea
Erythema marginatum.

Prolonged P-R interval on the
ECG
Raised ASO titre, or
streptococcal sore throat.

At least one major and two minor, or two major and one minor, criteria must be present to make the diagnosis. In practice difficulties of diagnosis arise in children who develop polyarthritis due to other causes. These are frequently associated with fevers, raised ESR and often with a raised ASO titre. As well as the ASO titre there are other tests for recent streptococcal infection; the most widely used is the antistreptozyme test (ASTZ). Other common causes of a febrile polyarthritis in children are Henoch[16]-Schönlein[17] purpura, Still's[18] disease, arthralgia of German measles and Reiter's syndrome in teenaged boys.

Treatment of Rheumatic Fever

The most important factor in assessing the prognosis is the state of the heart when the patient is first seen. If there is no evidence of carditis when first seen subsequent valve lesions are unlikely to develop. Evidence of mild carditis (prolonged P-R interval and pericardial friction rub) is associated with a low incidence of valve lesions. Recurrent attacks of rheumatic fever follow the same pattern as first attacks; carditis in a first attack is likely to be associated with carditis in subsequent attacks.

Several controlled trials have not shown that corticosteroids have a long-term advantage over salicylates in the treatment of acute attacks. However, other observers believe that steroids given early in the attack do prevent valve damage. Attacks of rheumatic fever associated with severe carditis should be treated with corticosteroids. Salicylates will relieve the fever and joint pain. The duration of treatment is variable; in the absence of carditis, six weeks' treatment will usually be sufficient. If there is carditis, twelve weeks' treatment is the rule, with a gradual reduction of the dose, provided the ESR and fever do not rise and the child continues to gain weight.

Prophylaxis

Following an attack of rheumatic fever associated with carditis patients should be kept on long-term antibiotic prophylaxis against subsequent streptococcal infections, either with oral penicillin taken *twice* daily or (more effectively) with monthly injections of benzathine penicillin. A previous attack of rheumatic fever not associated with carditis warrants continuous oral prophylactic penicillin. The age of 15 is the arbitrary age at which prophylaxis is stopped, provided there has not been an attack of rheumatic fever for five years. As to the treatment of sore throats in children who have not had rheumatic fever, mild sore throats should probably not receive routine penicillin unless there is bacteriological evidence of streptococcal infection, or the sore throat is likely to be part of an epidemic of streptococcal sore throats, or there are severe toxic manifestations (high fever, headaches, vomiting and difficulty in swallowing).

VALVE LESIONS

Mitral Stenosis

The mitral valve consists of two cusps, the larger is the aortic cusp and is situated close to the aortic valve, the smaller is the septal cusp. The cusps are prevented from inverting by the chordae tendinae, which are anchored to the ventricular wall by the papillary muscles. Narrowing of the valve orifice is due to inflammation of the cusps causing them to fuse. The normal size of the mitral orifice is 5 cm². The area must be more than halved before there is any significant haemodynamic effect. In the presence of stenosis the left atrium has to contract more forcibly to pump blood into the left ventricle, leading to the presystolic murmur during atrial contraction. However, most blood enters the ventricle passively in the middle of diastole; as blood flows through the narrowed orifice turbulence is produced which results in the mid-diastolic murmur. Other associated signs are the loud first sound and the opening snap.

The elevated left atrial pressure is transmitted back to the pulmonary veins, causing reflex vasoconstriction of the pulmonary arterioles, which may become fixed and irreversible. This happens in about 20 per cent of mitral stenotics and may occur when the stenosis is mild— it does not depend on the severity of the stenosis. The pulmonary artery pressure becomes elevated, resulting in right ventricular hypertrophy. Intermittent pulmonary oedema may occur due to the raised pulmonary venous pressure. As the disease progresses the left atrium dilates and fibrillates; this may be responsible for a sudden deterioration of symptoms; if the atrium contains clot the onset of fibrillation may cause a systemic embolus.

Haemoptysis is a common symptom of mitral stenosis and may be due to:

Rupture of a pulmonary vein
Rupture of a bronchial vein
Pulmonary infarction
Associated chronic bronchitis
Pulmonary haemosiderosis
Rarely, rupture of a pulmonary arteriole.

The assessment of a case of mitral stenosis involves consideration of symptoms, auscultatory findings, chest x-ray, electrocardiogram (to establish whether there is any evidence of right ventricular hypertrophy), screening of the heart (to detect valve calcification) and occasionally right heart catheterisation.

The purpose of right heart catheterisation is to measure the pulmonary artery pressure; this is normally done before and after exercise. The pressure may be normal at rest, but in the presence of increased pulmonary vascular resistance there is a sharp rise on exercise. The pulmonary artery pressure of normals does not rise more than a few millimetres of mercury after exercise. It is also important to measure the height of the left atrial pressure – this is possible by "wedging" the catheter firmly in a pulmonary arteriole; this will accurately reflect left atrial pressure changes. The rate of decline of the x and y descent are noted. There is a slowing of the rate of descent analogous to the appearances of the jugular venous pulse in tricuspid stenosis (see page 8).

In the plain x-ray of the chest, pulmonary hypertension is seen as an increase in the size of the heart and dilatation of the proximal pulmonary arteries. The peripheral pulmonary arteries end abruptly— "peripheral pruning". Elevation of left atrial pressure is suggested by left atrial enlargement, increased venous markings in the upper zones and decreased markings in the lower zone due to changes in regional pulmonary blood flow. Septal or Kerley's "B" lines at the bases are due to distended septal lymphatics associated with an elevated pulmonary venous pressure. Later, pleural effusions, pulmonary haemosiderosis and pulmonary fibrosis may occur.

It is important to realise that the auscultatory methods of assessing mobility of the valve cusps are sometimes misleading. The first heart sound may be loud and an opening snap present in a few cases in which the valve is calcified or very sclerotic. Furthermore, mitral incompetence may be present with a loud first sound and an opening snap—it used to be thought that these two auscultatory findings excluded significant mitral incompetence.

Mitral Incompetence

The mitral valve may become incompetent as a result of (i) damage to the valve cusps either by rheumatic fever or bacterial endocarditis, (ii) dilatation of the fibrous valve ring, and (iii) distortion of the cusps by malfunction of the papillary muscles by which the chordae tendinae are attached to the ventricles. The papillary muscles are part of the ventricular muscle and may be involved in any disease affecting the myocardium, particularly myocardial infarction, in which one papillary muscle may be infarcted. They are also affected in congestive heart failure, in which the papillary muscles may not function adequately, in common with the remainder of the myocardium. The functional mitral regurgitation which occurs in left ventricular failure is probably due to papillary muscle dysfunction, as it usually rapidly disappears when the failure is controlled. The alternative suggestion that the functional incompetence is due to dilatation of the valve ring is less likely because the fibrous ring is stiff and hard and is unlikely to be able to decrease rapidly in size. The murmur which occurs with dysfunction of one papillary muscle may occur in any part of systole; it is often high-pitched and ejection in type. Damage to a papillary muscle occurs particularly following posterior infarcts.

A murmur similar to that of mitral incompetence may also be produced by myocardial infarction causing rupture of the interventricular septum; this is commoner with anteroseptal infarcts. In this case the murmur is usually pansystolic, best heard at the left sternal edge, and frequently accompanied by a thrill and features of right heart failure if there is a significant left-to-right shunt.

Myxomas.—Clinical features which should alert one to the possibility of a left atrial myxoma simulating mitral valve disease are:

No history of rheumatic fever
Female patients in the second half of life
Unexplained episodes of severe congestive heart failure
Short history of "mitral stenosis" with an intermittent murmur
Absence of valve calcification
Attacks of syncope, particularly related to alterations of position
Systemic manifestation (fever, leucocytosis, raised ESR, anaemia and raised gamma globulin)
Systemic emboli in the presence of sinus rhythm.

Left atrial myxomas are much commoner than right; when myxomas do occur in the right atrium they may simulate lone tricuspid stenosis or constrictive pericarditis by causing signs of severe right-sided failure with a normal-sized heart.

Aortic Stenosis and Coarctation

Narrowing is commonest at the level of the valve (valvar stenosis) and is either congenital (bicuspid valve) or due to rheumatic fever. Narrowing below the valve is much rarer and is either due to a fibrous diaphragm or due to abnormal muscular hypertrophy—hypertrophic obstructive cardiomyopathy. Narrowing above the valve (supravalvar stenosis) is extremely rare, it is congenital and often associated with idiopathic hypercalcaemia and a characteristic facies.

Aortic sclerosis consists of atherosclerotic hardening and irregularity of the cusps of the aortic valve without gross narrowing. Clinically, the character of the pulse is vital in diagnosing the cause of an ejection murmur at the aortic area. Valvar aortic stenosis is associated with an anacrotic pulse, aortic sclerosis with a normal pulse, and hypertrophic obstructive cardiomyopathy with a "jerky" pulse with a rapid upstroke. Severe aortic stenosis is accompanied by angina which does not usually improve with trinitrin, syncope, particularly during exertion, and left ventricular failure. The murmur is conducted to the carotid vessels and to the apex and is accompanied by a diminished and delayed aortic second sound; excessive delay of the aortic second sound results in reversed or paradoxical splitting. Valvar stenosis is usually associated with an ejection systolic click, whether post-stenotic dilatation is present or not. Valvar stenosis of congenital origin does not usually cause calcification of the aortic valve whereas rheumatic valvar stenosis frequently causes valve calcification.

Indications for surgery.—Aortic stenosis in children and young adults may cause sudden death before any symptoms or ECG evidence of ventricular hypertrophy have developed. Operation on the aortic valve is usually considered if there is a systolic gradient of more than 50 mm Hg across the valve. In patients who have developed aortic stenosis later in life operation is not usually advised until moderate symptoms have developed or there is evidence of rapid deterioration of left ventricular function. There is evidence that calcific aortic stenosis developing in middle age affects valves which have been abnormal from birth.

Hypertrophic obstructive cardiomyopathy should be suspected if the pulse is "jerky", the murmur does not radiate into the neck, there is no ejection systolic click and the valve is not calcified. It is worth emphasising that aortic sclerosis is accompanied by the murmur of aortic stenosis but a normal pulse form.

Congenital aortic stenosis due to a bicuspid valve is frequently associated with coarctation of the aorta. Coarctation may occur at any level and may be multiple; however, by far the commonest site is immediately after the origin of the ductus arteriosus (adult type); narrowing above the ductus is usually more severe and is not often seen in adults (childhood type). The childhood type of coarctation is associated with a well-known but extremely rare feature, viz. cyanosis of the legs and clubbing of the toes with normal upper extremities. This is due to associated pulmonary hypertension, causing unsaturated blood to enter the lower aorta from the pulmonary artery through a patent ductus arteriosus. If the left subclavian artery originates below the patent ductus the left arm and hand will be cyanosed whereas the right will be normal.

Coarctation is much commoner in men and in Turner's syndrome than in otherwise normal women; it is frequently accompanied by other congenital abnormalities such as bicuspid aortic valves, mitral stenosis and berry aneurysms of the cerebral arteries. Berry aueurysms are due to congenital defects in the walls of the arteries which are usually situated at the bifurcation of the vessels; they do not usually enlarge until associated hypertension and atherosclerosis cause critical weakening.

The collateral arterial circulation which develops in severe coarctation results in palpable arterial pulsation on the back which is best seen with the patient leaning forward. The collateral arteries may cause a murmur which is indistinguishable from that of coarctation itself. Sometimes pressure on a palpable collateral artery will abolish the murmur if it is originating from the collaterals. Rib notching seen on the plain chest x-ray on the undersurface of the upper ribs is due to enlarged intercostal arteries eroding the ribs.

Other causes of rib notching are:

Neurofibromatosis and enlargement of nerves (amyloidosis and congenital hypertrophic polyneuropathy)
Inferior vena cava obstruction
Following a Blalock operation (left-sided only)
Rarely, congenital.

Coarctation may be associated with post-stenotic dilatation of the aorta and subacute bacterial endocarditis which usually affects the bicuspid aortic valve. The site of the coarct or the site where the stream of blood impinges on the arterial wall may be the seat of the subacute bacterial aortitis.

The causes of elevated blood pressure in coarctation have not been established with certainty. The simplest explanation is that the narrowed aorta and collaterals provide a greater resistance to flow to the lower limbs than the upper; however, in many cases of coarctation the diastolic pressure is the same in both upper and lower limbs. Another suggestion is that reduced renal blood flow or pulse pressure is responsible for generalised hypertension of renal origin but the lower limbs are protected by the narrowed aorta. A third suggestion is that the arterioles of the upper limbs have developed differently from those of the lower.

The usual causes of death in patients with coarctation are bacterial endocarditis, ruptured aorta, congestive cardiac failure and ruptured cerebral aneurysm. Twenty-five per cent of patients survive to old age. Malignant hypertension is said never to occur. The operative mortality of uncomplicated cases is low and, if discovered during childhood, surgical correction of uncomplicated coarctation is usually advised around the age of 15.

The real dilemma arises in patients who have coarctation which is not discovered until adult life and who are entirely free of symptoms. Having reached adult life they could so easily belong to the 25 per cent of *all* cases which survive to old age, furthermore there is no guarantee that correction of the coarctation will reduce the blood pressure, and thirdly, the commonest cause of death is subacute bacterial endocarditis (SBE). If the patients are carefully observed and follow the precautions against SBE the chances of developing subacute bacterial endocarditis are reduced. If the patient is entirely free of symptoms, operation in the adult is normally performed only if hypertension is severe and difficult to control, or if there is cardiac enlargement or left ventricular hypertrophy. I think there is a strong case for performing carotid angiograms on such patients and advising operation if a cerebral aneurysm is found.

Aortic Incompetence and Aortic Aneurysms

Aortic incompetence in the absence of any other valve lesions is likely to be due to syphilis. This is even more likely if there is coronary ostial stenosis which causes angina not relieved by trinitrin or if there is dilatation of calcified ascending aorta. Nonetheless, the commonest cause of aortic incompetence is rheumatic fever and it is usually associated with mitral stenosis. Severe aortic incompetence from any cause may be associated with a mitral diastolic murmur if the regurgitant jet causes roughening of the aortic cusp of the mitral valve (Austin Flint[19] murmur). Mitral incompetence may occur if left ventricular failure causes papillary muscle dysfunction or dilatation of the mitral valve ring.

Other causes of aortic incompetence are:

Bacterial endocarditis	Marfan's syndrome
Ruptured sinus of Valsalva[20]	Aortic aneurysm
Atherosclerosis	Lathyrism.

Aortic incompetence causes an increase in the stroke volume, and this increased volume of blood usually produces an ejection murmur of functional aortic stenosis; on rare occasions this functional aortic stenosis can cause a systolic thrill even though there is no organic narrowing at the valve.

Patent ductus arteriosus causes signs which can be similar to those of aortic incompetence. In patent ductus the systolic murmur occurs late in systole, is usually accompanied by a thrill, is often heard posteriorly and is loudest anteriorly on the left side.

Aortic aneurysm.—Aneurysm of the ascending aorta is known as the "aneurysm of signs" because compression of the superior vena cava is marked. Compression of the right main bronchus may cause collapse of the right lung. Aneurysm of the arch of the aorta is known as the "aneurysm of symptoms" (compression of trachea, oesophagus, recurrent laryngeal nerve and stellate ganglion resulting in cough, dysphagia, hoarseness and Horner's[21] syndrome). Dissecting aneurysms are associated with a tearing pain which may mimic ischaemic cardiac pain but unlike myocardial infarction hypertension is usual in the early stages. Enlargement of the aorta as seen on the chest x-ray may not occur for several days after the dissection. Dissection may occur anywhere along the length of the aorta and occlusion of any of the branches of the aorta may occur including the coronary, carotid, spinal, renal and mesenteric arteries, although it is exceptional in cases of dissection to be able to detect any difference between the femoral pulses.

Dissection of the aorta should be suspected if severe chest pain is accompanied by any neurological signs, hypertension, evidence of bleeding, or abdominal pain. There may even be a rise in serum transaminases and ECG changes of ischaemia.

Pulmonary Stenosis

Like aortic stenosis the narrowing may be valvar, subvalvar or supravalvar. Valvar pulmonary stenosis is almost invariably of congenital origin. The physical signs include a pulmonary ejection systolic murmur accompanied by an ejection click, wide splitting of the pulmonary second sound which is diminished in intensity. Later, severe stenosis is accompanied by signs of right heart failure. The loudness of the pulmonary systolic murmur is not a good indication of the severity of the stenosis as mild stenosis usually produces a soft murmur, moderate stenosis a loud murmur and severe stenosis a soft murmur due to right heart failure causing a diminution in cardiac output. There may be post-stenotic dilatation with valvar stenosis and an ejection click; a click is not heard in subvalvar infundibular stenosis.

Subvalvar stenosis is often associated with a ventricular septal defect which causes functional muscular hypertrophy of the infundibulum (or outflow tract) of the right ventricle.

Stenosis of the main pulmonary arteries and branches occurs but is very rare. Peripheral pulmonary artery stenosis causes a murmur which is heard in systole and diastole over a large part of the chest and is, therefore, one of the rare causes of a continuous murmur.

Indications for surgery.—If the patient has pulmonary stenosis alone, then symptoms and evidence of right ventricular hypertrophy are sufficient indications for resection even if the systolic gradient across the valve is small. In the absence of symptoms a systolic gradient approaching 100 mm Hg is the accepted indication for resection.

Pulmonary Incompetence

This is most frequently due to severe pulmonary hypertension—the resulting murmur is called the Graham Steell[22] murmur and is often surprisingly loud.

Tricuspid Incompetence

This is nearly always associated with lesions of other valves. However, lone tricuspid incompetence is being seen more frequently in drug addicts who develop bacterial endocarditis as a result of intravenous injection of unsterile drugs. It occurs in right-sided heart failure and is accompanied by a giant *v* wave in the JVP and systolic pulsation of an enlarged liver.

Tricuspid stenosis is almost always accompanied by some degree of incompetence. Characteristically, murmurs originating from the right heart increase on inspiration due to increased filling and hence output of the right heart.

SUBACUTE BACTERIAL ENDOCARDITIS (SBE)

The commonest organisms responsible for SBE are *Streptococcus viridans (Strep. salivarius), Strep. faecalis* and *Staphylococcus aureus.* Other causative organisms are pneumococci, *E. coli*, salmonella, brucella, haemophilus, *Candida albicans, Coxiella burnetii* and possibly some viruses and mycoplasmas.

The left side of the heart is involved in over 90 per cent of cases. The two commonest causes of involvement of the right side are intravenous injections with unsterile syringes, seen particularly in drug addicts in whom the tricuspid valve is frequently involved, and ventricular septal defects in which the endocarditis occurs in the right ventricle where the jet of blood from the left ventricle impinges on its wall. The practical importance of the predominance of left-sided involvement is that it may be necessary to culture arterial blood in order to grow the causative organism.

The main symptoms and signs are referable to cardiac involvement, septicaemia and embolic complications. There are two unexplained but well documented clinical observations with regard to the cardiac manifestations: the first is that SBE is uncommon in the presence of atrial fibrillation and the second is that the disease rarely occurs for the first time in the presence of heart failure, although heart failure is a common late complication.

Associated septicaemia is responsible for the fever, raised sedimentation rate, splenomegaly, clubbing, positive blood culture and anaemia. The anaemia is usually the anaemia of infection, in which there is toxic depression of the bone marrow resulting in a normocytic normochromic anaemia. A Coombs-positive haemolytic anaemia occurs occasionally. Leucocytosis usually occurs but is not invariable; occasionally there is a leucopenia. The gamma globulins are often raised and sometimes the rheumatoid and LE latex tests are positive in the absence of rheumatoid arthritis or SLE.

As a result of the septicaemia mycotic aneurysms may occur in any artery and abscesses in any organ. The embolism of fragments of the vegetations gives rise to some of the more exotic manifestations of SBE. Emboli are responsible for small renal infarcts which give rise to microscopic haematuria. In the skin emboli are seen as petechiae which characteristically occur in crops and have a white centre. Similar lesions occur in the conjunctivae, in the soft and hard palates and in the retina. Other manifestations of SBE are splinter haemorrhage under the nails and café au lait pigmentation of the skin. It is important to note that splinter haemorrhages may occur in 20 per cent of the normal hospital population.

Osler's[23] nodes are said to be pathognomonic, they consist of crops of raised reddish nodules which are always tender and usually occur in the pulp of the fingers and palms of the hands.

Arthralgia is common in SBE and may cause confusion with acute rheumatic fever. The nodules of rheumatic fever may be confused with Osler's nodes. However, the rheumatic nodule is not tender and is not in the skin, it is subcutaneous and the skin can be rolled over it. Rheumatic nodules usually last several weeks and the overlying skin is not red, they are often symmetrical in distribution and tend to occur over bony surfaces. The nodules of rheumatoid arthritis are similar to rheumatic nodules but are permanent and are associated with the characteristic joint deformity.

SBE is sometimes one of the most difficult diagnoses to make. It is important to appreciate that over a quarter of the cases occur in patients over the age of 60, that a cardiac murmur is not always audible, that a normal valve may become infected (particularly in children), that the disease presents with neurological signs and symptoms in approximately 20 per cent of cases and that infection is especially liable to occur following childbirth or urethral instrumentation.

Treatment of SBE

Prophylactic treatment consists of surgical correction of amenable congenital heart lesions, and adequate penicillin cover for dental extractions; other procedures such as cystoscopy and childbirth should be covered with penicillin plus gentamicin, as the most likely infecting organisms is *E. coli*. All the teeth should be x-rayed, and any which are very carious or associated with apical abscesses should be extracted. An aminoglycoside (gentamicin) is combined with penicillin for the treatment of resistant organisms. Gentamicin, like all the aminoglycosides, may be toxic to the vestibular branch of the eighth nerve.

The site of infection in SBE is usually avascular heart valves. Bacteriostatic antibiotics prevent organisms dividing and give the body's own defence mechanisms a chance to destroy organisms; however, in SBE the infection is out of reach of the host's defence mechanisms; hence as a general rule bactericidal drugs are preferable to bacteriostatic.

Streptococcus viridans is probably still the commonest cause of SBE and is usually sensitive to penicillin; however, the degree of sensitivity varies. Organisms which are highly sensitive are treated with 500 000 units of benzyl penicillin 6-hourly. For organisms which are relatively resistant to penicillin, much higher doses are required. Penicillin and gentamicin are both bactericidal and are synergistic. High doses of penicillin are best administered by continuous intravenous infusion. There are certain disadvantages of very high doses of penicillin: if the sodium salt is given, the high intake of sodium may precipitate heart failure—this can be overcome by giving the potassium salt. High doses of penicillin may cause cerebral oedema and haemolytic anaemia; they may also cause a slight fever, even in a patient who is not normally penicillin sensitive—this may be taken as indication that the infection is not controlled. Treatment is usually continued for six weeks or until signs of infection (fever, leucocytosis, raised sedimentation rate and weight loss) have subsided.

The dose of antibiotic should be adjusted according to the lowest concentration which is completely bactericidal for the infecting organism. As a working rule the lowest blood level of the antibiotic should be five times as high as the least concentration necessary to kill the organism *in vitro*.

If no positive blood culture is obtained and there is strong clinical evidence of SBE, penicillin and gentamicin are given, starting with 10–20 mega units of benzyl penicillin a day and increasing the dose if the patient remains febrile after 48 hours. SBE due to other infecting organisms should be treated with large doses of the most suitable bactericidal antibiotic to which the organism is sensitive.

Mixed infections sometimes occur and may give rise to difficulty if only one of the organisms has been grown from the blood, particularly if a fever remains when antibiotics are given in adequate amounts to control the one organism which has been isolated. Blood cultures should always be taken at the height of a spike of fever and from arterial blood if samples of venous blood are persistently sterile in the face of continuing infection.

Death in SBE most commonly occurs from the heart failure due to perforation of a valve cusp or rupture of a chorda tendinae. Perforation of an aortic valve cusp causes a rise in diastolic pressure in the left ventricle and early closing of the mitral valve with consequent fall in cardiac output and disappearance of the aortic diastolic murmur. There are three indications for emergency replacement of an infected valve:

1. The presence of drug-resistant organisms
2. The development of recalcitrant infection around a mechanical prosthesis
3. The development of intractable heart failure whatever the infecting organism or the stage of its treatment.

ISCHAEMIC HEART DISEASE

The myocardium may become ischaemic in the absence of narrowed coronary arteries, as in severe left ventricular hypertrophy, in which the myocardium outgrows its blood supply, and conditions in which the cardiac output is diminished, such as aortic stenosis, tight mitral stenosis and severe pulmonary hypertension. By far the commonest cause of narrowing of the coronary arteries is atheroma; however other conditions are occasionally responsible:

Syphilis may cause stenosis of the origin of the coronary arteries (ostial stenosis)

Polyarteritis nodosa and giant-cell arteritis

Coronary embolism—from valve vegetations; atrial thrombi, fat and air embolism

Congenital coronary artery fistula shunting blood from the myocardium into the right side of the heart or pulmonary arteries.

Narrowing of the arteries due to atheroma occurs principally within a few centimetres of their origin. Complete occlusion is due to thrombus formation in a narrowed segment, haemorrhage beneath an atheromatous plaque (intramural haemorrhage), or dislodgement of a plaque. The clinical features of narrowing of the coronary arteries sufficient to cause myocardial anoxia are:

Myocardial infarction   Arrhythmias
Heart failure   Sudden death.
Angina

It is now known that the myocardial muscle consists of at least two functional layers. The outer two-thirds, or epicardium, has a more efficient autoregulatory system than the inner endocardium.

The blood supply to the endocardium is much more susceptible to reduction in perfusing pressure than is the epicardium. The pressures generated during systole in the endocardial layer are higher, and the pressures generated during maximum blood flow (during diastole) are also higher because of reduced compliance in the endocardial layers. Thus, changes in blood viscosity and reduced oxygen-carrying ability, as in anaemia and ventricular hypertrophy, predispose to preferential ischaemia in the endocardium often without any cardiographic changes.

Factors Predisposing to Ischaemic Heart Disease

Age.—Although atheroma is found in the coronary arteries of children, it increases progressively with age.

Sex.—Ischaemic heart disease is rare in women before the menopause, although in negroes the sex incidence is the same at all ages.

Hypertension.—The incidence is increased in hypertensives, nevertheless, the disease occurs in the absence of hypertension. In Japan, where hypertension is common, severe coronary artery disease is rare.

Diabetes.—The incidence is high in diabetics and people with a family history of diabetes. The majority of young men with clinical coronary artery disease have an abnormal glucose tolerance test.

Obesity.—Life insurance statistics show an association between overweight and ischaemic heart disease; nevertheless the association is probably between obesity and hypertension. Obesity in the absence of hypertension is probably not a predisposing factor.

Heavy cigarette smoking.

Sedentary occupation.

Heredity.

Height of serum cholesterol and diet.

Aggressive temperament.

Mechanisms of Atheroma Formation

Mechanical.—This theory, originated by Virchow,[24] suggests that the plasma (including lipoproteins) is able to enter the endothelium and subintimal layer, and that the smooth-muscle cells trap these lipids. Hypoxia favours the development of smooth-muscle cells, which have a tendency to incorporate low-density lipoproteins (LDL), and explains why atheromatous plaques begin in the watershed zone between oxygen supplied from the lumen and that supplied from vasa vasorum.

Encrustation.—This hypothesis suggests that the primary event is the formation of thrombi on the endothelial surface, which becomes infiltrated with cholesterol and other lipids.

Haemodynamic.—This emphasises the importance of mechanical factors and the occurrence of atheroma at areas of bifurcation and narrowing. It is suggested that in such situations, turbulent as opposed to laminar flow occurs, and this increases the transfer of plasma into the intimal and subintimal layers. It is suggested that the turbulence exerts a suction effect which tends to lift the intimal off the subintimal layer.

Intramural capillary haemorrhage?—It is suggested that mechanical factors result in capillary haemorrhage into the arterial wall.

Lipophage migration.—This suggests that cholesterol-laden macrophages, which may originate in the Kupffer cells of the liver, migrate from the lumen into the arterial wall.

Causes of Atherogenesis

The notion that elevation of the plasma lipids is correlated with an increased incidence of coronary artery disease is now accepted; it is not, however, accepted that the correlation implies causation, nor that reducing the level of lipids reduces the risk. It is often suggested that the raised lipids and high incidence of coronary artery disease are both related to the primary cause or causes of the disease. Nonetheless, the relationship between the incidence of the disease and elevation of the lipids based on epidemiological studies and primary prevention studies, is widely regarded as being so important as to make the likelihood of cause and effect very great. This does not mean that other factors are not important, nor that the presence of other factors does not alter the relative importance of elevated plasma lipids as the causative factor of coronary artery disease in an individual case.

Plasma Lipids

The plasma lipids are insoluble in water and therefore have to be transported attached to a carrier; these carriers are the lipoproteins. There are four lipids and four lipoproteins. All four lipoproteins carry all four lipids, but in different proportions.

The lipids are:

Cholesterol
Triglycerides
Phospholipids
Free fatty acids.

The lipoproteins are:

Chylomicrons
Very-low-density lipoproteins (VLDL or prebeta lipoproteins)
Low-density lipoproteins (LDL or beta lipoproteins)
High-density lipoproteins (HDL or alpha lipoproteins).

The amount of each lipid attached to each lipoprotein is usually relatively constant. Normally most cholesterol is transported on the low-density or beta lipoproteins. There are many possible variations in the lipids and lipoproteins, for example:

The relative amounts of alpha and beta lipoproteins

The proportion of cholesterol attached to alpha and beta lipoproteins

The ratio of cholesterol to phospholipid attached to beta lipoproteins.

Other Factors Implicated in Atherogenesis

Several other factors may be involved in atherogenesis (with or without measurable changes in the blood lipids):

Diabetes	Obesity
Hypertension	Reduced intake of dietary fibre
Cigarette smoking	Increased sodium intake
Hyperuricaemia	Sucrose intake
Increased platelet aggregation	Level of some clotting factors.

Coronary artery disease, lipids and atheroma.—Epidemiological studies relating to the causes of coronary artery diseases fall into a number of groups:

Studies which show a significant relationship between average daily cholesterol consumption in the diet and the national incidence of coronary artery diseases.

International post-mortem comparisons which relate the degree of atheroma to the amount of fat in the diet (International Atherosclerosis Project).

Studies which relate dietary intake of fat to the subsequent development of coronary artery diseases (Seven Countries Study).

Studies on changing incidence of coronary artery disease in immigrant groups (Ni-Hon-Lan Study).

International studies involving different dietary habits of identifiable groups and their incidence of coronary artery disease, in relation to the incidence in the country as a whole.

All these studies demonstrate a clear relationship between the lipid content of the diet, the level of blood cholesterol, and the incidence of coronary artery disease.

One major paradox, which must be considered before accepting the clearly implied causal relationship between dietary lipids and an increased risk of coronary artery disease, is the paradox of group versus individual cholesterol measurements. Many series have shown a poor correlation between dietary lipid and level of serum cholesterol in different individuals. In an effort to resolve this paradox, the National Cooperative Pooling Project was established in the US, and it has found that the risk of developing symptomatic coronary artery disease is directly related to the level of serum cholesterol under the age of 55, but not over the age of 55. However it has now been established that even over the age of 55 the risk is clearly related to high levels of LDL and low levels of HDL, although not to cholesterol itself. However, little progress has been made in establishing why individual cholesterol levels vary so much even if the dietary lipid intake is the same.

For a full understanding of the problem, it is necessary to be aware that most of the epidemiological and animal experimental studies have been concerned with determining aetiology. Other studies have started from an acceptance of the hypothesis that the lipid content in the diet is a primary cause of atherosclerosis, and that other factors such as blood pressure are important but secondary causes. In order to test the hypothesis the American National Heart and Lung Institute tried between 1959–1971 to organise a large-scale single-factor primary prevention trial, but so formidable were the logistics that it was judged to be impossible. Instead, a Multiple Risk Factor Intervention Trial (MRFIT) was recommended. This should establish whether men in the upper 10 per cent of risk can reduce that risk by "multifactorial life-style and drug intervention" aimed at controlling serum cholesterol, blood pressure and cigarette smoking.

There have already been some important randomised and controlled primary and secondary prevention trials, involving modifications of dietary intakes, but unfortunately they are all open to valid criticisms with respect to randomisation, number of participants, and controls, and no consistent conclusions can be drawn.

The best known of these diet trials are:

> Chicago Coronary Prevention Program
> New York Anti-Coronary Club
> Helsinki Mental Hospital Study
> Los Angeles Veterans Administration Domiciliary Center Survey
> Minnesota Mental Hospital Study.

There are now serious reservations about the advice given by many national and professional bodies to governments concerning recommended dietary changes likely to lead to a decline in the incidence of coronary artery disease. A summary of the main evidence against dietary saturated-fat intake being the major determinant of coronary artery disease is as follows (McMichael, 1979):

> Animal feeding experiments induce fatty plaques which biochemically differ considerably from spontaneously occurring atheroma.
> Concepts of atheroma formation which fail to take into account the importance of repeated mural thromboses are misleading.

The Seven Countries Studies, on which the recommendations in the 1976 Joint Report of the Royal College of Physicians and the British Cardiac Society were based, includes a group of East Finns who were dissimilar in many respects other than blood cholesterol levels from the remainder of those included in the comparisons, and inclusion of this group disproportionately distorts the evidence, which even so is not overwhelming.

Studies in India among railway workers show a clear correlation between a high incidence of coronary artery disease and a *low* dietary fat intake.

Therapeutic induction of hypothyroidism, which raises blood cholesterol, does not result in an increase in coronary atheroma.

Trappist monks live on a low-fat diet but their coronary arteries are as bad as their less abstemious brethren, the Benedictines.

Two major secondary prevention trials, although showing a reduction in cholesterol, have not shown any reduction in recurrence of coronary thrombosis.

The incidence of coronary artery disease parallels the dietary intake of sucrose much more closely than that of fat. This weakens the arguments of a causal relationship.

Support for the reservation expressed about the over-enthusiastic introduction of steps to alter the national diet has come from other sources (Ahrens, 1979).

Myocardial Infarction

Infarction of the myocardium may occur when there is no demonstrable occlusion of the coronary artery by thrombus. When thrombosis does occur there is often evidence of a hypercoagulable state as measured by platelet stickiness, fibrinogen level and prothrombin time. Some of these factors are affected by the level of the circulating lipids.

Auscultatory Physical Signs of Myocardial Infarction

Pericardial friction rub
Gallop rhythm
Reversed splitting of the second sound (due to left ventricular dysfunction or left bundle-branch block)
Paradoxical systolic expansile pulsation of precordium
Soft first heart sound due to prolonged PR interval
Systolic murmur due to papillary muscle dysfunction or ruptured intraventricular septum.

Enzymes in myocardial infarction.—Damage to cells leads to leak of enzymes normally contained within the cells. The nomenclature and units of the commoner enzymes have been agreed by an International Convention. All enzymes are given a systematic name and a trivial name. The International Units of measurement describe the enzyme activity per litre which transforms a micromole of substrate per minute. The same figure will give the number of milliunits of enzyme per ml. Previously enzymes were expressed in spectrophotometric units.

Aspartic transaminase (glutamic-oxaloacetic transaminase).—Normal values 5–17 iu/l (or 10–35 spectrophotometric units per ml). This is the enzyme most frequently measured following myocardial infarction; the rise in serum glutamic oxaloacetic transaminase (SGOT) roughly corresponds to the size of the infarction. Following myocardial infarction the serum concentration rises to a peak after 12–48 hours and gradually falls to normal in 5–7 days; the rise does not start for at least 6 hours. Serial measurements should always be performed, for it may be the only method of identifying an extension of the infarction. A rise in enzyme concentration may be significant even though the initial value was within the normal range; for example, a rise from 10–40 spectrophotometric units may be as significant as one from 35–65. Note that there is a rise in this enzyme following pulmonary infarction particularly if the patient is shocked. It also rises in hepatocellular damage (e.g. liver congestion in congestive cardiac failure); there is also a slight rise in pancreatitis, dissecting aneurysm, and with opiates and coumarol anticoagulants. A rise in SGOT is, therefore, not diagnostic of myocardial infarction.

Alanine transaminase (glutamic-pyruvic transaminase—SGPT).— Normal values 4–13 iu/l or 8–25 units/ml measured spectrophotometrically. Contrary to popular misconception this enzyme may rise following myocardial infarction (this may be due to associated hepatic congestion) although the rise is not so high or consistent as with SGOT. It probably does not rise in pulmonary infarction.

Lactate dehydrogenase (LDH).—There are 5 different iso-enzymes of LDH—LDH_{1-5}. LDH_1 is the most likely iso-enzyme to rise in myocardial infarction. LDH_1 as well as catalysing lactate to pyruvate (hence its name) also catalyses hydroxybutyrate to oxobutyrate; hence LDH_1 measured by its effect on hydroxybutyrate is called serum hydroxybutyrate dehydrogenase (SHBD)—normal range 50–150 iu/l. The main value of LDH_1 (and SHBD) is the fact that following myocardial infarction it tends to rise more slowly than SGOT; it usually reaches a maximum at 48–72 hours and falls to normal in 7–14 days. It is important to note that LDH (even LDH_1) nearly always rises following pulmonary infarction. It also rises with damage to renal tissue, hence if it is measured in the serum it may be an indication whether urinary infection is causing renal damage.

Iso-citrate dehydrogenase (ICD).—This does not generally rise following myocardial infarction although it probably does so following pulmonary infarction.

Creatine phosphokinase (CPK).—This enzyme is specific for damage to muscle (voluntary and smooth). It may be raised due to the slight muscle damage of an intramuscular injection. This may have important practical implications if a patient with suspected cardiac pain is given an injection of analgesic before blood is taken. CPK is also raised in myxoedema.

TABLE I

EXPECTED SERUM ENZYME INCREASES IN CERTAIN CONDITIONS

Enzyme	Myocardial Infarction	Pulmonary Infarction	Hepatic Damage	Skeletal Muscle Damage
SGOT (AsT)	+ +	+ in the presence of shock or pneumonia	+ +	+ +
SGPT (AlT)	+ slightly	0 usually	+ +	+ +
LDH$_1$ (SHBD)	+ +	+ +	±	+ +
ICD	0	+	+ +	0
CPK	+ +	0	0	+ +

Other Disturbances Following Myocardial Infarction

Pulmonary congestion and reduced arterial Po_2 occur much more frequently than is usually appreciated; furthermore the Po_2 may remain subnormal for up to 4 weeks (Valentine *et al.*, 1966). Pulmonary congestion causing a reduced arterial Po_2 can usually be corrected with oxygen administration or diuretics.

Lactic acidaemia, again, is commoner than expected, and is present in over half of cases admitted to hospital; the acidosis results in a fall in plasma bicarbonate and a fall in the pH of the blood.

The output of cortisol from the adrenals is increased in most cases and the level of cortisol correlates well with the rise in white cell count and cardiac enzymes. The high cortisol is partly responsible for the rise in blood sugar and resistance to insulin which is also common.

The effect on the blood lipids is variable; the cholesterol and triglycerides often fall, particularly if they were elevated; however, there is a very close correlation between the rise in serum free fatty acids and the incidence of dysrhythmias. The high free fatty acids are probably due to the increased output of noradrenaline, the level of which may be related to the incidence of dysrhythmias.

From these observations it is suggested that patients at highest risk following myocardial infarction can be identified when other parameters of seriousness are not present (e.g. shock, prolonged chest pain, heart failure, dysrhythmias, bundle-branch block and bradycardia). If necessary high-risk patients can be identified by:

Evidence of pulmonary congestion
Reduced arterial Po_2
Reduced bicarbonate

High circulating free fatty acid
Increased blood sugar
Increased blood cortisol.

PROGNOSIS IN MYOCARDIAL INFARCTION

The mortality rises progressively with increasing age in men. In women the mortality is considerably greater than in men and remains relatively constant regardless of age.

Effects of Preceding Cardiovascular Disease

1. Hypertension.—The evidence is contradictory.

2. Previous angina.—Prognosis is undoubtedly worse if angina only developed a few weeks before the infarct; however, long-standing angina may not adversely affect prognosis.

3. Previous myocardial infarction.—Again, the evidence is conflicting: while commonsense suggests that a second attack of myocardial infarction must be more dangerous even if only because the chance of sudden death increases, careful studies have not confirmed that second and subsequent attacks have an increased mortality.

Prognosis of the Acute Attack

The reported series shows that the overall hospital mortality of acute attacks of myocardial infarction is 15–30 per cent, possibly varying with treatment. The true mortality of myocardial infarction is higher because an unknown number die before they can be admitted to hospital. Factors known to affect adversely the prognosis in the acute attack are:

Shock and hypotension
Congestive heart failure or left ventricular failure
Persistent fever and leucocytosis
Severity and duration of cardiac pain
Diabetes
Dysrhythmias including sinus bradycardia, atrial and ventricular ectopic beats and conduction defects
Systemic and pulmonary emboli.

The outcome of the acute attack is probably not related to the size or position as judged from the electrocardiogram, provided that there are no dysrhythmias or conduction defects. Subendocardial infarcts probably have a better prognosis than transmural infarcts. The slightly greater danger of posterior infarcts is due to their proximity to the conducting tissue; however, provided there is no evidence of conduction defects the risks are probably the same. Rupture of the interventricular septum is more common with anterior infarcts, rupture of the chordae tendinae and ensuing mitral regurgitation are more common with posterior infarcts.

Approximately 80 per cent of deaths from myocardial infarction will occur within the first 24 hours; the majority of the remaining deaths will occur during the following two weeks.

It should be noted that the ultimate prognosis is quite independent of whether the electrocardiogram returns to normal in terms of disappearance of Q waves, abnormal ST segments or T waves.

The risk of death following acute myocardial infarction is greater if the ECG shows right bundle-branch block and left axis deviation.

Coronary Prognostic Index

Using the method of discriminant analysis with a computer Norris and his colleagues have produced a list of early measurable factors which adversely affect the *hospital* mortality from coronary thrombosis. Although of some value in estimating the prognosis in individual patients the index is of greater value in the objective assessment of claims of new treatment of coronary thrombosis (Norris *et al.*, 1969). Factors which adversely affect the prognosis of *acute* myocardial infarction in order of importance are:

1 Hypotension   4 Transmural infarction
2 Old age   5 Cardiac enlargement
3 Pulmonary oedema   6 Previous angina.

They did not find that the prognosis was adversely affected by previous diabetes, hypertension, obesity or myocardial infarction.

Factors which adversely affect prognosis *after recovery from acute* myocardial infarction are (Norris *et al.*, 1971):

1 Old age   3 Heart size
2 Pulmonary oedema   4 Previous myocardial ischaemia.

Post-myocardial infarction syndrome.—Following an operation in which the pericardium has been opened, a syndrome sometimes develops three weeks to six months afterwards which consists in fever, pericardial pain, and pericardial effusion. There is a tendency to relapse for up to two years. An identical syndrome has been described following myocardial infarction and is known as Dressler's[25] syndrome or the post-myocardial infarction syndrome. The syndrome is usually treated with salicylates and steroids. Early treatment is desirable because arrhythmias and cardiac failure are frequent complications.

THE ANTICOAGULANT CONTROVERSY

The rationale for the administration of anticoagulants is based on:

The probability that thrombosis is less likely to occur if clotting of blood is impaired

Experimental evidence in dogs that extension of coronary thrombosis can be prevented with anticoagulants

The belief that much of the mortality from coronary thrombosis is due to peripheral venous thrombosis and embolism, and extension of mural thrombus within the coronary artery

Statistical evidence from series of clinical cases of myocardial infarction treated with and without anticoagulants

The belief that atheroma may be due to mural thrombosis on the wall of arteries which *subsequently* become infiltrated with lipids.

The problems about anticoagulants have arisen because:

It is not made clear whether anticoagulants are being used to treat the acute attack of "myocardial infarction"/"coronary thrombosis" or whether they are to prevent a second attack

Death in ischaemic heart disease is frequently due to nonthrombotic events

Antithrombotic agents other than anticoagulants may be of value in (a) preventing or slowing atheroma, (b) preventing thrombus formation and thus preventing coronary thrombosis.

There have been numerous controlled trials to evaluate the efficiency of anticoagulants; they nearly all suggest that anticoagulants are beneficial, but none of them is entirely free from criticism with regard to controls, allocation of patients, quality of treatment, diagnosis, follow-up and statistical analysis (Mitchell, 1981). Considerable support for the value of anticoagulants came from the Sixty-Plus Reinfarction Study.

Anticoagulants for the Acute Attack of Myocardial Infarction

No one denies that the anticoagulants reduce the risk of venous thrombosis and death from pulmonary embolism but the concept of anticoagulants preventing further thrombosis within the artery is seriously questioned. Several autopsy studies have failed to demonstrate arterial occlusion in unequivocal cases of fatal second myocardial infarcts following soon after a first infarct. The conclusion is that many second infarcts are not caused by further thrombosis. In a very large international collaborative series 25 per cent of deaths from myocardial infarction had no thrombotic occlusion of any of the coronary arteries.

As to the treatment of acute cardiac infarction with anticoagulants mortality figures have shown a definite reduction in thrombo-embolic complications but not necessarily of mortality. To some extent it is possible to predict those cases which will be prone to deep vein thrombosis and thrombo-embolic complications. These "bad risks" cases are characterised by:

Prolonged shock	Arrhythmias
Intractable pain	Diabetes
Obesity	Previous myocardial infarction
Heart failure	or deep vein thrombosis.

In 1969 the Medical Research Council Working Party published its findings on the value of short-term anticoagulants following myocardial infarction. It concluded that there was no significant reduction in mortality with 28 days' anticoagulants, although there was a marked reduction in thrombo-embolic complications, some of which were serious. This survey did not completely answer the problem as to the value of *short-term* anticoagulants—the level of anticoagulation was not high, some patients were transferred from control to treatment group, there was a small reduction in mortality in the treated group and a marked reduction in the number of thrombo-embolic complications.

The most rational course at present is to consider treating with short-term anticoagulants those patients who fall in the "bad risk" group who do not have a definitive contra-indication to anticoagulants.

Value of Anticoagulants in Preventing a Further Myocardial Infarction (Secondary Prevention)

There are innumerable trials showing that anticoagulants are beneficial; however, most of them have defects with regard to controls, allocation of patients and quality of treatment. Until 1955 anticoagulants were very widely used; however, some physicians remained sceptical. The most comprehensive survey in favour of anticoagulants was the report of the Committee on Anticoagulants to the American Heart Association (Wright *et al.*, 1954).

In an effort to clarify the situation, further controlled trials have been conducted. In 1964 the Medical Research Council trial concluded that while anticoagulants reduce the risk of reinfarction and perhaps of death under the age of 55, this effect largely disappears by the third year of treatment. It should be noted that this influential trial did not contain enough women for proper statistical analysis. It had come to be widely believed that any protection from anticoagulants only affects men. It has since been shown that women are protected to the same extent as men. Further support for a marginally beneficial effect in patients under the age of 55 is given by the International Anticoagulant Review Group (1970). The exact duration of protection is still an open question.

The controversy remains, particularly as there continue to be sporadic reports of benefit from anticoagulants (Modan et al., 1975; Tonascia et al., 1975). Generally these confirm that the benefit from anticoagulants lasts about one year following a myocardial infarction. The extent to which oral anticoagulants are still used varies, but in the United States 28 per cent of hospitals administer anticoagulants to most patients with myocardial infarction; in the United Kingdom 11 per cent of hospitals anticoagulate myocardial infarct patients, whereas in other Western European countries 85 per cent of hospitals still anticoagulate most patients (Bassan and Rogel, 1976), and are continuing to report considerable benefits from anticoagulants.

Despite the fact that most of the studies showed some improvement in mortality with oral antithrombotic agents, the majority of deaths following myocardial infarction may not be thrombotic in nature (e.g. they may be due to dysrhythmias or sudden heart failure). It is becoming clear that thrombus formation is not simply related to the conventional clotting factors, but may be initiated by disturbances in platelet function, such as their stickiness and tendency to aggregate and release initiators of the conventional fibrin-forming clotting factors. There are now world-wide trials in progress to establish the value of drugs which are known to modify platelet behaviour (Gautmacher, 1979). The main agents are:

Aspirin
Dipyridamole (Persantin)
Sulphinpyrazone (Anturan).

There are a number of secondary prevention trials to assess the value of these agents in reducing the frequency of thrombotic events, e.g.:

AMIS (Aspirin Myocardial Infarction Study)
PARIS (Persantin/Aspirin Reinfarction Study)
ART (Anturan Reinfarction Trial).

There is still no certainty as to how these anti-platelet-aggregation drugs work, but aspirin is known to inhibit an enzyme, cyclo-oxygenase, which is involved in the production of prostaglandins. The situation is complicated because one prostaglandin (thromboxane) in the platelets increases platelet aggregation while another prostaglandin in the wall of blood vessels (prostacyclin) reduces platelet aggregation. Aspirin inhibits the production of both the beneficial prostacyclin and the harmful thromboxane. However, it is believed that the thromboxane pathway may be inhibited by much lower doses than the prostacyclin pathway. The situation is further confused by the fact that dietary modification may influence platelet aggregation and prostaglandin production, in addition to its effect on the blood lipids. There are also factors, particularly in fish oil, which prevent Eskimos, who live almost entirely off animal fats and proteins, from having an unusually high incidence of coronary artery disease.

Coagulation and Anticoagulants

Thrombin formation forms fibrin from fibrinogen. Once formed, fibrin becomes stronger as a result of increasing the number of cross-linkages between fibrin molecules, a process which requires Factor XIII and calcium. The initiating event in the clotting cascade is activation of Factor X. Factor X can be activated by two mechanisms: firstly by tissue thromboplastins from damaged cells via Factor VII (extrinsic pathway), and secondly from contact with an abnormal surface, e.g. collagen (intrinsic pathway, so-called because the clotting cascade begins without requiring intrinsic thromboplastins). The intrinsic pathway activates Factor X through several other clotting factors (XII, XI, IX and VIII). The extrinsic pathway takes only a few seconds to activate thrombin; the intrinsic pathway takes several minutes; this is a safety mechanism against intravascular coagulation. Once activated, Factor X in the presence of Factor V produces thrombin from prothrombin.

Action of anticoagulants.—*Heparin.*—By itself, heparin has no effect on clotting, but in the blood there is a natural inhibitor of clotting called antithrombin III. Its action is normally slow but when it binds with heparin its conformity changes, so that it has a much greater affinity for thrombin and so prevents clotting. The heparin/antithrombin III complex also inactivates Factors XII, XI, VII and X. The action of low-dose heparin is mainly the inhibition of Factor X; hence in low doses it reduces the tendency to thrombosis without having an effect on the clotting time.

Coumarin anticoagulants.—These act by inhibiting the action of vitamin K, which is a co-factor concerned in the manufacture of clotting factors. Coumarin anticoagulants interfere with the resynthesis of vitamin K. The effect of inhibiting vitamin K will depend on the normal half-life of the affected Factors II, VII, IX and X. The first to fall is Factor VII (proconvertin), the last is Factor II. Longer-term administration of coumarin anticoagulants (or deficiency of vitamin K) leads to the overproduction of clotting factor precursors, some of which themselves inhibit blood clotting and are called Proteins

Induced by Vitamin K Absence (PIVKAS); they may be relevant to the tests used to monitor the dose of anticoagulants.

Tests of coagulation. *Prothrombin time.*—This measures the extrinsic pathway (tissue thromboplastin, Factors VII, X, thrombin, and fibrin formation).

Activated partial thromboplastin time (APTT).—This measures the *intrinsic* pathway (XII, XI, IX, X, thrombin, and fibrin formation). A standardised platelet thromboplastin is used (hence "partial") as is a standard "surface", in the form of kaolin (hence "activated").

Thrombotest.—This is a commercial test made of all clotting factors except those affected by vitamin K, so that it is sensitive to the presence of those factors dependent on vitamin K; it also takes account of the presence of PIVKAS. Its main value however is that it can be made on capillary blood, unlike the prothrombin time and APTT.

Heparin.—A steady-state blood level of heparin may not be achieved until 48 hours after infusion, because of uptake by the reticulo-endothelial system. The half-life of infused heparin is about 1½ hours. This is prolonged in renal failure. The normal intravenous loading dose is 10 000 units with an average infusion rate thereafter of 1000 units per hour. There is some evidence that prolonged heparin therapy leads to a *reduction* in anti-thrombin III levels and a decreased binding capacity of antithrombin III for thrombin, so that antithrombin III neutralises less thrombin which may lead to an increased tendency to clot.

Control of heparin dose.—The partial thromboplastin time should be kept at approximately twice the normal (about 50–100 seconds is the therapeutic range). Heparin has less effect on the "Thrombotest" method because of the dilution involved in performing the test. The APTT and Thrombotest can also be used for controlling heparin dosage if the heparin in the sample is first neutralised by protamine.

Coumarin anticoagulants.—The most widely used is warfarin (named after the institution in which it was isolated and which holds the patents—Wisconsin Alumni Research Foundation coumarin).

Withdrawal of Anticoagulants

It is suspected that cessation of anticoagulant therapy is associated with an increased number of thrombic incidents. There are clinical statistical surveys which both confirm and refute this clinical impression. Nevertheless there is good laboratory evidence of increased coagulability of the blood in *some* patients when anticoagulants are stopped. The question then arises whether this "rebound hypercoagulability" can be mitigated by more gradual withdrawal. Again the clinical statistical evidence is conflicting, but there is laboratory evidence that hypercoagulability is reduced when anticoagulants are withdrawn slowly. There seems to be a special risk of thrombotic complications in patients who have been on anticoagulants for more than two years. From a practical point of view it is wise to "tail off" anticoagulants gradually when this is being done as an elective procedure. When patients have been controlled on anticoagulants for more than two years, "tailing off" should be done very gradually.

TREATMENT OF HEART FAILURE

The treatment of heart failure first concentrated on attention to the pumping function of the heart with inotropic drugs, and then progressed to reducing the preload on the heart by reducing fluid load by diuretics; it has now progressed to the logical step of giving attention to reducing the afterload or peripheral resistance. Part of the physiological response to heart failure is to increase peripheral resistance, and once the pump is working optimally as a result of inotropic drugs it is logical to try to reduce peripheral resistance. The drugs which produce peripheral arterial dilatation are hydralazine, prazosin, minoxidil and phenoxybenzamine. Drugs such as isosorbide dinitrate act principally on the venous capacitance vessels, and so primarily reduce congestion at the heart. In the presence of heart failure these drugs do not usually result in hypotension and tachycardia, which may be a feature when the same drugs are used for the treatment of essential hypertension.

Related to the more rational approach to the management of heart failure are questions concerning the routine use of inotropic drugs. The use of digoxin was questioned first in patients with cor pulmonale, some of whom had a high cardiac output. The use of continued digoxin administration in patients who have had heart failure, but who are now out of failure and in sinus rhythm, has been challenged as unnecessary. It is known however that digoxin can impove cardiac output in heart failure when sinus rhythm is present, and clinical deterioration may occur in up to a third of patients if their digoxin is stopped, even though they are in sinus rhythm and their heart failure has been controlled previously.

Angina

Other drugs should be considered in the treatment of angina if beta blockers in optimum doses do not sufficiently relieve symptoms, or if there are contra-indications to them such as bronchospasm or heart failure. Some patients are unwilling to take trinitrin because of the severe transient headaches it may produce. Isosorbide dinitrate for some patients is better than trinitrin—it has a longer half-life and acts as quickly if the tablets are chewed before being swallowed. There is no convincing evidence that the longer-acting nitrates or sustained-release preparations are effective. Perhexiline (Pexid) acts as a peripheral and coronary vasodilator, but is generally considered too toxic for routine use. Nifedipine (Adalat) is a potent calcium antagonist which causes a reduction in myocardial oxygen demand. It has no antidysrhythmic properties and can be used in conjunction with beta blockers. Occasionally angina is *worsened* by the drug. Prenylamine (Synadrin) depletes catecholamines from the sympathetic system and this may delay its beneficial action for 1–2 weeks. It should *not* be used with beta blockers or other negative inotropic drugs, because there is a risk of ventricular tachycardia. For this reason it should be used with caution if drugs liable to cause potassium depletion are also being administered.

Prinzmetal's Syndrome (variant angina)

The syndrome is due to spasm of the coronary arteries and was first described in 1959. It consists of chest pain at rest or on slight exercise, with transient elevation of the ST segments in the electrocardiogram, which return to normal as soon as the pain recedes. The chest pain, which resembles that of angina, may last longer than a classical anginal attack, and may not have nearly such a clear relationship to exercise and rest. In classical angina the ST segments usually become depressed during an acute attack or during an exercise test. When angina is due to spasm, long-acting vasodilators such as isosorbide are more logical than beta blocking drugs.

CORONARY ARTERY BYPASS GRAFTING

Coronary Angiography

Selective coronary angiography was introduced in 1958. It is now a relatively safe procedure; the associated mortality varies but it is probably about 1 per cent, with a similar significant morbidity. The indications are still debatable and are partly dependent on availability. Generally speaking, several attacks of proven myocardial infarction under the age of 60, and first attacks at a young age, particularly if primary risk factors are absent or eliminated (e.g. weight reduction and cessation of smoking), and angina which is poorly responsive to conventional medical treatment, are indications for angiography.

The decision whether or not to proceed to bypass surgery depends on a number of factors:

The severity of symptoms of angina are no guide to the extent of the disease of the coronary arteries
Medical treatment of angina, particularly with beta blockers, probably has no effect on survival—only on symptoms

The results of coronary artery surgery (or any other therapy) are bad if there is severe ventricular failure (ventricular dyskinesia) Surgery is indicated for:

(a) Ventricular septal defects caused by septal infarction
(b) Papillary muscle dysfunction causing mitral incompetence
(c) Ventricular aneurysm

Prevention, both primary and secondary, is also essential (smoking, hypertension, hyperlipidaemia, diabetes).

The present position about coronary artery bypass can be summed up as follows:

Persistent significant angina remains the basic indication for the operation

In selected cases angina is relieved in 80 per cent of patients

Relief of angina may not be accompanied by improvement of left ventricular function

The bypass may become occluded in 20 per cent of patients, leading to a deterioration in left ventricular function

The underlying coronary disease is not improved by coronary artery bypass grafting

The effect on prognosis is still undetermined, but it is reasonable to suppose that operation may improve prognosis in patients with 3-vessel disease, and probably with significant 2-vessel disease; prognosis may not be improved in single-vessel disease

Whether or not surgery is advised, constant attention must be given to risk factors, especially cigarette-smoking and hypertension

The figures for surgical results quoted tend to reflect the results in the best centres

The place of coronary artery bypass grafting in unstable or intermediate angina (also called crescendo angina, acute coronary insufficiency or pre-infarction angina) is still controversial, but unstable angina is more often associated with single-vessel disease and is an indication for early coronary angiography.

Problems in Management of Myocardial Ischaemia

Coronary artery bypass surgery
The value of coronary-care ambulances
The value of coronary-care units and hospital treatment for patients with myocardial infarction
The risks of early mobilisation and early discharge from hospital
The value of beta blockers and other drugs in reducing mortality after myocardial infarction.

Mobile Coronary-Care Units (MCCU)

The majority of deaths from myocardial infarction occur in the first hour, and there is now evidence from many countries that mobile coronary-care units can reduce this mortality. The best known units are in Belfast, Brighton and Seattle, and the introduction of MCCUs was recommended in 1975 by the Royal College of Physicians. However, consideration of cost-effectiveness and serious problem about staffing and equipment have prevented their more widespread introduction in the UK.

Home Versus Hospital Treatment of Coronary Thrombosis

In 1971, Mather in Bristol suggested that mortality was similar whether or not patients with myocardial infarction were admitted to hospital; however this study has been severely criticised for the following reasons:

> It did not contain any women
> Only 25 per cent of patients were included in the trial
> The cases were seen relatively late and were relatively mild, all the more serious ones having been already admitted to hospital.

Early Mobilisation or Early Discharge

Recently evidence has been produced in favour of so-called early mobilisation, but it should be noted that the two most important trials in this respect referred to 7 and 10 days as "early" mobilisation. Other trials have suggested that early discharge from hospital may be as safe as keeping the patient in, but following early discharge there is roughly a 7 per cent readmission rate and a 7 per cent mortality after discharge in the first 6 weeks, and it is debatable whether some of these deaths would not have occurred if the patients had remained in hospital.

Beta Blockers following Myocardial Infarction

In patients receiving the discontinued beta blocker oral practolol, there was a reduction in sudden death in those with an anterior myocardial infarct, but no effects were found on other manifestations of myocardial infarction. However, recent evidence suggests that beta blockers are beneficial following myocardial infarction.

The Use of Prophylactic Antidysrhythmic Drugs

Prophylactic lignocaine, mexiletine and disopyramide have all been advocated as soon as the diagnosis of myocardial infarction is suspected; however, the general feeling is against giving antidysrhythmic drugs without adequate monitoring facilities.

DYSRHYTHMIAS

Atrial fibrillation.—This is the commonest. P waves are always absent and the ventricular rate is always totally irregular. *Atrial tachycardia* occurs when the sinus node or an ectopic atrial focus fires off impulses and the ventricles contract very rapidly. Some of the atrial impulses may be blocked at the atrioventricular node and the ventricles only respond to the impulses which are not blocked (atrial tachycardia with block). The ventricles usually respond to atrial impulse with a normal QRS complex; sometimes, however, conduction of the impulse in one of the branches of the bundle of His is disturbed and the ventricular QRS complex is abnormal or "aberrant".

At a normal rate an atrial ectopic focus may discharge prematurely, giving rise to an atrial extrasystole, in which case the P wave is abnormal in shape and the P-R interval abnormally short.

Atrial flutter.—This consists of regular rapid atrial discharges some of which are regularly blocked by the atrioventricular node so that the ventricular rate is slower. Because of the difficulty in distinguishing different types of tachycardia arising from the atria or atrioventricular node such tachycardias are frequently called "supraventricular" tachycardias.

Junctional or atrioventricular nodal rhythms.—The shape of the ventricular QRS complex is usually normal. Electrical impulses may be conducted upwards towards the atria from the A-V node giving rise to an inverted P wave. This P wave may precede, be lost in, or follow the ventricular QRS complex.

Ventricular ectopic beat.—Conduction of the QRS complex is always abnormal and usually resembles the complexes of either right or left bundle-branch block. They may occur singly or in groups as a ventricular tachycardia; there are no preceding P waves.

Distinction between Supraventricular and Ventricular Tachycardias

No P waves in ventricular tachycardia

Supraventricular tachycardia is usually perfectly regular whereas a ventricular tachycardia is usually slightly irregular

In ventricular tachycardia the first heart sound varies in intensity due to the slight irregularity causing variations in length of the diastolic pause

Shape of QRS complexes will be normal in supraventricular tachycardia unless there is associated aberration

The shape of the complexes in ventricular tachycardia will resemble any previous ventricular ectopic beats—if a previous ECG is available

Carotid sinus compression may slow a supraventricular tachycardia but not a ventricular tachycardia.

A-V block.—First degree: prolongation of the P-R interval. Second degree: some dropped beats, i.e. every P wave is not followed by a QRS complex. The Wenckebach[26] phenomenon is a particular type of second-degree block in which the P-R interval becomes progressively longer before one beat is dropped. The P-R interval then becomes short and the cycle is repeated.

Third degree A-V block occurs when none of the P waves trigger off ventricular complexes (complete heart block), which may lead to Stokes[27]-Adams[28] attacks.

The Electrophysiological Basis for Dysrhythmias

The fundamental difference between the various pacemaker tissues of the heart, and the remainder of the myocardium, is their ability to depolarise spontaneously (automaticity). The pacemaker which normally controls the heart rate is the one which depolarises and repolarises most rapidly. The depolarisation wave from the main pacemaker thus depolarises all other cells capable of acting as pacemakers *before* they are ready to depolarise spontaneously. Once all the cells have depolarised, they are refractory to further stimuli unless subjected to a stimulus of greater intensity. Normally the interior of a pacemaker cell is negatively charged with respect to the outside, the resting transmembrane potential being about 90mV (see Fig. 19). The remainder of the myocardial cells are non-automatic, and will maintain their transmembrane potential until a wave of depolarisation lowers it below the threshold potential; thereafter depolarisation inevitably occurs. The rate of automatic impulse formation decreases from the sino-atrial node through the conducting system to the Purkinje[29] fibres, which means that normally the sino-atrial node is the controlling pacemaker.

The gradual spontaneous lowering of resting potential to approach the threshold potential, which characterises all pacemaker cells, is due to a leak of sodium ions into the cell. This property does not occur with non-automatic cells unless they are damaged, in which case they can develop pacemaker properties of their own. The spread of an electric impulse involves alterations in adjacent cell membranes so that sodium ions can leak inwards, raising the resting potential beyond the threshold level, and so causing these cells to depolarise. Thus the spread of the depolarisation wave throughout the heart takes a finite length of time (unlike electrical conductivity). The ability to maintain a voltage difference between the inside and outside of a healthy, resting cell depends on preventing leakage of sodium and potassium ions into it, and this involves the cell in energy production. If the cell is deprived of oxygen, the energy supply fails, the transmembrane potential is lost or declines, and the process of repolarisation takes longer, resulting in a slowing of the rate of conduction through the injured tissue. Following a myocardial infarct, normally non-automatic cells may develop automaticity, leading to the production of ventricu-

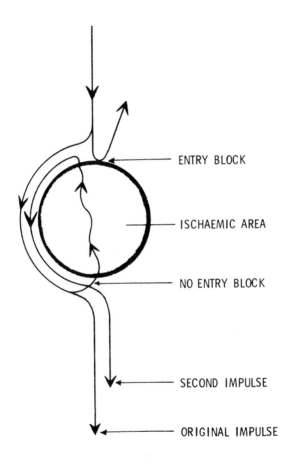

ENTRY BLOCK

ISCHAEMIC AREA

NO ENTRY BLOCK

SECOND IMPULSE

ORIGINAL IMPULSE

FIG. 18.—Re-entry phenomenon or unidirectional (one-way) block. The impulse arrives at the ischaemic area but is unable to pass through because of the unidirectional block. It therefore passes around the area and is partly propagated onwards; but because the block is only one way, the impulse can pass *back* slowly through the area. If then it arrives at the original site of attempted entry after the refractory period caused by the original impulse, a further impulse can be propagated through the original pathway, giving rise to repeated impulses, tachycardia and arrhythmias. The effect may be abolished by drugs which either completely block entry to the ischaemic area (thus preventing re-entry as well) or by enhancing conduction through the ischaemic area.

lar tachycardias. In the muscle fibres of the heart, depolarisation results in an inflow of calcium ions, which is the fundamental trigger of mechanical contraction, involving the contractile proteins actin and myosin.

Current of injury.—If a damaged cell does not repolarise completely it remains at a less negative potential than an adjacent, normal, fully repolarised cell, and a current known as the current of injury flows. This causes the characteristic ST-segment elevation in the ECG following a myocardial infarct.

Excitability or vulnerability.—A depolarisation stimulus arriving at a normal cell during repolarisation does not cause further depolarisation, but an injured cell may depolarise before being fully repolarised; this state of abnormal excitability or vulnerability is greatest at a stage of depolarisation which coincides with the T wave of the electrocardiogram.

Re-entry and unidirectional block.—This refers to the phenomenon whereby damaged tissue conducts the depolarising impulse differently depending on the extent of the damage. Depending on circumstances it may completely block the entry of an impulse, or it may slow the conduction of an impulse once the impulse has entered, so that it may emerge from the damaged area *after* the refractory period due to the initiating depolarisation, leading to a rapid stimulus to further depolarisation. This can occur in two separate ways (see Fig. 18).

After-potentials.—This refers to the property of damaged cells to have a small, spontaneous, secondary afterswing when repolarisation is complete. If this afterswing should reach the threshold potential, the cell will again spontaneously depolarise.

Temporal dispersion of recovery of excitability.—This refers to the effects of the autonomic nervous system on the normal depolarisation/repolarisation timing, and the effects of the autonomic system on the re-entry phenomenon.

Unfortunately, knowledge of the electrophysiological changes in normal and injured cells, and the theoretical ways in which antidysrhythmic drugs could alter action potentials to limit their automaticity, is not matched by an availability of drugs capable of altering action potentials in specific and beneficial ways.

Antidysrhythmic drugs exert a beneficial effect by:

1 1 Action on action potentials reducing automaticity (Figure 19): (a) Prolonging phase 4, and so increasing cycle length; (b) raising the threshold potential, i.e. the voltage at which inevitable depolarisation will occur; (c) Lowering the resting potential so that with a depolarisation stimulus it takes longer for the threshold potential to be reached.
2. Reducing after-potentials

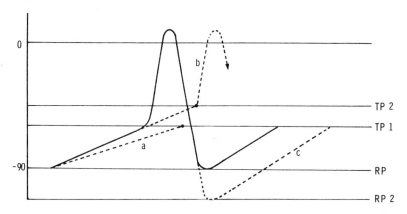

Fig. 19.—Diagram of electrical changes in a pacemaker myocardial cell during depolarisation, with theoretical possibilities for the actions of drugs in slowing the rate of depolarisation.

TP1 First Threshold Potential.

TP2 Threshold Potential with drug which raises threshold potential (and therefore slows rate) by mechanism "b".

RP1 Resting Potential at rapid rate.

RP2 Resting Potential with drug which lowers resting potential (and therefore slows rate) by mechanism "c". Line "a" shows the mechanism of drugs which slow the rate by increasing cycle length.

3. Limiting re-entry and converting unidirectional block into bidirectional block

4. Limiting harmful autonomic influence.

The mechanisms of action of the antidysrhythmic drugs have been classified electrophysiologically and clinically (Vaughan Williams, 1978):

> *Drugs of Class* 1.—These reduce the rate of depolarisation without affecting resting potential or without increasing the duration of the action potential. They prolong the refractory period. Examples are lignocaine, procainamide and mexiletine.

> *Drugs of Class* 2.—These reduce sympathetic drive, either by beta adrenergic blockade, e.g. propranolol, or by interfering with the release of neurotransmitters. An example is bretylium.

> *Drugs of Class* 3.—These prolong the duration of the action potential and the refractory period. An example is sotalol.

> *Drugs of Class* 4.—These block the movement of calcium from the cell membrane to the contractile system of the muscle, and so prevent an electrical stimulus resulting in muscle contraction. An example is verapamil.

Treatment of Dysrhythmias

Many drugs have the property of slowing the heart rate. Practically all the available drugs have been used to treat all the dysrhythmias. However, certain drugs, whose effects are well known and which work in the majority of patients with a particular dysrhythmia, are generally used before other "second line" drugs.

When confronted with a patient who has a tachycardia, the first thing to decide is whether the tachycardia is causing:

Heart failure
Low cardiac output, poor peripheral perfusion or hypotension.

The commonly recommended drugs in particular dysrhythmias are shown in Table II.

TABLE II (A)
TREATMENT OF DYSRHYTHMIAS

	Factors modifying treatment	First-line management	Second-line management
Supraventricular			
Sinus tachycardia	If LVF present	digoxin	
	If due to excess catecholamine drive	beta blockers	
Atrial extrasystoles		procainamide phenytoin	beta blockers disopyramide
Paroxysmal tachycardia	Pacing if resistant to drugs or if LVF is caused by tachycardia	digoxin beta blockers procainamide	phenytoin verapamil
Atrial fibrillation	Digoxin if LVF present	digoxin procainamide	DC conversion disopyramide
Atrial flutter	DC shock if LVF	digoxin	beta blockers
A-V junctional tachycardia	Verapamil (not to be injected for 8 hours after giving beta blocker)	verapamil	procainamide digoxin
Sick sinus syndrome		pacing	
Ventricular			
Extrasystoles	If rate is slow: atropine If rate is rapid: beta blockers	lignocaine procainamide	mexiletine disopyramide
Tachycardia		lignocaine procainamide	mexiletine disopyramide

N.B.—Disopyramide is negatively inotropic; therefore, if heart failure is present, digitalis should be considered first.

Phenytoin is especially useful in digitalis-induced arrhythmias.

Phenytoin may be used in either supraventricular or ventricular dysrhythmias.

Lignocaine may also be effective in supraventricular tachycardia.

Table II (B)
Drugs

Drug	Proprietary name	Ampoule size	Amount of drug per ml	Recommended maximum dose
Digoxin	Lanoxin	2 ml	0·25 mg	1 mg
Practolol	Eraldin	5 ml	2 mg	5mg repeat after 5 minutes
Procainamide	Pronestyl	10 ml	100 mg	1 g 2 mg/minute maintenance
Phenytoin	Epanutin	5 ml	50 mg	250 mg over 5 minutes, repeat 10 minutes later if necessary
Disopyramide	Rythmodan	5, 10, 15 ml	10 mg	150 mg/hr (conversion within 10 min) 800 mg/day maintenance
Verapamil	Cordilox	2 ml	2·5 mg	5 mg i.v. over 1 hour 100 mg/day maintenance
Mexiletine	Mexitil	10 ml	25 mg	25 mg/minute as a bolus 50–100 mg/hour infusion maintenance
Lignocaine	Xylocard	5 ml	20 mg 200 mg	100 mg as a bolus 5 mg/minute as maintenance

ECG Patterns of some Specific Disorders of Rhythm and Conduction

Captured beats refers to A-V dissociation in which some of the atrial impulses successfully pass through the A-V node and result in a ventricular complex.

Escape beat refers to a beat occurring after an interval longer than the usual cycle length. It refers to the fact that if an atrial beat is not conducted normally through the A-V node, the A-V node or other tissues assumes the pacemaker function.

Reciprocal rhythms or beats refers to the phenomenon of an impulse arising in the A-V node and causing a nodal ventricular contraction, following which the impulse is retrogradely conducted back through the A-V node and gives rise to a further ventricular beat. It will generally be detected as inversion of some of the P waves.

Parasystole refers to the coexistence of two pacemakers each of which is responsible for an independent rhythm. In other words, the dominant pacemaker fails to suppress an ectopic pacemaker. The ectopic pacemaker is said to have "entrance or protection block".

Intraventricular conduction defect.—QRS complex width may vary with different heart rates. The resulting QRS pattern usually approximates to right bundle-branch block because the right bundle usually has the longest refractory period. Occasional sinus-conducted beats may be prolonged or abnormally shaped because of the simultaneous occurrence of an ectopic ventricular beat, which becomes fused with the QRS complex arising from the sinus beat.

Fusion beats.—The fusion of ventricular complexes which originate from different foci; they occur in parasystole.

Exit block refers to a sudden decrease in heart rate (usually halving) with an atrial or nodal tachycardia, and is an explanation for the sudden reduction in rate based on the concept of *reduced exit* of impulses from the pacemaker.

Entry block refers to parasystole and is an explanation of why the dominant pacemaker impulse fails to suppress the impulse from an ectopic pacemaker: the normal impulse is unable to *enter* the ectopic pacemaker.

Ectopic beat or extrasystole refers to a beat originating from any pacemaker other than the sinus node.

Premature beat refers to the early occurrence of an ectopic impulse.

Pre-excitation refers to the bypassing of normal A-V junctional tissue, which results in a short PR interval and usually abnormal ventricular conduction; the most common variety is the Wolff-Parkinson-White syndrome, although there are many ECG variants of the classical syndrome.

Fascicular block.—The bundle of His divides into right and left branches, with the left branch further dividing into anterior and posterior branches. Complete heart block may occur when, (a) the bundle of His is damaged by a single lesion (unifascicular block), (b) both main branches are damaged by two lesions (bifascicular block), and (c) all three branches are damaged (trifascicular block). The right bundle and left anterior bundle share a common site in the upper part of the interventricular septum, and the left anterior bundle has a long subendocardial course and is therefore especially liable to damage. Blockage of the anterior branch of the left bundle results in extreme left axis deviation with a normal QRS width. Blockage of the posterior bundle results in extreme right axis deviation, but is almost never seen alone.

Atrioventricular dissociation refers to the independent beating of atria and ventricles; usually the rate is over 60 per minute. Atropine and exercise will usually allow the atrial impulse to be conducted through the A-V node, and results in captured ventricular beats. It should be distinguished from complete A-V block (complete heart block), in which the ventricular rate is below 40 per minute and exercise or atropine have no effect in increasing the ventricular rate. A-V dissociation is not usually an indication for pacing unless it causes Stokes-Adams attacks.

His Bundle Electrogram

This technique is not available outside specialist centres, but an awareness of its implications is important in appreciating the pathophysiology of A-V block. It is possible by placing intracardiac electrodes in relation to the bundle of His to record potentials from the bundle (H deflection). By noting whether the H deflection occurs late in cases of heart block it can be ascertained whether the cause of atrioventricular block is above the bundle or below it. There is an approximate correlation between the site of a block and the width of the QRS complex. Higher or proximal blocks have narrow QRS complexes and are associated with a better prognosis.

Elective DC Conversion

Atrial fibrillation or flutter which is rapid and not causing heart failure or hypotension should be controlled initially with digoxin. When the rate is controlled, the use of elective DC conversion should be considered. The digoxin should be stopped for 48 hours before the attempted conversion of the fibrillation or flutter. It is customary to give anticoagulants for at least 3 weeks before the conversion, to lessen the likelihood of dislodging a clot from the atrial wall. Anticoagulants prevent new thrombus formation in the left atrium, which allows time for organisation of old thrombus to occur. If possible the period of anticoagulation should be more than three weeks—there is evidence that complete organisation of a recent atrial clot takes longer than three weeks in some patients. Inspection of the atria in patients operated on for mitral stenosis frequently shows recent and friable clot, even though the patients have been fully anticoagulated for several months. It is wise to anticoagulate patients for at least two months, if possible, before elective DC conversion. DC conversion should always be considered for atrial flutter and atrial fibrillation. But there are some definite *contra-indications* to conversion:

Atrial fibrillation due to thyrotoxicosis (until the patient is euthyroid)
Mitral incompetence
Mitral stenosis (conversion should be attempted after a successful mitral valvotomy)
Ischaemic heart disease

Previous arterial emboli
Large left atrium
Fibrillation of more than 6 months' duration.

Following successful DC conversion to sinus rhythm the patient should be given oral procainamide 250–500 mg q.d.s. for one month—this lessens the likelihood of relapse. Occasionally pulmonary oedema develops after a successful DC conversion, probably because of improvement in output from the right side of the heart. The left atrium being smaller and less expansile when it is functioning normally and not fibrillating, it is probably unable to accommodate the increased venous return from the lungs, leading to pulmonary oedema.

The sick sinus syndrome describes a situation in which function of the sinus node is intermittent. The patient usually has both a bradycardia and a tachycardia. On the same cardiogram the patient may have sinus rhythm, sinus bradycardia, nodal rhythm, supraventricular ectopic beats, or tachycardia. If symptoms are present long-term pacing is indicated.

CARDIAC ARREST

Sudden failure of the heart to pump blood (cardiac arrest) may be due to:

Complete cessation of electrical and mechanical movement within the heart (asystole);
Rapid but ineffective electrical and mechanical movement of the heart (ventricular tachycardia and fibrillation).

The vital priority is speed in diagnosing cardiac arrest—establishing the cause can come later. The initial treatment is the same whatever the cause.

Diagnosis

The diagnosis of cardiac arrest is based on:

The history of sudden collapse
Unconsciousness
Absent or diminished carotid pulses and heart sounds.

In addition the patient may be cyanosed, apnoeic, have widely dilated pupils, or someone may already be doing external cardiac massage.

Treatment

A patent airway should be ensured. The patient should be lying on his back preferably on a hard surface (either on the floor or on a mattress under which a fracture board has been placed). To ensure a patent airway the neck should be extended and the mandible drawn forwards—this stops the tongue flopping backwards into the airway.

A Brook airway should be inserted, and mouth-to-mouth respiration started if the patient is not breathing spontaneously. If an anaesthetist is present he should insert an endotracheal tube, when the patient can be inspired from an Ambu bag and given oxygen at the same time.

It should be ensured that effective external cardiac massage is being performed.

An intravenous infusion should be set up and 100 ml of 8·4 per cent sodium bicarbonate (1 ml contains 1 mEq or mmol) run in, to prevent acidosis due to accumulation of lactic acid in the anoxic tissues.

An ECG machine should be set up and a definitive diagnosis made. Now is the time to assess the situation fully.

Definitive diagnosis is the stage most frequently mismanaged. The number of possible diagnoses from the ECG are only 4, and the correct treatment of each is more or less agreed. The function of the heart is to pump and the function of the ECG is to record electricity—it should be emphasised that normal electrical complexes on the ECG do not mean that the heart is pumping blood; on the other hand, the heart can be effectively pumping blood even though the ECG records abnormal electrical impulses. Both the ECG electricity and the functioning of the pump must be assessed by feeling peripheral pulses, inspecting the pupils and listening to the heart sounds, and noting whether or not the skin remains cyanosed.

The four abnormalities of the electrocardiogram and their emergency treatments are:

1. Asystole.—Only a few or no ventricular complexes are seen.

Treatment: Injection of 5 ml of 1 in 10 000 adrenaline into 1 cardiac chamber. The needle should be inserted into the chest where it is thought the apex beat should be and a point 5 cm deep to the sternal angle aimed for. If this fails an injection of 5 ml of 10 per cent calcium chloride should be given into the heart. Injection of adrenaline and/or calcium chloride should produce ventricular fibrillation.

2. Ventricular or supraventricular fibrillation or tachycardia.—Ventricular complexes occur as a series of regular or irregular troughs and peaks.

Treatment: Intravenous lignocaine or procainamide 100–500 mg, followed by DC defibrillation. It should be ensured that both electrodes are well covered with contact jelly but that the jelly does not extend beyond the electrodes; one is held on the upper sternum and the other over the apex—several shocks can be delivered if necessary.

3. Heart block.—Ventricular complexes may look relatively normal, but are slower than 40 per minute. P waves may or may not be present.

Treatment: Isoprenaline 1–5 μg intravenously very slowly, followed later by external or internal pacing.

4. Sinus bradycardia.—Normal-shaped complexes with preceding P waves, but at a much slower rate than normal.

Treatment: Atropine sulphate 0.6 mg intravenously or intramuscularly, followed by isoprenaline if necessary.

VENOUS THROMBOSIS

Over 50 per cent of patients with deep vein thrombosis have no physical signs. Deep vein thrombosis and pulmonary embolism are more common than is generally realised in healthy people with no predisposing cause. The site of *origin* of thrombosis is frequently not the site from which a pulmonary embolus originates; thus a pulmonary embolus in the presence of unilateral signs of deep vein thrombosis is *equally* likely to have arisen from the leg *without* physical signs. The sites of *origin* of venous thrombosis in order of frequency are:

Deep veins of the calf
Posterior tibial veins
Common femoral vein
Popliteal vein
External iliac vein.

Although these are the sites in which deep vein thrombosis begins, the pelvic veins are by far the most frequent *source of pulmonary emboli*.

Physical Signs

It must be assumed that the physical signs of deep vein thrombosis, such as Homans'[30] sign, are insensitive guides, and that the incidence of thrombosis is more common than they indicate. However, this applies to most other diseases, and is not a reason for abandoning the signs but a spur to improving them.

The deep veins possess valves, and drain from the muscles of the calf into the anterior and posterior tibial veins; these unite just below the popliteal fossa to form the popliteal vein, which continues upwards to form the femoral vein medial to the femoral artery under the mid-point of the inguinal ligament. Because the femur slopes inwards and forwards from the hip to the knee, the vein lies behind the femur at the lower end, medial to it in the middle third, and anterior to it at the top. The deep veins of the plantar surface of the foot drain mainly into the posterior tibial vein, which is situated deep to the tendo-Achilles. The anterior tibial vein runs in the groove between the tibia and fibula in the lower two-thirds of the lower leg, and then penetrates the interosseous membrane to join the popliteal vein.

The *superficial* veins of the lower leg are in communication with the deep veins and with each other. The short saphenous vein runs up the back of the calf from behind the medial malleolus to enter the *popiteal* vein behind the knee, while the long saphenous vein runs up from in front of the malleolus on the medial side of the leg to enter the femoral vein in the femoral triangle. The femoral vein becomes the external iliac vein, which is situated near the rectum. The majority of the deep veins in the calf are within the soleus muscle, which is deep to the gastrocnemius. These anatomical points are important because they help in the appreciation of a number of significant signs of deep vein thrombosis which are frequently ignored.

1. Thrombosis of the plantar veins causes pain and tenderness on palpation in the soles of the feet.

2. Thrombosis affecting the posterior tibial vein causes tenderness on palpation behind the tendo-Achilles.

3. Thrombosis of the anterior tibial vein causes tenderness in the groove between tibia and fibula in front of the lower leg.

4. Because the veins in the soleus muscle are more often affected than those in the more superficial gastrocnemius, palpation of the calf should be done in such a way that the *deep* muscles of the calf are palpated; this is best done using both hands. The debonair, token clasping of the calf without removing the bedclothes, which sometimes passes for palpation of the calf, should be deprecated.

5. Blockage of the deep intramuscular veins of the lower leg, or of the tibial veins, results in more blood flowing in and between both superficial saphenous veins. Small dilated communicating veins, particularly from the short to the long saphenous veins, can be seen just below the knee or above the ankle; these veins slope upwards and are more pronounced on the anterior and lateral aspects of the lower leg.

6. Obstruction of the deep intramuscular veins, and associated local inflammation cause fluid to accumulate locally. If this is severe, it is seen as oedema or increase in circumference of the leg; however, it can be detected at a stage earlier than this by careful examination. The knee is flexed to the 90° position with the foot resting on the bed—this completely relaxes the calf muscles; the flat *palm* of the hand is used gently to lift those muscles up and down, trying to assess two things; firstly, the weight of the muscles, and secondly, their hardness as compared with the opposite side.

7. Careful palpation of the popliteal vein in the popliteal fossa and posterior part of the lower thigh.

8. Careful palpation of the adductor muscles on the medial side of the mid-thigh.

9. Careful palpation of the femoral vein medial to the femoral artery below *and* above the inguinal ligament. Tenderness above the inguinal ligament indicates extension to the external iliac vein.

10. Rectal examination, to discover whether there is tenderness of the veins within the pelvis. In a woman, vaginal examination may be indicated, particularly as a base-line observation.

In a case of suspected deep vein thrombosis all the above signs should be systematically looked for in addition to the more orthodox signs, viz.:

Oedema
Increased warmth
Homans' sign
Difference in circumference of the two legs
Diminished arterial pulsation of the affected side
Superficial thrombophlebitis
Slight elevation of the temperature.

Causes of Deep Vein Thrombosis

Virchow's triad of the known predisposing factors to vascular thrombosis is:

1. Damage to the vessel wall. This may be mechanical trauma such as a blunt injury, or may occur if there is hypoxia of the circulating blood, or if the veins are compressed when empty of blood. Damage to the endothelium can cause thrombosis even when blood flow is normal. Certain drugs, hormones, and toxins also damage vascular endothelium, e.g. adrenaline, serotonin, dextran, ACTH, bacterial endotoxins and cholesterol.

2. Reduced blood flow. This is particularly important in patients who are kept in bed, thus reducing or eliminating the venous pump mechanism which is partly responsible for blood flow in the veins. The movement of the diaphragm is probably an important factor in aiding venous return; this movement is of course reduced following abdominal or thoracic surgery.

3. Increased coagulability of the blood. This occurs following bed rest and operations. It may also occur following fatty meals or in the presence of hypercholesterolaemia.

Factors Predisposing to Deep Vein Thrombosis

Immobility and trauma
Surgery, pregnancy, parturition and oestrogen contraceptives
Congestive cardiac failure
Age—there are conflicting reports about effect of increasing age on
the incidence of deep vein thrombosis

Sex—there is probably no increased risk in women if pregnancy, etc, are excluded

Obesity

Race—the incidence is said to be low in Africans and Indians

Climate—the incidence is probably increased in cold weather

Malignant diseases, polycythaemia, anaemia and dehydration

Pelvic tumours.

Confirmatory Investigations

Phlebography. Contrast dye is injected into the superficial veins of the feet. Thrombi are seen as *constant* filling defects; recent thrombus is usually only attached at one point, hence there may be a thin line of contrast between the filling defect and the wall of the vein. Complete occlusion of a vein is assumed if the filling of the veins above and below the non-opacified vein is seen.

^{125}I-labelled fibrinogen. Fibrinogen is incorporated into both recent and old clots. Radioactive counts are made at fixed points on both legs. The counts overlying thrombus will be increased. This technique can only be used to detect venous thrombosis below the mid-thigh level; above this the background radiation is too high for meaningful results.

Ultrasound flowmeter. This detects slowing of blood flow in partially occluded *large* veins such as the femoral and iliac veins. It is an extremely simple technique.

Treatment

Analgesics for local pain.

Elastic bandaging of the leg, beginning at the feet and working upwards; care should be taken to see that the elastic bandage does not locally constrict any part of the leg. The purpose of the bandage is to compress the superficial veins and so encourage increased flow through the deep veins.

Positioning of the leg.—When the legs are horizontal the veins still drain upwards (from the posterior tibial vein at the heel to the femoral vein in the front of the thigh). The rate of flow in the veins may be increased if the foot is elevated so that the blood is then flowing horizontally or even slightly downhill; this is probably the optimum position once venous thrombosis has occurred. However, for the *prevention* of deep vein thrombosis, elevation of the *head* of the bed may be better, because when the feet are raised there is a tendency for the veins to collapse and this may offset any increased flow; total blood flow to the legs is *reduced* with the leg elevated. An additional advantage of raising the *head* of the bed is that the patient tends to slip to the foot of the bed, and has to use his leg muscles to keep himself in the proper place in the bed; this constant muscular activity promotes venous return.

Prevention of further clotting.—Heparin 10 000 iu intravenously is given immediately the diagnosis is made. An intravenous drip should then be set up and heparin given at a rate which keeps the clotting time between 15–20 mins. Heparin affects every stage of the clotting process, and in particular it inhibits thromboplastin generation, the action of thrombin on fibrinogen, and the conversion of prothrombin to thrombin. Heparin is a cumulative drug, especially in the presence of renal failure, and it also has some fibrinolytic, antihistamine and anti 5-hydroxytryptamine properties; it also decreases platelet stickiness. All these properties are valuable in deep vein thrombosis and pulmonary embolism. Oral anticoagulants are given at the same time—usually warfarin or nicoumalone (starting dose 20 mg, maintenance dose approximately 4 mg daily).

Preservation of venous valves.—Thrombolytic treatment to preserve venous valves has been successfully used. Following deep vein thrombosis, recanalisation of veins usually occurs, but the valves are completely disorganised by the fibrosis within the clot. Damage to the veins may have long-term unpleasant effects, such as the post-phlebitic syndrome, chronic leg oedema, induration and ulceration; any measures which can preserve the valves may be of value. To be of value treatment must be started within five days of the thrombosis developing or recent non-adherent clot should be demonstrated by phlebography. However the treatment is expensive and time-consuming and most physicians doubt whether it is reasonable to use it on a wide scale for deep vein thrombosis alone.

Prevention of recurrent pulmonary emboli.—There is considerable evidence that fatal pulmonary emboli nearly always arise from the ileofemoral (proximal) veins; clinical evidence of involvement of these veins may not be present. In the case of recurrent pulmonary emboli which are not prevented by adequate anticoagulation, the only hope used to be vena cava ligation or plication. With the advent of phlebography it is usually possible to outline the clot in the iliofemoral veins, or to demonstrate occlusion of the veins; if a clot is seen, or obstruction is demonstrated, femoral and/or pelvic venotomy and thrombectomy can be performed, while infusing heparin continuously through a catheter in the femoral vein. The phlebography should always be performed on *both* sides since a fatal pulmonary embolus frequently comes from the side in which there are no clinical signs. Occasionally vena cava ligation or plication are still required when thrombectomy fails to remove all the thrombus or is followed by further thrombosis despite full anticoagulant therapy.

Following a pulmonary embolus for which the patient has been fully anticoagulated, a second embolus occurs with surprising frequency. In one series, 14 per cent of patients had a second and fatal embolus and 26 per cent had a second but not fatal embolus (Browse, 1969). This is why these sophisticated methods of investigation and treatment with thrombectomy can be so important to an individual patient.

Prevention of deep vein thrombosis.—Many series have confirmed the value of anticoagulants given prophylactically in preventing venous thrombosis following major surgery (including thoracotomy, hip, abdominal and gynaecological operations). Surgeons who have experience of operating on patients who are well controlled on anticoagulants generally affirm that bleeding during and after operation is not a problem (Sevitt, 1968). It is a shame that local N.H.S. exigencies usually preclude such time-consuming but life-saving measures as prophylactic anticoagulation. Without anticoagulants the incidence of venous thrombosis following major surgery in patients over the age of 40 is 35 per cent. This alarming incidence *cannot* be lessened by intensive prophylactic physiotherapy to the legs postoperatively. There is now firm evidence that 5000 iu heparin given every 12 hours subcutaneously will lessen the incidence of deep vein thrombosis following most major operations and after myocardial infarction.

Low-dose heparin.—Subcutaneous doses of 5000 units of heparin have an antithrombotic effect without affecting whole blood clotting time. It is now know that heparin in low doses exerts its action by stimulating the production of antithrombin III; much higher doses of heparin are necessary to inhibit the thrombin-fibrinogen reaction. There is now a great deal of evidence showing that low-dose heparin is of value in preventing post-operative deep vein thrombosis and deep vein thrombosis following myocardial infarction.

CONGENITAL HEART DISEASE

The development of the heart and great vessels is completed after two months gestation, thereafter only increase in size occurs. This is important with regard to infections or drugs known to interfere with the development of the heart and great vessels. Rubella occurring in the first two months of pregnancy is a potential cause of cardiac malformation (usually patent ductus arteriosus and pulmonary stenosis); when rubella occurs after two months there is much less danger. Other conditions known to be associated with a higher-than-normal incidence of congenital heart disease are mongolism (the commonest lesion is an ostium primum atrial septal defect), Turner's[31] syndrome (coarctation and pulmonary stenosis), gargoylism (fibroelastosis), Marfan's[32] syndrome (dissecting aneurysms and atrial septal defects), and drugs such as thalidomide (atrial and ventricular septal defects).

The commonest congenital heart diseases in order of frequency are ventricular septal defect, atrial septal defect (secundum type), patent ductus arteriosus and Fallot's[33] tetralogy. Fallot's tetralogy is the commonest congenital heart disease of adults, causing clubbing and cyanosis.

Ventricular Septal Defects (VSD)

The defect is nearly always in the membranous part of the septum. The size of the defect does not necessarily reflect its haemodynamic severity, since the defect may partly close during systole due to contraction of the muscular part of the ventricular septum; spontaneous closure of small defects is the rule. When the defect is large, more blood may be passing through it than is pumped into the systemic circulation. There are two mechanisms which tend to reduce the left-to-right shunt with large defects: one is an increase in pulmonary arteriolar resistance, and the other is hypertrophy of the pulmonary outflow tract causing functional muscular hypertrophic subvalvar pulmonary stenosis. The characteristic murmur of a VSD is pansystolic and best heard in the third and fourth left intercostal spaces; it radiates over the precordium and is frequently accompanied by a thrill (mitral incompetence is less commonly accompanied by a thrill, and the murmur radiates into the axilla). If the muscular part of the septum contracts, the murmur may only be present early in systole. There is often a third heart sound due to the extra volume of blood entering the ventricle because of diversion of a portion of the stroke volume through the defect. The maladie de Roger[34] is a ventricular septal defect which is causing no symptoms and is not accompanied by any alteration of the electrocardiogram or chest x-ray. Small septal defects frequently close spontaneously.

In larger defects the output of the right ventricle may be double that of the left ventricle into the aorta (i.e. half the cardiac output passes through the defect—a 50 per cent shunt). The increased volume of blood flowing through the pulmonary and mitral valves may cause functional mitral diastolic and pulmonary systolic murmurs. This is important because a pulmonary ejection systolic murmur does not necessarily indicate organic stenosis of the valve or functional stenosis of the infundibulum. The presence of a mitral diastolic murmur gives an indication that the shunt is fairly large.

At higher flow rates the right ventricular pressure increases due to functional infundibular narrowing or pulmonary hypertension. The elevated right ventricular pressure will diminish the flow through the defect, leading to disappearance of the mitral diastolic and lessening of the pulmonary systolic murmurs. As the right ventricular pressure rises further it exceeds the systemic pressure, and venous blood from the right ventricle flows through the defect into the left ventricle causing central cyanosis (Eisenmenger's[35] syndrome).

Treatment.—Operation is generally indicated if the pulmonary to systemic flow rate is more than 3:1, especially if the right ventricular systolic pressure exceeds 50 mm Hg. Operation is contra-indicated when the Eisenmenger situation has developed. Polycythaemia commonly develops in congenital heart disease; it increases the viscosity of the blood and this offsets any advantage of increased oxygen capacity. If cyanotic congenital heart disease is associated with severe polycythaemia (Hb greater than 17 g per cent or PCV more than 65 per cent) venesection should be considered. The risk of thrombosis *in situ* is considerably increased in the presence of polycythaemia and if this is occurring anticoagulants may be indicated.

Atrial Septal Defects (ASD)

In the embryo the atria are at first separated by a crescentic septum (septum primum) which grows downwards to fuse with the atrioventricular rings; the gap between the two limbs of the crescent is the ostium primum. As the ostium primum closes a hole develops in the upper part of the septum—the ostium secundum. A second septum (the septum secundum) develops in the right atrium. In the fetus the lungs are not functioning and the right heart is responsible for pumping blood through the patent ductus arteriosus into the aorta; the blood entering the right heart comes from the umbilical vein of the placenta, and is rich in oxygen and nutrients. At birth the lungs expand, the pressure in the right heart falls so that the pressure in the left atrium is higher than in the right. The septum primum is pressed against the septum secundum, the ostium secundum is obliterated, and blood flow ceases. A small oval portion of the ostium secundum may remain patent and forms the foramen ovale. A secundum ASD is due to persistence of the whole of the ostium secundum (i.e. the second hole in the septum primum is not blocked off by the septum secundum). A primum ASD is due to the persistence of the ostium primum. The septum primum is associated with the atrioventricular valve rings, hence primum defects are complicated by incompetence of the atrioventricular valves. The physical signs of a secundum ASD are an elevated *a* wave in the JVP (due to the stronger left atrial contraction being transmitted through the defect to the right atrium), a diastolic murmur at the tricuspid area, and an ejection systolic murmur at the pulmonary area due to increased blood flow through the tricuspid and pulmonary valves. The pulmonary component of the second sound is widely split because the already overloaded right atrium and ventricle are unable to accommodate more blood during inspiration: splitting is already maximum in expiration (fixed splitting).

Right bundle-branch block usually occurs. The chest x-ray may show enlargement of the right atrium and large pulmonary arteries due to increased blood flow (pulmonary plethora). A primum ASD is also accompanied by a pansystolic murmur due to incompetence of the atrioventricular valves. The electrocardiogram may show right bundle-branch block with left axis deviation, the explanation for which is not known. In contrast, the right bundle-branch block of a secundum defect is accompanied by right axis deviation.

Treatment.—Surgical correction is indicated if the pulmonary to systemic flow rate is 2 or 3:1, or there is evidence of increasing pulmonary hypertension. Patients in whom the diagnosis is made in adult life pose a special problem. They usually remain symptom-free until 30–40, the average age of death of unoperated cases being around 50. Operation is usually not performed in adults over the age of 45 or if the pulmonary vascular resistance is at systemic levels.

A patent ductus arteriosus results in a collapsing pulse and a murmur heard in systole and diastole, since the systolic and diastolic pressures in the aorta exceed those in the pulmonary artery throughout the cardiac cycle.

Congenital heart defects which are unimportant haemodynamically are often the cause of subacute bacterial endocarditis. The defect itself need not be affected and associated lesions are frequently the only sites infected, e.g. SBE develops in the right ventricle in a mild VSD where the stream of blood impinges on the wall of the ventricle, or it develops on the bicuspid aortic valve associated with coarctation.

HYPERTENSION

The average blood pressure of most, but not all, *populations* of *healthy* people increases slowly with age. However the blood pressure of many individuals in the population remains the same throughout their lives. Rise in blood pressure with age seems to be proportional to the starting blood pressure (Miall and Lovell, 1967). The distribution curve of blood pressure in the general population does not show two peaks, one for normal people and one for people with hypertension. However the controversy is still not resolved as to whether essential hypertension is a distinct disease or whether blood pressure is a variable, like height, which means that no particular level of blood pressure can be said to be abnormal and thereby indicate the *disease* "hypertension". Some workers feel that essential hypertension is a distinct disease determined by a single pair of genes, and that the distribution curve for blood pressure in the general population may show a bimodal distribution. It is thought that other pieces of evidence suggest an important role for inheritance in the development of essential hypertension: namely, the occurrence of hypertensive complications in pairs of identical twins, the fact that populations do exist in which blood pressure does not rise with age, and the frequent strong family history of hypertension or hypertensive complications in patients with hypertension. Blood pressure, like height, is different in individuals, and the complications of high blood pressure are not determined solely by inheritance but by environmental factors as well.

The South Wales epidemiological surveys involving urban (Rhondda Valley) and rural (Vale of Glamorgan) populations support both polygenetic inheritance *and* environment as causes of raised blood pressure. The evidence favours shared genes (i.e. widespread occurrence of genes influencing blood pressure), so that environmental factors are likely to be more important in causing the development of a high pressure or change of pressure in healthy individuals and their relatives (Miall and Oldham, 1963).

Two clear conclusions can be drawn from life-insurance statistics and the Framingham and Veterans Administration surveys: *mortality* from *most* hypertensive complications is related to the height of the diastolic pressure, and the same level of raised diastolic pressure is more serious the younger the person. What may still be uncertain is whether lowering the blood pressure to normal in borderline hypertension restores or even improves the outlook. It is agreed that treatment may not improve outlook, because the hypertension may have been present for some time and may already have caused its damage. This problem is still unresolved and large trials are in progress in the UK and USA to try to establish whether borderline hypertension should be treated.

THE CONTROL OF BLOOD PRESSURE AND ITS DERANGEMENT IN HYPERTENSION

The precise causes of most cases of hypertension are usually not known. The situation is complicated for the following reasons:

Should hypertension develop, the normal controlling mechanisms may behave differently from when hypertension is not present

Should hypertension develop, other controlling mechanisms assume a much greater importance than they do in normals

Different controlling mechanisms are important, depending on the duration of the hypertension

Only rarely is a discrete disturbance of any one of the controlling mechanisms ever responsible for the development of hypertension.

The Control of Blood Pressure in Normals

Blood pressure is dependent on:

1. Cardiac output
2. Peripheral resistance
3. Circulating blood volume.

1. **Cardiac output** is dependent on
   (a) Venous return
   (b) Autonomic control of heart rate and contractility
   (c) The ability of the myocardium to respond appropriately.

2. **Peripheral resistance** is dependent on the length and bore of the main resistance vessels; both of these criteria are influenced by systemic and local factors. The blood flow in different organs is affected by modulation of autonomic alpha- and beta-receptor stimulation, and accumulation of local metabolites (e.g. CO_2 and lactic acid), which result in local vasodilatation.

The bore of arterioles is affected by:

(a) *Intrinsic tone of arterioles*. This may be an important factor; it is known that a very slight increase in arteriolar smooth muscle may have a profound effect in reducing the distensibility of arterioles, leading overall to an increase in peripheral resistance and to hypertension (this phenomenon is sometimes referred to as the Folkow concept).

(b) *Autonomic regulation*. Most vascular smooth muscle contains alpha receptors which tend to produce *vasoconstriction*; the beta receptors, which are fewer, tend to produce vasodilatation. However, beta receptors predominate in the interface between autonomic sympathetic fibres and the target organ (often wrongly called a synapse); thus beta blockers work mainly by reducing noradrenaline release from the synapse, and therefore prevent stimulation of alpha receptors in the vessel wall. This explains why both alpha and beta blockers may work in hypertension. Autonomic nervous system regulation is mediated by carotid artery and aortic baroreceptors. These in turn modulate hypothalmic sympathetic outflow, as well as directly affecting the heart and possibly the adrenal medulla. Some vascular beds, e.g. brain and kidney, do not behave as the rest of the body; they have their own autoregulation and preferential blood flow.

(c) *Circulating hormones*
   (i) Angiotensin II
   (ii) Catecholamines

Angiotensin II. In addition to its direct action on blood vessels, it also stimulates ACTH production and some of the enzymes involved in adrenal steroid production, particularly the 18-hydroxylation reaction which results in production of 18-deoxycorticosterone, which itself has vasoactive and salt-retaining properties.

3. **Control of blood volume.** This is mediated through aldosterone, antidiuretic hormone, and renal blood flow, all of which are in turn affected by the development of hypertension. Sodium retention and increased blood volume may develop an important role in the regulation of blood-pressure levels once the general level of blood pressure is raised.

The main factors invoked to restore a fall in blood pressure vary according to the duration the restoring influences are required for:

(a) Rapid restoration (few seconds to 12 hours):
Baroreceptors
Chemoreceptors
Brain ischaemia (resulting in stimulation of vasomotor centre)
(b) Less rapid (30 minutes to 2 days):
Renin/angiotensin stimulation (via direct effect on blood vessels)
(c) Slow (2 days onwards):
Renin/angiotensin stimulation (via aldosterone production and sodium retention)
Direct renal control via sodium excretion.

The extent to which the various mechanisms control the blood pressure varies under different circumstances: for example, a relatively low sodium intake leads to an increase in control due to angiotensin and aldosterone, and so an angiotensin antagonist may well result in a fall in blood pressure, but this is not to prove that angiotensin output is either excessive or pathological; it merely shows that under certain circumstances one of the normal controlling mechanisms is quantitatively more important than the others.

The known actions of many of the drugs effective in treating hypertension indicate that to a variable extent in different patients all the mechanisms may be implicated.

An unresolved controversy in the pathophysiology of sustained hypertension is whether the changes in peripheral resistance due to abnormalities of the arteriolar walls are more important than the kidneys in sustaining hypertension. It is not now thought that an increase in cardiac output is generally of major importance in the development of hypertension.

PRINCIPAL HYPOTHESES ABOUT THE INITIATION OR PERPETUATION OF ESSENTIAL HYPERTENSION (Peart, 1980)

Altered sodium excretion by the kidneys
Increased salt intake

Altered renin production or failure to suppress renin
Altered peripheral resistance and increased sensitivity of the
    arterioles
Resetting of baroreceptors
Increased cardiac output and/or blood pressure
Altered function of total system
Increased production of aldosterone or adrenal intermediaries
Overactivity of the sympathetic system
Increased catecholamine production.

PRIMARY CAUSES OF HYPERTENSION

Hyperaldosteronism
Renal disease
Phaeochromocytoma
Cushing's disease (see p. 421)
Coarctation of the aorta (see p. 44)

Renin and Hyperaldosteronism

It was demonstrated in 1898 that crude extracts of kidney caused
elevation of the blood pressure; in 1934 Goldblatt showed that
constricting one renal artery led to hypertension which could be
relieved by removing the *opposite* kidney. It was demonstrated in 1940
by Page and Helmer that the kidney produces an enzyme, (renin)
which acts on a circulating globulin (angiotensinogen) to produce
angiotensin I and II. Renin is also a potent stimulator of aldosterone
production, and acts as the trophic hormone for aldosterone production, and is in turn inhibited by aldosterone; angiotensin II also
stimulates aldosterone production. The enzyme which converts angiotensin I to angiotensin II can be selectively inhibited by captopril;
this leads to a rise in renin but a fall in aldosterone and blood pressure,
showing that angiotensin has inherent blood-pressure-raising activity
(Fig. 20).

There are some forms of hypertension associated with low levels of
renin. The best known of these is Conn's syndrome of excess
aldosterone production from the adrenals.

It is now recognised that there are four main types of
hyperaldosteronism:

1. Adrenal adenoma
2. Bilateral adrenal hyperplasia
3. Hyperaldosteronism which can be suppressed with deoxycorticosterone
4. Hyperaldosteronism which can be suppressed with glucocorticoids (i.e. ACTH-dependent).

THE RENIN / ALDOSTERONE SYSTEM

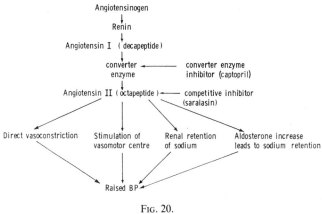

Fig. 20.

All types of primary hyperaldosteronism are associated with hypertension, hypokalaemia, raised aldosterone levels and low renin levels. If adenoma is present the aldosterone levels are much higher in one renal vein; in addition, adenomas are partially under ACTH control (unlike bilateral hyperplasia), so that there is more of a diurnal variation in aldosterone production in patients with an adenoma. A rare disorder which can give rise to confusion is Liddle's syndrome, which is a primary renal tubular disorder with the biochemical abnormalities of aldosteronism but with low levels of aldosterone. Spironolactone has no effect in this disorder, but triamterene, which inhibits tubular transport, may reverse the tendency of the kidneys to conserve sodium and lose potassium even though aldosterone secretion is low.

There are now several reports of hypertension in association with the production of excess amounts of weakly salt-retaining intermediary mineralocorticoids (e.g. deoxycorticosterone, 18-hydroxy,11-deoxycorticosterone, corticosterone, and dehydroepiandrosterone). In these cases the renin levels are also low; the blood pressure can sometimes be lowered in low-renin hypertension with aminoglutethimide, which interferes with the conversion of cholesterol to pregnenolone, a precursor of adrenal mineralocorticoids. Nevertheless, there is still considerable doubt as to the validity of the hypothesis that *idiopathic* hypertension can be meaningfully subdivided into high- and low-renin groups. It is sometimes held that high-renin hypertensives are particularly prone to vascular complications, and that they are more responsive to beta blockers and spironolactone than the low-renin groups.

In primary aldosteronism, hypokalaemia may be missed if blood is taken with the vein occluded, if the blood is not immediately separated, or if the patient has been on a low-sodium diet. The effect of posture on the aldosterone level may be helpful in distinguishing adenoma from hyperplasia; in the erect posture (4-hours standing) the aldosterone level falls in adenoma but rises in hyperplasia and in normals. This is supposed to reflect the fact that adenomas are partly responsive to ACTH, and thus the output of aldosterone falls along with the normal morning fall in ACTH levels (check cortisol at the same time to demonstrate that ACTH output has fallen as it should). The effect of spironolactone on the blood pressure can be used as a confirmatory test (it has to be given in large doses (400 mg/day) for at least 4 weeks before a beneficial effect may be observed). Additional tests for aldosteronism include failure to suppress aldosterone levels with saline infusions, and failure of renin levels to rise with frusemide injections, which produce hyponatraemia and a potent stimulus to renin secretion.

Stimulation or Suppression of Renin and Aldosterone in Normals

Increase:
    Sodium restriction
    Diuretic
    Upright posture.

Decrease:
    Sodium excess
    Recumbent posture.

The Assessment of Hyperaldosteronism

Diagnosis is substantiated by:

> Failure of renin to rise with frusemide (because renin is already suppressed by uncontrollable aldosterone excess)
> Failure to suppress aldosterone with saline (because aldosterone production is more or less autonomous)
> Failure to suppress aldosterone with recumbency (which is the normal response).

If the diagnosis is substantiated, the cause (either adenoma or hyperplasia) has to be established. This can be done by:

> Adrenal-vein sampling
> Labelled iodocholesterol scan, which may show concentration in hyperplasia (this effect can be increased by ACTH stimulation of the adrenal)
> The effect of aldosterone-inhibiting drugs such as spironolactone on the blood pressure (the effect is greater usually in hyperplasia)

The effect of posture on aldosterone levels may help. Adenomas are partly under ACTH control. ACTH output is low in the morning and therefore there is a drop in aldosterone level; however, in normals the effect of standing upright on *increasing* aldosterone is more than sufficient to overcome the ACTH effect, therefore aldosterone output increases in normals but not in adenomas. In hyperplasia there is a more variable response but generally there is a slight rise.

Treatment

Most centres advise removal of an adenoma since some may become malignant, and in order to control the blood pressure, unacceptably large doses of spironolactone may be required. Removal of an adenoma results in improvement in the blood pressure in the majority.

Renal Hypertension

Renal artery stenosis results in an increase in renin secreted by the juxtaglomerular apparatus situated in the walls of the afferent glomerular arteries. Renin leads to an increase in angiotensin, which has a direct effect on the kidney, promoting sodium retention; it also causes the secretion of aldosterone, which itself causes sodium retention. The retention of sodium leads to expansion of the plasma volume, and so to increased cardiac output and redistribution of sodium by changes in the distensibility of the extravascular space. The raised angiotensin levels also have a neurogenic effect, as well as raising aldosterone levels. In the later stages of hypertension due to unilateral renal disease, irreversible changes occur in the opposite kidney, leading to sustained hypertension (vicious-circle hypertension), because of continued renal ischaemia or reduced pulse pressure continually stimulating renin production.

Renal Artery Stenosis

At post-mortem, renal artery narrowing is common in normotensive people, and in life there may be arteriographic evidence of renal artery stenosis in normotensives. Nevertheless, severe unilateral renal artery stenosis results in hypertension which is curable by repairing the stenosis. Unilateral renal artery stenosis is probably responsible for 2 to 5 per cent of cases of hypertension.

Narrowing of the renal arteries may be due to an atheromatous plaque, fibromuscular hyperplasia, embolism or external compression. Fibromuscular hyperplasia is much commoner in women between the ages of 30–40, the stenoses are frequently multiple, tend to occur in the more distal parts of the arteries, and to be accompanied by aneurysm formation (often multiple). Arteriosclerotic narrowing usually occurs in the proximal part of the artery, near its origin from the aorta. Clinical features which should lead to a suspicion that renal artery stenosis may be present are sudden acceleration of previously mild hypertension, severe hypertension below the age of 35, the development of hypertension following an episode of renal pain suggesting embolism or infarction, and malignant hypertension. Careful auscultation may reveal a renal-artery bruit.

Suggestive features in the IVU are a difference in size of more than 2 cm between the two kidneys, and a delayed appearance time of the dye in one kidney with subsequent increased density of the dye on that side. The appearance time is delayed because of the decreased blood flow, and the concentration is increased because slower blood flow results in slower excretion. The next diagnostic step is usually a renal arteriogram to confirm the presence and location of the stenosis. The presence of stenosis does not necessarily mean that the hypertension is due to the stenosis or that it is causing any alteration in the function of the kidney. In order to decide if the narrowing is likely to be responsible for hypertension it is usual to demonstrate a difference in function between the two kidneys. The easiest method of doing this is by noting the rate of uptake and excretion by the kidneys of a radioactive substance. A narrowed renal artery will delay uptake and excretion if the blood flow is significantly diminished. A gamma-ray scintillation counter is used to count simultaneously over both kidneys. The two radioactive substances commonly used are ^{131}I-labelled hippuran, and a diuretic labelled with ^{203}Hg.

Circulating renin activity and renal vein renin is almost invariably raised in the presence of renal artery stenosis. Saralasin, a competitive inhibitor of angiotensin II will lower the blood pressure if the renin and angiotensin II levels are raised, and if vicious-circle hypertension has not supervened.

Phaeochromocytoma

Tumours of the adrenal medulla produce catecholamines, resulting in hypertension which at first is paroxysmal but later becomes sustained. Hypertension causes damage to the arterioles of the kidney, resulting in localised areas of renal ischaemia. These ischaemic areas cause further hypertension by stimulating renin formation and secondary hyperaldosteronism, and a vicious circle is established. This is a feature of all forms of hypertension, and is the mechanism by which the episodic hypertension of phaeochromocytoma becomes sustained. There are usually other features of catecholamine release, such as palpitations, pallor, severe headaches, perspiration and anxiety. There is often glycosuria. The metabolites of the circulating catecholamines are excreted in the urine and the one most conveniently measured is vanillylmandelic acid (VMA). Certain drugs interfere with the estimation of VMA; these are barbiturates, salicylates and methyldopa. Drugs which block the effects of the circulating catecholamines may be used to confirm the diagnosis; phentolamine will block the alpha adrenergic activities of adrenaline and noradrenaline and cause a lowering of the blood pressure (a fall of 35 mm Hg in the systolic pressure is a positive response). The test must not be performed if the patient has taken antihypertensive drugs in the previous ten days. Surgical removal of the tumour is the treatment of choice. Both adrenals should be inspected because the tumours are bilateral or multiple in 10 per cent of cases, and may occur in extra-adrenal sites, including thorax, bladder and sympathetic ganglia. Medical treatment is used pre-operatively or if the tumours are malignant (10 per cent), and recur. The alpha effects of adrenaline and noradrenaline can be controlled with a long-acting alpha-blocking drug such as phenoxybenzamine, and the beta effects with a beta blocker such as propranolol.

TREATMENT OF HYPERTENSION

Definition of Hypertension

It is common to use the WHO definitions which are:

Definite hypertension systolic pressure over 160
diastolic pressure over 95
Borderline hypertension systolic pressure over 140
diastolic pressure over 90
Normal systolic pressure below 140
diastolic pressure below 90.

Two clear conclusions can be drawn from the Framingham and Veterans Administration Surveys (VA 90 and VA 115), and life-insurance statistics: namely, that mortality and morbidity from most hypertensive complications are directly related to the level of the blood pressure, and that the same level of pressure is more serious the younger the person. It is also clear that:

Both systolic and diastolic pressures rise with age
There is no level at which complications suddenly increase in frequency, i.e., there is no threshold for the development of hypertensive complications
The risk of complications are the same in men and women
The elderly with raised blood pressure are also at risk of developing complications

With treatment, the greatest reduction is in strokes and heart failures; the benefits in reduction of myocardial infarction are less impressive

Borderline hypertension develops into established hypertension, particularly in the young

A family history of hypertension is associated with an increased risk of developing a hypertensive complication in the presence of hypertension.

A number of other factors concerned with the *aetiology* of hypertension have also emerged from epidemiolgical studies:

The prevalence of hypertension may be related to the level of salt intake of the population studied

There is an increased incidence of hypertension in negroes, the frequency of hypertensive complications is also greater in negroes

There is some good evidence of an association between soft water and the incidence of hypertension and sudden death

Obesity has a complicated inter-relationship with hypertension; however, hypertensive complications are more common in the presence of obesity, and hypertension is more likely to develop in the obese; weight reduction in obese hypertensives is associated with a reduction in blood pressure.

What is still uncertain is whether lowering the blood pressure to normal in borderline hypertension improves the outlook. This problem is still unresolved and there are large trials in operation in the US and UK to establish the criteria for treating borderline hypertension.

Management of Hypertension

The important steps in management are:

Exclusion of primary causes
The decision to treat.

Primary causes to be excluded are:

Coarctation of the aorta	Phaeochromocytoma
Cushing's syndrome	Adrenal disease
Renal disease	Pregnancy.

Treatment of Hypertension

The decision to treat will be affected by the level of blood pressure. There is no controversy in severe and established hypertension and in the presence of cardiovascular hypertrophy (left ventricular hypertrophy, fundal changes, lacunar strokes and cardiac enlargement). The difficulties arise in patients with borderline hypertension, and the decision to treat will be influenced by:

The presence of complications of hypertension despite the borderline nature of the blood-pressure readings

The presence of other risk factors involved in the pathogenesis of atherosclerosis, such as diabetes, hyperlipidaemia, polycythaemia, hyperuricaemia, smoking habits, family history, obesity, and race.

TABLE III

SITES OF ACTION OF ANTIHYPERTENSIVE DRUGS

Central actions	Beta blockers
	Clonidine (also an α stimulator)
	Methyldopa
Sympathetic postganglionic blockers	Bethanidine
(preventing release of noradrenaline from	Guanethidine
sympathetic postganglionic fibres)	Debrisoquine
Peripheral target organ α-receptor blocker	Labetalol
	Prazosin
	Phenoxybenzamine
	Phentolamine
Postsynaptic β-receptor blocker	Beta blockers
	Labetalol
Direct action on vascular smooth muscle	Hydralazine
	Minoxidil
	Diazoxide
	Sodium nitroprusside
Circulating hormone antagonists	
Angiotensin competetive inhibitor	Saralasin
Renin/angiotensin blocker	Captopril
Aldosterone blocker	Spironolactone

Initial Treatment of Hypertension

It is now agreed that beta blockers and a thiazide diuretic should be the drugs of first choice in the treatment of most cases of hypertension, but there is still debate about the best drug to add to this regime if the blood pressure is not adequately controlled. The most usual second-line drugs, in the order of frequency with which they are used, are hydralazine, methyldopa, prazosin, clonidine and bethanidine (Ramsay, 1980).

Mechanism of Action of Antihypertensives

Diuretics.—Diuretics induce sodium depletion, and thus reduce extracellular fluid volume. However this effect is only transient and cannot account for the continued antihypertensive action of diuretics. They may cause their effect by reducing the sodium content of smooth muscle in the arterioles; this causes the cells to be less excitable—an effect which may be mediated by decreased intracellular calcium concentration. Even a mild reduction of vessel-wall sodium reduces the vasoconstrictor effect of angiotensin II. Diuretics also enhance the action of other antihypertensive drugs, possibly by abolishing the slight tendency to fluid retention which some of them cause.

Beta blockers.—The antihypertensive action of beta blockers was found accidentally. They all act by competitive inhibition. The side-chain which they all contain is identical to that of isoprenaline. The aromatic ring to which the side-chain is attached differs for different beta blockers, and gives each of them other minor properties which may be advantageous or not, depending on the circumstances. The mode of action of beta blockers in hypertension is complex and debatable; some of the mechanisms are:

> Reduced cardiac output—this is variable and cannot be the main mechanism
>
> Blockade of beta adrenergic receptors in vessel walls—this is an unlikely mechanism, since beta adrenergic receptors mediate a vasodilator effect, i.e. beta blockade of these receptors should produce vasoconstriction
>
> Blockade of preganglionic beta receptors—this is probably the main mechanism of action
>
> Inhibition of renin. Once a fashionable hypothesis, this is no longer thought to be a likely mechanism. Beta blockers may be effective when renin levels are low, and some have no effect on renin secretion
>
> Central action. This is probably an important mechanism of action; the drugs concentrate preferentially in the hypothalamus and produce a hypotensive effect when instilled directly into the cerebrospinal fluid.

Which Beta blocker?

There is no difference in antihypertensive action between any of the beta blockers when given in equipotent doses. There is therefore no point in changing from one beta blocker to another if the first is ineffective. There is an advantage from the point of view of compliance in prescribing a long-acting preparation which needs to be given only once a day.

Beta blockers may reduce the blood sugar but more importantly, because they block the effects of adrenaline, they may remove many of the premonitory symptoms of hypoglycaemia. There are a number of minor physical and pharmacological differences between beta blockers, e.g.:

Lipid solubility.—Some beta blockers are more lipid-soluble than others, and therefore should be present in higher concentrations in the central nervous system, and have a longer plasma half-life. Neither of these properties is thought to be have any clinical relevance.

Cardioselectivity.—Some beta blockers have a greater effect on the heart than other smooth muscle, leading to the concept that the heart contains so-called beta-1 receptors and the remainder of the body has beta-2 receptors. Even the cardioselective blockers may have an effect on beta-2 receptors, causing some bronchoconstriction, but in this case the effects on the airways can be reversed by a beta-2 stimulant such as salbutamol. The use of a cardioselective beta blocker has less of an effect on the hypoglycaemic action of beta blockers, and produces less masking of the hypoglycaemic symptoms. In some patients beta blockers act as partial alpha-receptor agonists. This can lead to peripheral vasoconstriction and Raynaud's phenomenon. Paradoxically, they may still retain their hypotensive action while producing clinical evidence of vasoconstriction. Vasoconstriction may be very severe and lead to gangrene. There is no real evidence that cardioselective beta blockers are any better in this regard than the other beta blockers.

Partial agonist activity (PAA).—This refers to the fact that some beta blockers do not reduce the heart rate as much as others with the same blood-pressure-lowering effect. This may be an advantage if a beta-blocker-induced bradycardia lowers cardiac output and causes symptoms.

Membrane stabilising activity (quinidine or local anaesthetic property).—This is only present in very high non-clinical doses and has no clinical relevance.

Drug	Proprietary name	PAA
Cardioselective		
Atenolol	Tenormin	0
Acebutolol	Sectral	+
Metoprolol	Betaloc	0
	Lopresor	
Non-cardioselective		
Propranolol	Inderal	0
Oxprenolol	Trasicor	+
Pindolol	Visken	+
Nadolol	Corgard	0
Sotalol	Sotacor	0
Timolol	Blocadren	0

Alpha Adrenergic Blockers

These drugs are used when catecholamine excretion is increased, as in phaeochromocytomas, or when clonidine is being discontinued. Phenoxybenzamine was the first drug in the group to be used, but it produces a marked postural hypotension. There are two newer drugs with some alpha blocking effects; these are:

Labetalol which can have both alpha- and beta-blocking properties. The alpha-blocking effect acts on peripheral blood vessels, the beta-blocking effect acts on the heart, preventing the reflex tachycardia which normally follows a fall in blood pressure. The beta blockade on the heart is insufficient to prevent the rise in cardiac output with exercise, which may occur with other beta blockers. It does not produce a marked postural fall, but does have some of the side-effects, such as impotence, associated with alpha blocking drugs. It should not be used with hydralazine.

Prazosin is another drug with alpha- and beta-blocking properties. It is very important to remember that many patients develop severe postural hypotension at the start of treatment. This drug should therefore be started after the patient has retired to bed. It also acts directly on blood vessels, causing vasodilatation.

Centrally Acting Drugs

Clonidine.—Clonidine is an interesting drug which can be termed a "selective alpha-receptor agonist", i.e., it stimulates some alpha receptors more than others and the alpha receptors it stimulates most are those in the hypothalamus, which results in *reduced* sympathetic outflow and increased parasympathetic outflow. Given intravenously, clonidine has a transient *hypertensive* effect, because it stimulates peripheral alpha receptors. It reduces catecholamine synthesis, but on cessation of clonidine there is often a severe rebound increase in catecholamines that can lead to dangerous hypertension. This can be made *worse* by beta blockers because in addition to blocking synaptic beta receptors they also block vessel-wall beta receptors which mediate a *vasodilator* response. If these receptors are also blocked, vasodilatation cannot occur and the hypertension is made worse. The treatment of clonidine-cessation hypertension is an alpha blocker such as phenoxybenzamine.

Methyldopa.—The site of action is central, like clonidine. The substrate alphamethyldopa is converted by a noradrenaline-producing enzyme into alphamethylnoradrenaline, which, like clonidine, stimulates hypothalamic alpha-receptors, leading to a reduction in sympathetic outflow. Alphamethyldopa may lead to sedation and loss of concentration; it may also cause a fever and positive Coombs' test several months after it is started. Occasionally it causes hepatocellular damage. Its hypertensive action is cancelled by tricyclic antidepressants (the main mechanism of which is to *increase* dopa and dopamine in the brain, in contrast to alphamethyldopa, whose action is to increase methyldopa and methyldopamine and hence divert precursors away from noradrenalin synthesis to methylnoradrenaline synthesis.

Postganglionic adrenergic blocking drugs (guanethidine, bethanidine, debrisoquine).—Rather than blocking receptor sites, these drugs act by preventing the release of the neurotransmitter noradrenaline. This increases the sensitivity of the circulation to circulating noradrenaline. These drugs are not effective if chlorpromazine or tricyclic antidepressants are given at the same time.

Vasodilators.—The main drugs are hydralazine, diazoxide, minoxidil and sodium nitroprusside. They produce direct vasodilatation, with no effect on the autonomic nervous system, and therefore compensatory tachycardia in response to a fall in blood pressure is common. They have no effect on venous capacitance vessels, but increase flow on the arteriolar side and hence capillary pressure is increased and may lead to oedema. Because venous pressure is maintained they do not produce postural hypotension.

Hydralazine in doses above 400 mg/day may produce a lupus-like syndrome with positive ANF, which may persist indefinitely. The drug is acetylated in the liver, and the side-effects are most likely with slow acetylators. Acetylator status is easily tested by measuring free and conjugated sulphonamide in the urine after a test dose of sulphadimidine. A reflex tachycardia is almost invariable if the blood pressure is reduced, and hydralazine should only be given with a beta blocker. As with isoniazid, a peripheral neuropathy may occur which responds to pyridoxine.

Minoxidil should also be used only in combination with a beta blocker and diuretic; a major disadvantage is the fact that, like diazoxide, it increases the growth of body hair to an extent that is usually unacceptable in women.

Diazoxide is not routinely used for the long-term treatment of hypertension; fluid retention, diabetes and postural hypotension, which are common, preclude its use except when the blood pressure needs to be controlled rapidly.

Sodium nitroprusside is only used intravenously to control malignant hypertension, or occasionally to reduce after-load on the heart in severe left ventricular failure. It has a number of potentially serious side-effects and should generally be used only as a third- or fourth-line drug. The drug is metabolised to cyanide and thiocynate. Cyanide accumulation occurs if there is liver impairment, and this may lead to impairment of red-cell function. If this occurs, large doses of hydroxycobalamin (50–100 mg, i.v.) should be given. If renal failure is present, thiocyanate may accumulate; this leads to mental confusion

TABLE IV
ANTIHYPERTENSIVE DRUGS

Antihypertensive drug	Proprietary name	Tablet size	Starting dose (daily)	Maximum daily dose	Dose increments (daily)	Interval between increments
Bethanidine	Esbatal	10 mg 50 mg	30 mg	200 mg	15 mg	3 days
Clonidine	Catapres	100 μg 300 μg	150–300 μg	1·2 mg	100 μg	3 days
Debrisoquine	Declinax	10 mg 20 mg	20 mg	60 mg	10 mg	3 days
Hydralazine	Apresoline	25 mg 50 mg	75 mg (1st dose at night)	200 mg	25 mg	3 days
Labetalol	Trandate	100 mg 200 mg 400 mg	300 mg	2400 mg	300 mg	1–2 weeks
Minoxidil	Loniten	2·5 mg 5 mg 10 mg	5–10 mg	50 mg	5–10 mg	3 days
Prazosin	Hypovase	0·5 mg 1 mg 2 mg 5 mg	1·5 mg	20 mg	1·5 mg	3–5 days
Propranolol	Inderal	10 mg 40 mg 80 mg 160 mg	160 mg	2·5 g	160 mg	7 days

and hypothyroidism. It is possible to monitor blood cyanide and thiocyanate levels.

Malignant Hypertension and Hypertensive Encephalopathy

Hydralazine.(Apresoline. 1 ml ampoule contains 20 mg hydralazine.) Hydralazine should be given by slow intravenous injection in a dose of 20–40 mg. It can be given by intravenous infusion but should NOT be diluted with 5 per cent dextrose. It should be diluted with 5 per cent sorbitol or Ringer's solution. Its duration of action is relatively short, but it may cause tachycardia and should therefore be preceded by a parenteral beta-blocker.

Labetalol. (Trandate. 20 ml ampoule contains 100 mg labetalol.) Labetalol is a peripheral alpha-blocking drug which also acts as a beta-blocker on the heart. This effect on the heart is important because it abolishes the normal sympathetic induced tachycardia which follows peripheral vasodilatation. Labetalol should be given in a dose of 25–50 mg over 1 minute; if necessary 50 mg can be given at 5-minute intervals. The total dose should not exceed 200 mg. The drug is usually effective in 5–10 minutes and the effects last 12–18 hours. Alternatively, the drug can be infused at 2 mg/minute. The patient should be kept flat, as postural hypotension may be severe.

Diazoxide. (Eudemine. Tablets 50 mg; 20 ml ampoules contain 300 mg diazoxide.) Diazoxide injection should only be used intravenously and be given rapidly over about 10 seconds. A response should occur within 5 minutes; the effect lasts for up to 4 hours. Over 24 hours up to 1200 mg may be given. Diazoxide may cause tachycardia and angina and it is advisable to give an intravenous injection of propranolol in a dose of 7·5–10 mg *before* giving diazoxide. (Propranolol [Inderal]. 1 ml ampoule contains 1 mg; the manufacturers recommend giving atropine 1 or 2 mg *before* giving propranolol although this *may* not be necessary.) Diazoxide is liable to cause hyperglycaemia and often severe salt- and water-retention and it should be used in combination with a loop diuretic such as frusemide or ethacrynic acid. These drugs may worsen the hyperglycaemia. The diazoxide regime is probably the best one to use if there is significant renal failure.

Sodium nitroprusside. (Nipride. 50 mg ampoules.) Sodium nitroprusside acts immediately but only for so long as it is administered. The maximum dose must not exceed 800 μg/min. The average dose is 100–200μg/min depending on whether the patient is already taking antihypertensive drugs. Great care is needed if there is renal or liver impairment. 50 mg of sodium nitroprusside is made up to 1·0 l with 5 per cent dextrose, giving 50 μg/ml.

Trimetaphan. (Arfonad. 5 ml ampoules contain 250 mg trimetaphan.) Trimetaphan is a ganglion-blocking drug which also has a direct vasodilating action on the peripheral blood vessels. Two 5 ml ampoules (500 mg) are diluted with 500 ml of dextrose-saline. This gives a concentration of 1 mg per ml. The drug is then administered at a dose of 3–4 mg per minute. Patients vary greatly in their response, so that care is needed, particularly when the drug is first administered.

HYPERVENTILATION

Hyperventilation often produces a wide variety of non-specific symptoms long before tetany develops, e.g. dizziness, paraesthesia, cramp, feelings of unreality, excessive sweating, and general exhaustion. Although the blood Pco_2 level may not be reduced, symptoms are caused by rapid changes in Pco_2 and can usually be reproduced if the patient is made to hyperventilate. Adaptation to prolonged lower levels of blood Pco_2 can occur (e.g. in those who live at high altitudes). In normals the end-tidal Pco_2 remains relatively static; in hyperventilators there are much wider fluctuations in end-tidal Pco_2 (Lum, 1981).

ARTERITIS

When confronted with a lesion due to arterial disease it is worth considering whether the affected artery is large, medium or small. Certain conditions have a predilection for arteries of a certain size; in practice this is not rigid, but may be useful (Table V).

Buerger's Disease (Thrombo-angiitis Obliterans)

The evidence is now strong that the condition is not a distinct disease. The disease was variously considered to be a combination of peripheral arterial gangrene accompanied by thrombophlebitis, commoner in the lower limbs of young men who smoked heavily. Specific histological features were claimed. However, the evidence is against Buerger's disease being a distinct entity because:

> The histological changes in the veins thought to be specific for the disease occur also in otherwise uncomplicated phlebothrombosis;
>
> Histological changes in the arteries thought to be specific for the disease occur also in otherwise uncomplicated arteriosclerotic gangrene;
>
> All cases in which the diagnosis can be considered clinically have evidence of arteriosclerosis. Buerger himself said that for the diagnosis to be considered, evidence of arteriosclerosis should be absent;

In severe atherosclerosis, perivascular fibrosis occurs and is often severe enough to involve venae comitantes, causing venous thrombosis.

TABLE V

LESIONS ASSOCIATED WITH ARTERY SIZES

Size of artery	Main lesions
Large	Arteriosclerosis
	Syphilis
	Embolism (due to clots, rarely to tumour or fungus emboli)
	Takayasu's disease
Medium	Polyarteritis nodosa
	Moenckeberg's sclerosis
	Giant-cell arteritis
	Buerger's disease
	Arteritis of severe infection and malignancy
	Embolism
	Arteriosclerosis
Small arteries and arterioles	Hypertension
	Dermatomyositis
	Scleroderma
	Raynaud's phenomenon
	Rheumatoid arthritis
	Ergotism

EFFORT SYNDROME (DA COSTA'S[36] SYNDROME)

The patient has a large number of symptoms referable to the cardiovascular system. None of the symptoms are classical or characteristic of organic disease, although they may be sufficiently similar to cause diagnostic confusion—this is particularly so if the effort syndrome is superimposed on known organic heart disease. The hallmark of the syndrome is that physical exertion seems to require an excessive amount of effort and seems to produce exaggerated reactions. Physical examination usually reveals no abnormality. There are a number of simple tests which may be useful in diagnosing and assessing the condition. All these tests are based on demonstrating that autonomic reflexes are modified by higher centres of the brain. The autonomic reflex may be suppressed, e.g. when reflex apnoea is absent after hyperventilation; the reflex may be exaggerated, e.g. excessive tachycardia in response to hyperventilation. Four simple tests for evaluating the effort syndrome are:

1. Absence of reflex apnoea after 2 minutes' hyperventilation

2. Inability to hold breath for 30 seconds
3. Orthostatic and hyperventilation tachycardia of more than 100
4. Slow return of pulse rate to normal after standard exercise.

CARDIOMYOPATHIES

The cardiomyopathies are a heterogeneous group of diseases in which the heart muscle is primarily involved. By convention, the group does not include heart muscle damage secondary to coronary artery disease, hypertension and valvular disease. In the American literature myocardiopathy, myocardosis and primary myocardial disease are synonymous. There are many classifications; one of the earliest was:

Congestive: with features of congestive heart failure
Constrictive: with features of constrictive pericarditis
Obstructive: with features of functional obstruction of the ventricular outflow tracts.

TABLE VI

CLASSIFICATION OF CARDIOMYOPATHIES

Primary		Secondary	
Infective	Viral	Nutritional	Starvation
	Bacterial		Kwashiorkor
	Parasitic		
		Toxic	Alcohol
Obstructive			Drugs
Endomyocardial fibrosis		Infiltrations	Amyloidosis
			Haemochromatosis
			Glycogen storage disease
Fibroelastosis			Sarcoidosis
Puerperal			Fat
Idiopathic	Familial	Collagen disease	Rheumatoid arthritis
	Non-familial		SLE
			Scleroderma
			Polyarteritis nodosa
		Endocrine	Myxoedema
			Acromegaly
			Myasthenia gravis
		Congenital	Friedreich's ataxia
			Muscular dystrophies
			Gargoylism

The accepted definition of cardiomyopathy (Goodwin, 1970) is: "A subacute or chronic disorder of heart muscle of unknown or unusual cause, often with associated endocardial and sometimes pericardial involvement." The functional classification into congestive, constrictive and obstructive has since been modified. Constrictive (restrictive) cardiomyopathy is rare, the most usual cause being amyloid infiltration. Hypertrophic cardiomyopathy may occur without obstruction to the outflow tract, but the main haemodynamic disturbance may be difficulty in ventricular filling due to decreased compliance of the hypertrophied ventricle. Obliterative cardiomyopathy refers to those cases in which there is encroachment on the cavity of the ventricles and usually endocardial thickening.

The diagnosis of cardiomyopathy should only be made when the commonest cause of myocardial damage (i.e. ischaemia due to coronary artery disease) has been excluded. Exclusion of coronary artery disease can be extremely difficult.

Occasionally patients with a congestive cardiomyopathy have hypertension or develop angina. Rarely hypertrophic obstructive cardiomyopathy can follow left ventricular hypertrophy due to some other cause such as hypertension. In obstructive cardiomyopathy the β-blocking drugs successfully lower the end-diastolic pressure. Anticoagulants are indicated if a dysrhythmia (usually atrial fibrillation) is present. Bacterial endocarditis in association with obstructive cardiomyopathy has been described.

PRIMARY CARDIOMYOPATHIES

Infective

Viral.—The commonest cause of viral myocarditis is the Coxsackie B virus. The illness is often biphasic—initial malaise is followed about ten days later by fever, tachycardia, cardiac dilatation and arrhythmias. Virus may be isolated from throat swab and stool; however, Coxsackie virus is often found in the stools of healthy children, so that virus isolated from the stools after the third week of the illness may have been acquired coincidentally. Neutralising antibodies to the virus are found in the serum, a fourfold rise in titre between acute and convalescent sera is confirmatory.

Myocarditis is occasionally seen in other viral infections such as poliomyelitis, influenza, mumps and glandular fever.

Bacterial.—The best known bacterial myocarditis is diphtheria, in which the myocarditis usually presents in the third week of the illness, with cardiac enlargement, ECG changes and circulatory collapse. Complete recovery in non-fatal cases is the rule. True myocarditis may occur with tuberculosis and probably occurs with miliary spread of the disease. Active carditis occurs in rheumatic fever, streptococcal infections and meningococcal septicaemia. Other bacterial infections which may be complicated by a myocarditis are Weil's[37] disease, toxoplasmosis and trypanosomiasis (particularly in South America, where the organism is *Trypanosoma cruzi* and the disease is known as Chagas'[38] disease).

Hypertrophic Obstructive Cardiomyopathy (HOCM)

During systole, the ventricle contracts progressively from apex to infundibulum. If this sequence is abnormal, and the infundibulum contracts before the end of systole it will obstruct the flow of the blood from the ventricle. Abnormal infundibular contraction may occur in either ventricle; it may be congenital or acquired.

There is a day-to-day variability of the symptoms, which include angina, syncope and dyspnoea. The pulse is characteristically jerky, with a rapid upstroke unlike the anacrotic pulse of aortic stenosis. There is an ejection murmur which is late in onset and best heard at the apex and left sternal edge. The rapid upstroke of the pulse is due to early rapid emptying of the ventricle; the functional narrowing of the outflow tract occurs late in systole, which corresponds with the late onset of the ejection murmur. Abnormal contraction of the ventricular muscle may interfere with the function of the papillary muscles, tending to distort the cusps of the mitral valve, and so cause mitral regurgitation. There is often a double impulse at the apex during systole, which may be due to a palpable atrial impulse or to forward displacement of the apex when the hypertrophied muscle of the outflow tract contracts. Drugs which improve the efficiency of myocardial contraction, such as isoprenaline and digitalis, tend to make the obstruction worse; beta adrenergic drugs such as propranolol decrease the obstruction.

Endomyocardial Fibrosis (EMF)

As its name implies both the endocardium and myocardium are involved. The endocardium becomes thickened and stiff, leading to constriction of the ventricular cavity and distortion of the papillary muscles, which causes incompetence of the atrioventricular valves. The myocardium becomes thickened and fibrotic. The disease occurs only in the tropics, but expatriates as well as the indigenous population may be affected. The onset is sometimes a febrile illness accompanied by malaise, dyspnoea and tachycardia. Occasionally there is an accompanying eosinophilia, but no other evidence of an infecting organism. The disease is usually complicated by intractable heart failure, pulmonary hypertension, or emboli, both pulmonary and systemic.

Fibroelastosis

The endocardium may become thickened at the site of excessive turbulence, as in the McCallum patch seen in the left atrium in mitral incompetence, where the blood impinges on the atrial wall. Endocardial thickening also occurs secondary to myocardial disease, for example EMF and myocardial infarction and in congenital heart disease, especially in the presence of desaturated blood. Nevertheless, excessive fibrosis of the endocardium occurs in the absence of any known causes. Primary fibroelastosis usually presents in the first few months of life as intractable heart failure; rarely the disease presents in adult life. The majority of children with fibroelastosis have a positive skin test to mumps antigen at an age when a positive reaction is unusual.

SECONDARY CARDIOMYOPATHIES

Nutritional

Congestive cardiac failure is frequently seen in severe malnutrition and is probably related to dietary deficiency of B_1 (thiamine), electrolyte imbalance if associated pellagra causes severe diarrhoea, or protein deficiency as in kwashiorkor. (Kwashiorkor—red boy—is a reference to the characteristic brown hair and skin pigmentation; another interpretation is "disease of the jealous child," referring to the occurrence of the disease in children who have been prematurely weaned because the mother is again pregnant.)

Toxic

Alcoholic cardiomyopathy.—Excessive consumption of alcohol to the exclusion of adequate vitamin intake, may result in beri beri and high-output heart failure because of widespread peripheral vasodilatation. However, a congestive type of cardiomyopathy may occur in alcoholics in the absence of the signs of beri beri. Alcoholic cardiomyopathy should be considered in anyone who has drunk continuously, for ten years or more, a bottle of spirits or ten to fifteen pints of beer a day. The ECG findings are variable but specific abnormalities have been described (Evans, 1959). These are the "spinous" T waves, in which left ventricular T waves become heightened and pointed; "cloven" T waves in which the upright T wave has a small depression near its summit, and the "dimple" T wave in which the normal T wave is absent and is replaced by a small dimple in an otherwise isoelectric S–U period. Treatment of the heart failure, prolonged bed rest and total abstinence from alcohol may result in a complete cure in the early stages.

Drugs.—Emetine hydrochloride, used to treat amoebiasis, and sodium or potassium antimony tartrate, used to treat bilharzia, both cause a myocarditis. The myocardium may be involved in sensitivity reaction to drugs.

Infiltration of the Myocardium

Amyloidosis.—The heart is a common site for deposition in primary amyloidosis, other common sites being muscle, skin and gums. The heart usually is small, and restricted by the amyloid tissue (an example of a "constrictive" type of cardiomyopathy). The heart is rarely involved in secondary amyloidosis, the main sites of deposition in which are kidney, liver and spleen. Curiously, the distribution of the amyloid deposits secondary to myelomatosis resembles that of primary amyloid.

Haemochromatosis.—Excessive absorption of iron due to lack of the normal "mucosal block" or a congenital deficiency of the iron-carrying beta globulin (transferrin) results in excessive storing of iron in the tissues. The stored iron acts as an irritant, causing fibrosis which, in the heart, leads to congestive failure; usually both sides of the heart are involved and conduction defects are common.

Fat.—Extreme obesity may be associated with infiltration of fat into the myocardium, hampering ventricular contraction. Rarely, the heart may be the site of deposition of the lipoid material in histiocytosis X.

Sarcoidosis.—The heart is frequently involved in cases of sarcoidosis severe enough to come to autopsy. This may lead to cardiomegaly, arrhythmias and congestive cardiac failure.

Glycogen storage disease.—In this disease there is excessive deposition of glycogen in different tissues, especially the heart, liver and skeletal muscles. There may be increased glycogen in the blood and urine. The affected infant usually presents with cardiomegaly or hypoglycaemia.

Collagen Diseases

Rheumatoid arthritis.—Cardiac involvement in rheumatoid arthritis usually causes a pericardial effusion. Rarely a rheumatoid nodule may cause fibrosis of the myocardium and congestive heart failure.

Systemic lupus erythematosus.—The most usual cardiac manifestations of SLE are sterile pericarditis and effusion, and the verrucous non-embolising endocarditis of Libman[39]-Sacks[40]. SLE may also cause widespread fibrosis of the myocardium and congestive cardiac failure without valvular or pericardial involvement.

Scleroderma.—The commonest organs involved are the gastro-intestinal tract, skin, lungs and peripheral nerves; involvement of the arteries results in Raynaud's phenomenon and ischaemia. Myocardial fibrosis is fairly common, and causes congestive failure or conduction defects if the bundle of His is involved. Cor pulmonale may occur secondary to pulmonary hypertension, due to lung fibrosis.

Polyarteritis nodosa.—Polyarteritis nodosa may cause heart failure secondary to associated hypertension or myocardial infarction due to involvement of the coronary arteries. In addition there is frequently pericardial involvement and focal myocardial fibrosis, which may result in heart failure out of proportion to the severity of the hypertension or the degree of coronary artery involvement.

Endocrine Diseases

Myxoedema.—Cardiac enlargement in myxoedema is usually due to the presence of a pericardial effusion, and angina to coexisting coronary artery disease. However, myxoedema may cause heart failure due to infiltration with mucoprotein. The ECG changes of myxoedema usually revert to normal promptly with thyroxine, suggesting that they are due to a rapidly reversible cause such as electrolyte disturbance of the myocardial cells.

Acromegaly.—The heart is usually large in acromegaly, as part of the general splanchnomegaly, or as a result of associated hypertension. However, there is also an increase in myocardial fibrosis, which leads to heart failure more readily than would be expected from the associated hypertension alone.

Myasthenia gravis.—In heart muscle, changes identical to those in voluntary muscles may occur, i.e. lymphorrhages, atrophy of muscle fibres and necrosis.

Congenital

Friedreich's ataxia.—This hereditary disease, appearing before adolescence, and characterised by degeneration of the spinocerebellar tracts, posterior columns, and pyramidal tracts and by skeletal deformity (kyphoscoliosis and pes cavus), also affects the heart. There may be cardiac enlargement, arrhythmias and conduction defects.

Muscular dystrophies.—All the muscular dystrophies may be accompanied by myocardial involvement, but it is most frequently seen in the pseudohypertrophic type and dystrophia myotonica. ECG abnormalities are common.

Gargoylism.—The myocardium may be involved in the widespread deposition of mucopolysaccharide characteristic of this condition.

REFERENCES

AHRENS, E. H. (1979) *Lancet*, **2**, 1345.
BASSAN, M. A. & ROGEL, S. (1976) *Heart Lung*, **5**, 742.
BROWSE, N. L. (1969) *Brit. med. J.*, **4**, 676.

Evans, W. (1959) *Brit. Heart J.*, **21**, 445.

Gautmacher, M. L. (1979) *J. roy. Soc. Med.*, **72**, 513.

Goodwin, J. F. (1970) *Lancet*, **1**, 731.

International Anticoagulant Review Group (1970) *Lancet*, **1**, 203.

Lum, L. C. (1981) *J. roy. Soc. Med.*, **74**, 1.

McMichael, J. (1979) *Brit. med. J.*, **1**, 173.

Medical Research Council (1964) *Brit. med. J.*, **2**, 837.

Medical Research Council (1969) *Brit. med. J.*, **1**, 335.

Miall, W. E. & Lovell, H. G. (1967) *Brit. med. J.*, **2**, 660.

Miall, W. E. & Oldham, P. D. (1963) *Brit. med. J.*, **1**, 75.

Mitchell, J. R. A. (1981) *Lancet*, **1**, 257.

Modan, B., Shani, M., Schor, S. & Rodan, M. (1975) *New Engl. J. Med.*, **292**, 1359.

Norris, R. M., Brandt, P. W., Caughey, D. E., Lee, A. J. & Scott, P. J. (1969) *Lancet*, **1**, 274.

Norris, R. M., Caughey, D. E., Deeming, L. W., Mercer, C. J. & Scott, P. J. (1971) *Lancet*, **2**, 485.

Peart, W. S. (1980) *J. roy. Coll. Phycns Lond.*, **14**, 141.

Ramsay, L. E. (1980) *J. roy. Coll. Phycns Lond.*, **14**, 249.

Sevitt, S. (1968) *Proc. roy. Soc. Med.*, **61**, 143.

Sixty-Plus Reinfarction Study (1980) *Lancet*, **2**, 980.

Tonascia, J., Gordis, L. & Schmerler, H. (1975) *New Engl. J. Med.*, **292**, 1362.

Valentine, P. A., Fluck, D. C., Mounsey J. P., Reid, D., Shillingford, J. P. & Steiner, R. E. (1966) *Lancet*, **2**, 837.

Vaughan Williams, E. M. (1978) *Brit. Heart J.*, **40** (Supplement), 52.

Wright, I. S., Marple, C. D. & Bock, D. F. (1954) *Myocardial Infarction*. New York: Grune & Stratton.

EPONYMS

1. KARL EWALD KONSTANTIN HERING (1834–1918)
Hering succeeded Carl Ludwig as Professor of Physiology in Vienna. In 1868 he and Breuer described the vagal reflex control of breathing—the first "feed-back" reflex to be described. His son Heinrich Hering (1866–1948) discovered the carotid sinus reflex.

2. JOSEF BREUER (1842–1925)
Breuer and Hering described the vagal reflex control of breathing in 1868. Freud acknowledged that Breuer was the originator of psychotherapy. With the famous patient "Ann O" Breuer realised that hysterical symptoms could be abolished if the unconscious causes could be determined.

3. ALEXANDER TIETZE (1864–1927)
Tietze was a surgeon who qualified and worked in Breslau. He contributed chapters to several surgical texts, including one on disease of the rectum and anus.

4. PIERRE CHARLES ALEXANDRE LOUIS (1787–1872)
Louis succeeded Laënnec at la Charité. He had a high reputation, particularly in the US, which was significantly influenced by French medicine as a result of many French doctors becoming US citizens with the Louisiana purchase in 1803. Louis was one of the first to recognise that tuberculosis usually originates from a primary focus.

5. NIKOLAUS FRIEDREICH (1825–1882)
Friedreich succeeded Virchow at Wurzburg, but then went to Heidelberg as a clinician and wrote extensively on the heart and nervous system. During the Franco-Prussian war of 1870 he studied the epidemiology of several diseases affecting the German armies.

6. ADOLF KUSSMAUL (1822–1902)
Kussmaul qualified in Heidelberg, becoming Professor of Medicine successively in Heidelberg, Erlangen, Freiburg and Strasbourg. His achievements included: attempted gastroscopy (on a sword swallower), the invention of the stomach pump, antemortem diagnosis of mesenteric embolism and coining the term "polyarteritis nodosa".

7. NIKOLAI SERGEYEVICH KOROTKOFF (1874–1920)
Korotkoff qualified in Moscow and specialised in vascular surgery. During the Russo-Japanese War of 1904–5 he discovered the auscultatory method of measuring the blood pressure when studying the arterial flow following injury. He communicated his discovery to the St Petersburg Military Academy in 1905 (in a communication of only 271 words). After the Revolution he became physician at the Metchnikoff Hospital, Leningrad. He "disappeared" in 1920.

8. JAMES HOPE (1801–1841)
Hope learned "stethoscopy" from Laënnec. He was the first to describe the origin of cardiac murmurs and wrote the world's first textbook of cardiology, which went to three editions in his short lifetime.

9. WILLEM EINTHOVEN (1860–1927)
Einthoven was Professor of Physiology at Leyden when he invented his low-inertia silver-plated string galvanometer. The production of electricity by the heart had already been demonstrated by John Burdon-Sanderson and Augustus Waller the younger.

10. WILHELM HIS (JUNIOR) (1863–1934)
He discovered the atrioventricular bundle while working in his father's anatomy department in Leipzig. Although born Swiss he joined the German army, and while on the Russian front described trench (or Volhynia) fever.

11. PETER JAMES KERLEY
Radiologist, Westminster Hospital, London.

12. SVEN IVAN SELDINGER
Swedish radiologist.

13. ADOLF EUGEN FICK (1829–1910)
Fick qualified in Marburg and then went with Carl Ludwig to Zurich, eventually becoming Professor of Physiology at Wurzburg. In addition to his method of calculating cardiac output, he introduced the aneroid manometer for studying blood pressure, and a tonometer for measuring intra-ocular pressure.

14. THOMAS DUCKET JONES (1899–1954)
American cardiologist.

15. THOMAS SYDENHAM (1624–1689)
Sydenham was born in Dorset; his family were ardent Puritans and fought with the Parliamentary armies during the Civil War. Sydenham was a cavalry officer for four years, having briefly attended Oxford first; after the war he returned there to resume his studies. By this time the Chancellor of the University was the parliamentarian Duke of Monmouth, who awarded Sydenham his medical degree more for his services as a cavalry officer than for his medical studies.
Sydenham's influence was largely due to the fact that he wrote and taught in English, that he believed in rational therapy so far as it was possible, and that he also recognised disease patterns clearly, especially of individual febrile illnesses.

16. EDUARD HEINRICH HENOCH (1820–1910)
Henoch qualified in Berlin, where he ran the neurology department; he studied under Schönlein and eventually became a paediatrician.

17. JOHANNES LUCAS SCHÖNLEIN (1793–1864)
Schönlein qualified and became Professor of Medicine in Warzburg but because of his liberal political views he was dismissed; he eventually became Professor of Medicine successively in Zurich and Berlin.

18. SIR GEORGE FREDERIC STILL (1868–1941)
London paediatrician. Still was the first Professor of Paediatrics in Britain. He qualified in Cambridge and worked at King's College Hospital, London.

19. AUSTIN FLINT (1812–1886)
Flint was co-founder of the Buffalo Medical College; he subsequently accepted appointments in New Orleans and New York, and was a frequent visitor to Europe.

20. ANTONIO MARIA VALSALVA (1666–1723)
In Bologna, Valsalva was a pupil of Malpighi. His great interest was the ear; he named the Eustachian tube and discovered and named the labyrinth. His manoeuvre was introduced to remove foreign bodies from the ear. At the age of 43 he married a 17-year-old girl; he survived 14 years.

21. JOHANN FRIEDRICH HORNER (1831–1886)
Horner qualified in Zurich in 1854 and studied with Carl Ludwig, who was still then at Zurich. Horner specialised in ophthalmology, and his syndrome was described by several others at more or less the same time. Horner himself acknowledged that Claude Bernard had beaten him to it (just).

22. GRAHAM STEELL (1851–1943)
Graham Steell was born and educated in Edinburgh, and practised medicine in Manchester.

23. SIR WILLIAM OSLER (1849–1919)
Osler qualified in Montreal and became Professor of Medicine successively in Montreal and Baltimore, eventually succeeding Sir John Burdon-Sanderson as Regius Professor of Medicine at Oxford. He had a profound influence on British medicine as a clinician (emphasising careful personal observation), as a man (being industrious, questioning and inspiring confidence) and as an educationist (being responsible for professorial departments of medicine, and the pre-registration houseman year).
His textbook of medicine "The Principles and Practice of Medicine" is arguably still the most famous single-author medical book ever to have been produced; it was first produced in 1892 and ran to 16 editions, the last of which appeared in 1945.

24. RUDOLF LUDWIG KARL VIRCHOW (1821–1902)
Virchow qualified in Berlin and was early influenced by Henle and Schwann. He took part in the Revolution of 1848 and for this was dismissed from his professorial post in Berlin, but was immediately offered a similar post in Wurtzburg in Bavaria. However, he was recalled to Berlin in 1856 and there published his influential work on cellular pathology. Later he turned to politics, sitting for many years in the Reichstag. He died after jumping off a tram. Virchow's views were to dominate medicine for several decades, largely because he was a good teacher and made his work comprehensible to practising clinicians. Virchow's view on atheroma as being a disorder affecting the walls of blood vessels, rather than the organisation of mural encrustations, (which was the theory of his rival Rokitansky), and his rejection of Koch's ideas of the pathogenesis of infectious diseases, should not overshadow the enormous contributions he made. His additional claims to fame include his work on the pathology of the nervous system (Virchow-Robin perivascular spaces), his studies of inflammation and white blood cells (he coined the name "leukaemia"), and his study of connective tissue.

25. WILLIAM DRESSLER
American cardiologist.

26. KAREL FREDERIK WENCKEBACH (1864–1940)
Wenckebach qualified in Utrecht and became Professor of Medicine successively in Groningen, Strasbourg and Vienna. An anglophile, he made many visits to Britain, including one to McKenzie who was still then a GP in Burnley. From the observations of an astute patient Wenckebach discovered the therapeutic value of quinine in atrial fibrillation.

27. WILLIAM STOKES (1804–1878)
Stokes' father was Regius Professor of Medicine in Dublin, but Stokes qualified in Edinburgh. In 1825 he published the first book in English on the use of the stethoscope. He became physician to the Meath Hospital, where he and Robert Graves were powerful influences for the improvement of clinical teaching. He eventually succeeded his father as Professor of Medicine and with William Crampton he founded the Dublin Zoo.

28. ROBERT ADAMS (1791–1875)
Thrice President of the Royal College of Surgeons of Ireland.

29. JOHANNES EVANGELISTA PURKINJE (1787–1869)
Purkinje was born in Bohemia and first studied philosophy, but later became Professor of Physiology in Breslau. His work led to Helmholtz's development of the ophthalmoscope. Purkinje discovered ciliary movement, finger-prints, and the Purkinje cells in the cerebellum.

30 JOHN HOMANS (1877–1954)
Homans qualified in The Harvard Medical School, where he became Professor of Surgery in 1928.

31. HENRY HUBERT TURNER (1892–1970)
Turner qualified in Louisville (Louisiana) and worked as chief of the Endocrine Clinic in Oklahoma.

32. BERNARD-JEAN ANTONIN MARFAN (1858–1942)
Marfan qualified in Paris in 1887 where he became Professor of Paediatrics. He was interested in infant feeding and congenital diseases, and was among the earliest to realise that if the primary tubercle has fully developed by the age of 15, there will be life-long immunity. At one time this was known as Marfan's law.

33. ÉTIENNE-LOUIS ARTHUR FALLOT (1850–1911)
Fallot qualified in Marseilles and became Professor of Hygiene and Legal Medicine there. He described the "maladie bleue" in 1888.

34. HENRI LOUIS ROGER (1811–1891)
Roger qualified and worked in Paris. He wrote several paediatric textbooks including one on auscultation. In 1861 he noted at the post-mortem of a child the defect in the interventricular septum which had not caused any cardiac symptoms in life.

35. VICTOR EISENMENGER (1864–1932)
German physician.

36. JACOB MENDES DA COSTA (1833–1900)
Da Costa qualified in medicine in Philadelphia, and studied in Paris, and eventually became Professor of Medicine in Philadelphia. His work on "soldiers heart" or "effort syndrome" was conducted during the American Civil War while he was in charge of a military hospital in Philadelphia.

37. ADOLF WEIL (1848–1916)
Weil qualified in Heidelberg and worked with Friedreich and Arnold. He eventually became Professor of Medicine in Heidelberg. He described in 1886 four cases of infectious jaundice; the cause was not known until identified in 1916 by Hans Reiter.

38. CARLOS CHAGAS (1879–1934)
Chagas qualified in Rio de Janeiro and worked on malaria erradication in the Amazon; he was Director of Public Health in Rio and then Professor of Tropical Medicine, becoming much involved with medical commissions attached to the League of Nations.

39. EMANUEL LIBMAN (1872–1946)

Libman qualified and eventually became Professor of Medicine in Columbia University. He was the first to describe aneurysms arising from impact, also the features of bacterial growth on a sugar and serum medium. He and Benjamin Sacks described Libman-Sacks endocarditis in 1924.

40. BENJAMIN SACKS (1896–1944)

Sacks was born of German parents in Baltimore but came to Europe to qualify in Strasbourg in the new medical school established there by the Germans after the Franco-Prussian War. At that time Waldeyer (the ring), Kussmaul and von Recklinghausen were all there. Sacks then studied with John Hughlings Jackson (epilepsy) in London, Charcot in Paris and Westphal (the nucleus) in Berlin. He became Professor of Neurology in New York. He and Libman described their endocarditis in 1924.

2

RESPIRATORY SYSTEM

RESPIRATORY ADVENTITIOUS SOUNDS

There are two separate conventions for naming the main varieties of adventitious sounds arising from the lungs and airways. Laënnec,[1] in his *Treatise on Mediate Auscultation* published in 1819, used "râle" (death-rattle) to describe the sound made by patients dying of advanced tuberculosis, but for humanitarian reasons he used the Latin translation, "rhonchus", in front of patients. Thus he used râle and rhonchus interchangeably to describe *all* adventitious sounds. His treatise was quickly and poorly translated into English and "râle" and "rhonchus" came to signify different types of sound.

The two main types of adventitious sound either continue more or less throughout one or both phases of the respiratory cycle or are an interrupted series of short sounds. The two nomenclatures are:

Adventitious sounds (râles) { crepitations (interrupted sounds)
{ rhonchi (continuous sounds)

Adventitious sounds { râles (interrupted sounds)
{ rhonchi (continuous sounds)

Thus, interrupted sounds are either called "râles" or "crepitations". Synonyms sometimes used are:

crepitations (râles)	*rhonchi*
moist sounds	dry sounds
crackling	musical sounds
explosive sounds	wheezes
discontinuous sounds	continuous sounds

Crepitations (râles) were believed to be caused by air bubbling through fluid in the alveoli and/or airways and that fine and coarse crepitations (râles) depended on the size of the airways through which the air was thought to be bubbling through fluid. High-pitched and low-pitched rhonchi (wheezes) were believed to correspond to the size of the airways which are narrowed—high-pitched rhonchi (wheezes) being produced by the smaller airways. Recently these widely held views of the origins of the adventitious sounds have been disputed and plausible alternative explanations produced (Forgacs, 1978). The reasons that the traditional explanations for adventitious sounds are unlikely to be correct are:

1. The viscosity and surface tension of secretions in the small airways cannot be overcome by physiological pressure gradients.

2. Crepitations (râles) are common during inspiration alone—sounds caused by air bubbling through fluid should be heard in both phases of breathing.

3. Recordings of crepitations show that individual crackles recur constantly in each respiratory cycle—this would not be the case if air was bubbling through fluid.

4. Crepitations occur constantly in localised and diffuse fibrosis of the lungs when no excess fluid is present.

5. Crepitations heard over dependent parts of the lungs sometimes disappear in the *next* breath following a change of posture, long before fluid could have had a chance to move to the new dependent part.

Crepitations are probably a sign of abnormal deflation, and are due to an alteration in the elastic properties of the lungs. Air bubbling through fluid only occurs in the larger airways, and then randomly in both phases of breathing.

6. Rhonchi (wheezes) do not vary in pitch when a low-density gas (such as helium) is breathed, whereas the pitch of wind instruments depends on the density of the vibrating gas; however, the pitch of instruments containing a vibrating reed is independent of the density of the vibrating gas. This suggests that a closer analogy to explain the generation of wheeze is a vibrating reed rather than a vibrating column of air. Furthermore, attempts to recreate wheeze by blowing through post-mortem airways have failed.

The vibrating reed analogy explains why some patients with severe airway obstruction do not have rhonchi (wheezes). The velocity of gas necessary to vibrate a reed is fairly high; if ventilation is reduced or hyperinflation is severe, exhaled air will not reach a sufficient velocity to cause the obstructed airways to vibrate. Wheeze is also sometimes absent due to collapse of the large airways or poor sound conduction through hyperinflated lungs. It follows that the pitch of the wheeze is not an indication of the size of the airway obstructed—this is supported by the fact that a high-pitched wheeze is sometimes heard when a tumour or foreign body obstructs a large airway.

RADIOLOGY OF THE LUNGS

X-ray films are the records of shadows cast by structures between the film and the source of x-rays. The shadows may be distorted by variations in technique. An exact diagnosis is usually not possible on a single x-ray; the shadow thrown by a radio-opaque mass will not disclose the composition of the mass. Past experience and training will suggest the probability of a shadow being due to a known cause. Sometimes there is virtual certainty, as in the case of Kerley's "B" lines being due to engorgement of septal lymphatics, at other times diagnosis involves discussion of possibilities and probabilities.

The following routine of examining a chest film is essential in order to avoid missing obvious abnormalities:

1. **Degree of penetration.**—Normally it should be just possible to see individual intervertebral discs behind the heart shadow, and the division of trachea into the main bronchi.

2. **Centring of the film** and whether it has been taken in full inspiration.

3. **Name of the patient.**—This avoids mistakes like diagnosing coalminers' pneumoconiosis in a woman. Check the nationality of the name—in a Greek patient, a solid, round opacity is likely to be hydatid cyst; in a Welshman, fine, nodular opacities may be due to pneumonconiosis. If the patient is a female, check that both breast shadows are present. If one breast has been removed, check for secondary deposits in the bones. An absent breast shadow will cause increased translucency in the lower zone. Check also for shadowing suggesting past irradiation, viz. lung fibrosis and associated periosteal calcification.

4. **Check the right and left side of the film.**—The heart shadow is a poor guide, as dextrocardia may be present. Right and left markers should be seen on the film.

5. **Bone abnormalities** such as rib fractures, rib notching, periosteitis, rib erosions or congenital fusion of the ribs. Note whether there is any kyphosis, scoliosis, or calcification of the ligaments of the spine.

6. **Soft tissues** for abnormal swellings or calcification.

7. **Size and silhouette of the heart shadow,** paying particular attention to shadows behind the heart. A double shadow behind the heart may be due to hiatus hernia, collapsed left lower lobe, paravertebral abscess or mediastinal tumour.

8. **Diaphragm.**—The right diaphragm in full inspiration is normally at the posterior end of the tenth rib and the anterior end of the sixth rib. The left diaphragm is about half an inch lower. Costophrenic angles should be acute in the absence of pleural effusion.

9. **Gastric gas bubble.**—If not under the left diaphragm, check whether it is on the other side or in the mediastinum (hiatus hernia). It may be absent if there is a large abdominal mass, splenomegaly or a full stomach.

10. **Trachea** should be central and not indented (by an external mass). It is usually possible to see its division into the main bronchi at the anterior end of the second rib.

11. **Mediastinum.**—Note widening or displacement. Any shadow

continuous with the mediastinum may arise from it even though it extends well out into the lung fields.

13. **Lung fields.**—The "lung markings" of normal lungs are vascular shadows. Note whether the markings are normal and regularly distributed, or if they are crowded together anywhere suggesting collapse of a lobe. The radiotranslucency of both sides should be the same. The lung markings should extend to the edge of the chest wall. If a pneumothorax is anticipated, a chest film should be taken in expiration—the volume of the lung will decrease but the volume of air in the pleura will stay the same, so that the lung is pushed further away from the chest wall during expiration.

Each lung field is conventionally divided into zones:

Upper zone: above the anterior end of the second rib

Middle zone: from the level of the anterior end of the second rib to the level of the anterior end of the fourth rib

Lower zone: below the anterior end of the fourth rib.

The horizontal fissure of the right lung may be seen in a normal film; it runs from the middle of the hilar shadow to meet the sixth rib in the axilla. Occasionally, an azygos lobe is present in the right upper zone; a fold of pleura may be seen extending to a small protrusion at the upper right hilum, the azygos vein. An azygos lobe occurs in approximately 1 in 1000 chest x-rays.

The size, number, homogeneity, density and distribution of abnormal shadows in the lung fields should be noted.

Terms Used to Describe Shadows (Simon, 1978):

Homogeneous opacity.—Uniformly radio-opaque opacity.

Patchy shadow.—Non-homogeneous opacity. Each of these may be well- or ill-defined; the size and location should be stated.

Bullous area.—An area of hypertranslucency.

Ring shadow.—An area of hypertranslucency surrounded by an opaque wall.

Honeycomb shadowing.—Numerous small ring shadows.

Oval or circular shadows.—1. *Fine or miliary mottling:* shadows less than 2 mm in size. 2. *Coarse mottling:* shadows 2 mm to 2 cm in size. 3. *Large circular shadow:* measuring 2 cm or more.

The presence of cavitation or calcification of all shadows should be noted. Lung shadows may be associated with other abnormalities in the chest x-ray, for example an ill-defined area of patchy shadowing in the right middle and lower zones may be due to aspiration pneumonia which may have occurred as a result of a dilated oesophagus. This may be seen as a well-defined opacity parallel to the right upper mediastinum in which there may be a fluid level or food residue.

Causes of Miliary Mottling

Miliary tuberculosis   Previous bronchogram
Sarcoidosis   Haemosiderin
Pneumoconiosis   Histoplasmosis
Secondary deposits   Pulmonary oedema.

To locate a shadow anatomically it is essential to have a lateral film; it is most unwise to attempt an anatomical diagnosis unless two views are available. In the lateral film the main fissure may be seen separating lower from middle and upper lobes on the right, and lower from upper lobe on the left. On the left side there is no middle lobe, it is represented by the lingula, whose bronchus comes off anteriorly from the upper lobe bronchus. The fissures may be the sites of accumulation of fluid, which may remain in the fissures after it has cleared elsewhere, particularly following left ventricular failure. The main fissure runs roughly in the line of the sixth rib; on the right side it is met by the horizontal fissure.

Aspiration or inhalation pneumonias are associated with shadowing in particular lobes depending on the position of the patient during aspiration:

Apical segment of right lower lobe, or less commonly the apical segment of the left lower lobe if the patient was on his back

Axillary subsegments of anterior or posterior segments of right upper lobe with the patient lying on his right side, depending on whether the patient was lying more on his back or on his face

Axillary subsegments of anterior and apicoposterior segments of the left upper lobe if the patient was lying on his left side

Right middle lobe and lingula if the patient was prone (as in swimming breast-stroke; seen particularly in shipwrecked sailors who have swum in oil-covered water)

Posterior or lateral basal segment of either lower lobe if aspiration occurs while the patient is sitting upright as in the dentist's chair.

The sites from which material may be aspirated are:

Upper respiratory tract and mouth, fauces, sinuses and septic teeth

Lower respiratory tract: blood and pus can be aspirated into healthy bronchi from areas of bronchiectasis or bleeding

Oesophagus: pharyngeal diverticula, achalasia of the cardia, hiatus hernia and neuromuscular inco-ordination as in bulbar palsy.

Diffuse Pulmonary Opacities

A large number of conditions may cause diffuse bilateral opacities within the lungs on x-ray. There are a number of clinical correlations which are helpful in grouping the diseases known to cause diffuse pulmonary opacities. These are (Crofton, 1978):

> Fever as the presenting sign
> No symptoms
> Cough, malaise and loss of weight
> Dyspnoea as the main symptom.

The main causes in each group are:

Fever
> Miliary tuberculosis
> Bronchopneumonia
> Extrinsic allergic alveolitis
> Sarcoidosis
> Polyarteritis and SLE
> Hodgkin's[2] disease.

No symptoms
> Sarcoidosis
> Pneumoconiosis
> Tuberculosis
> Fibrosing alveolitis
> Pulmonary microlithiasis.

Cough, malaise and loss of weight
> Carcinoma
> Tuberculosis
> Lymphomas
> Leukaemia.

Dyspnoea
> Idiopathic fibrosing alveolitis
> Extrinsic allergic alveolitis
> Rheumatoid disease
> Honeycomb lung
> Metastases
> Lymphomatosis
> Idiopathic pulmonary haemosiderosis
> Pneumoconiosis
> Sarcoidosis.

THE CONTROL OF BREATHING

The rhythmicity of normal breathing is controlled by the respiratory centre; the rate and depth of breathing are affected by a number of feedback loops, the best known of which is the Hering-Breuer reflex. During inspiration, stretch receptors in the airways stimulate an inhibitory system via the vagus which limits inspiration; then expiration occurs as a passive process. There are in addition local inhibitory impulses in the medullary respiratory centre which also inhibit inspiration. Cutting the vagus leads to breathing at a slower rate, but at increased depth. The main control of breathing at normal tidal volumes is the medulla, and as the tidal volume increases the Hering-Breuer reflex becomes an additional controlling mechanism. Tidal volume will increase as the medullary centre is stimulated by chemical changes in the blood. In addition to the stretch receptors in the airways, there are:

Cough receptors
J receptors in the alveoli, which lead to increased frequency and depth of breathing
Lung irritant receptors in the bronchioles, which may play a part in the deflation reflex, resulting in an increased rate and depth of breathing if the lung is deflated
Proprioceptive receptors in chest-wall structures.

Diseases of the lungs and airways result in abnormal or inappropriate stimulation of some of these receptors, leading to changes in the rate and depth of breathing, which may in turn lead to hyperventilation, tachypnoea, hypoventilation or dyspnoea before there are any changes in the blood gases or blood pH.

Other Mechanisms Controlling Breathing

Changes in blood gases.—Hypoxia stimulates chemoreceptors in the carotid sinus and aorta; a raised Pco_2 stimulates the respiratory centre directly. Increased ventilation is not stimulated until Po_2 drops from 100 mm Hg to 60 mm Hg, but a rise of only 2–3 mm Hg of CO_2 has an immediate effect on ventilation. The sensitivity to a small rise in Pco_2 increases at lower Po_2 levels. Raised levels of Pco_2 are a sensitive guide to alveolar hypoventilation; levels of Pco_2 below normal do *not* give a good indication of alveolar hyperventilation which, if still accompanied by a low Po_2, may be critically dangerous. Loss of responsiveness of carotid sinus hypoxia receptors by chronic hypoxia reduces the responsiveness of the respiratory centre to raised Pco_2 levels.

Changes in blood pH.—The changes in ventilation are greater with a respiratory acidosis than metabolic acidosis, even though the blood pH is the same; similarly, the rate of change of ventilation is slower with a metabolic than a respiratory acidosis. These differences do *not* apply in *chronic* respiratory acidosis.

TESTS OF RESPIRATORY FUNCTION

Disorders of respiratory function.—It is convenient to consider the various abnormalities of respiratory function in terms of the way in which oxygen must pass from the ambient air to the tissues. The normal volume of air which can enter the chest may be reduced, resulting in disorder of *ventilation*. The reasons that the lungs are unable to accept a normal volume of air are, broadly:

Reduced ability to expand the thoracic cage, resulting in *restrictive* disorders

The airways may be narrowed, impeding gas flow and resulting in *obstructive* disorders

The lungs may be too stiff, resulting in failure of ventilation due to altered *compliance*.

Even if the correct volume of air is able to enter the lungs, this volume may not be correctly distributed, resulting in disorders of *distribution*. Despite normal ventilation and distribution of air, there may be failure of gas to pass across from the alveoli to haemoglobin contained in the lung capillaries, due to an abnormality of the alveolar walls—so-called *diffusion* or *transfer* defects. The correct functioning of the respiratory system also requires that blood as well as gas should be distributed correctly; disorders of blood distribution are *perfusion* defects.

The transfer of gases from alveoli to haemoglobin and vice versa takes a finite length of time, and too rapid a flow of blood (as in exercise) results in insufficient time for the complete transfer of gases to take place; and likewise, flow rates which are too slow (as in severe heart failure or polycythaemia) result in inadequate amounts of blood coming into contact with alveoli. Furthermore, disorders affecting the gas-carrying capacity of haemoglobin, or its quantity, may also result in insufficient gas exchange. Similarly, alterations in the haemoglobin dissociation curve can also result in reduced uptake by haemoglobin of oxygen, and in the tissues a reduced ability to give up oxygen. Thus severe anaemia and haemoglobinopathies, pyrexia and acidosis may all affect the ability to supply oxygen to, and remove carbon dioxide from, the tissues.

The function of the respiratory system is to provide an adequate supply of oxygen and to remove carbon dioxide from the blood. Air is moved in and out of the chest by a bellows-like action—expansion of the rib cage by intercostal muscles and active descent of the diaphragm. During normal breathing (tidal breathing) about 500 cc of air is inhaled and exhaled at each breath (tidal volume). The maximum amount of air which can be blown out after maximum inspiration is about 5 litres (vital capacity). Air enters the chest through the trachea and is distributed to all parts of the lungs through the bronchi and bronchioles. Thus, without considering the lungs themselves we have three functions of air movement that can be measured:

1. Ability to cause air to move in and out of the chest or bellows function (ventilation)
2. The ability to allow this volume of air through the airways (obstruction)
3. The equality of distribution of this air to different parts of the lungs (distribution).

The ability to move air in and out of the chest is measured by recording the volume of air which can be blown out after a maximum inhalation (vital capacity or VC). This does not take into account the speed of breathing; this is measured by recording the volume of air blown out in one minute when breathing as fast as possible (maximum breathing capacity or MBC—normally 120 litres per minute).

The ability to allow air through the airways depends on their bore. It takes a longer time for a given volume of air to flow through a narrow tube than a wide one. Similarly, there is less air flow in a given time. These two facts form the basis of the tests for narrowing or obstruction of the airways. The FEV_1 is the volume of air flowing in the first second of a forced expiration. In diseases causing obstruction to the airways, the forced expiratory volume in the first second (FEV_1) is reduced. Furthermore, the ratio of FEV_1 to VC is also reduced; normal people can usually exhale 75 per cent of their vital capacity in the first second. In obstruction of the airways, the FEV_1 to VC ratio is less than 75 per cent. Another method of measuring volume of air flow in a given time is to record the maximum rate of flow (volume per minute), which is known as the peak expiratory flow rate (PEFR). It is measured with a Wright peakflow meter. The units of measurement are litres per minute and the normal is 400–600 litres per minute— note that this is a maximum *rate* of flow and does not indicate the actual volume flowing in one minute. The FEV_1 and PEFR measure volume flowing in a given time. It is also possible to measure the time taken to displace a given volume of air. The tidal volume is about 500 ml, and by listening over the trachea the length of time taken to exhale this volume of air during quiet respiration can be noted. Obstruction to the airways will prolong expiration time.

Distribution of Inspired Air

Despite being drawn into the chest, the inspired air may not be distributed or mixed correctly within the lungs. These parameters can be tested by nitrogen washout; that is, the patient breathes 100 per cent oxygen, and the time taken for all the nitrogen already in the lungs to be washed out is recorded; this is normally less than 7 minutes.

In a patient with maldistribution of air it takes longer to wash out the nitrogen from the underventilated parts of the lung. Another method of measuring equality of distribution is the "helium wash-out time" which is based on the same principle as the nitrogen wash-out time except that only a single breath of helium is taken whereas in the nitrogen wash-out time 100 per cent oxygen is inspired continuously.

The equality of distribution can be measured by adding a small amount of radioactive gas to the inspired air and counting the radioactivity over each part of the lung; the part of the lung receiving less radioactive gas will emit less radioactivity. The radioactive gas used is an isotope of xenon (^{133}Xe).

Restriction of ventilatory movement due to increase in residual volume (air trapping).—Occasionally it is necessary to obtain more information than is available from the more simple tests. The most useful additional static lung volumes are the residual volume (RV); this is the volume of air remaining in the chest after a forced exhalation. The implication of an increased RV is in younger patients with asthma, whose tests of vital capacity, FEV_1, and peak flow may have returned to near normal, but who still have evidence of "air trapping". The RV can only be measured by helium-dilution techniques or whole-body plethysmography.

Restriction of ventilatory movement due to decreased movement of the thoracic cage.—This can occur because of neurological disorders affecting the respiratory muscles, e.g. poliomyelitis, chest injuries, pain, ankylosing spondylitis, kyphoscoliosis, etc. In practice, most causes of restricted ventilation are assessed clinically, although it is possible to quantify the restrictions due to disorders of the thoracic cage, if it is thought that part of the restrictive defect is due to disease of the lung or pleura.

Diffusion Defects

It was formerly believed that defects in the transfer of gases from alveoli to red corpuscles were often due to interference with the diffusion of gases caused by a thickening of the "alveolar capillary membrane." Furthermore, these defects were not thought to affect carbon dioxide because it has a much greater diffusibility than oxygen, and thus diffusion defects only affected oxygen transfer. It is now believed that pure diffusion defects are relatively rare and that the majority of cases thought to have diffusion defects in fact have disturbed ventilation/perfusion ratios as well. Carbon monoxide has diffusing properties similar to oxygen, and the avidity with which haemoglobin takes it up makes it a reasonable assumption that the main limiting factor to removal of carbon monoxide is its transfer from alveoli to blood, and that this is equivalent to defects of oxygen diffusion. The uptake by the blood of a known amount of carbon monoxide gives a rough measure of "diffusion" and it is known as the "transfer" factor for carbon monoxide, or TCO. Disorders which affect the interstitial space will cause a reduction of the partial pressure of oxygen in the blood. Patients compensate for anoxia by increasing the rate of respiration; this hyperventilation usually results in a reduction of the amount of carbon dioxide in the blood. Diffusion defects are, therefore, characterised by an increased respiratory rate, a low Po_2 and a low Pco_2—other tests of respiratory function are usually normal. The rate of uptake of carbon monoxide depends on its partial pressure in the inspired air. The normal uptake is about 15 ml/min/mm Hg at rest; this should approximately double after exercise, due to an increase in ventilation and an increase in the blood supply to the lungs.

Disorders of Compliance

In practice it is rarely necessary to perform tests to quantify disorders of compliance, although as a concept lung compliance is important to clinical practice. Studies of compliance have helped to clarify significant aspects of pulmonary physiology. In simple terms, compliance can be deduced from the air volume which can be sucked into the lungs with a given change in intrathoracic negative pressure. The intrathoracic pressure is measured by a balloon in the oesophagus. The elasticity of the lungs will be reduced by pulmonary fibrosis, pulmonary venous congestion, and left-to-right shunts in which increased pulmonary artery blood flow causes the arteries to be turgid and stiff and to hold the lungs outwards like the spokes of an umbrella. Diseases which cause stiffening and deformity of the chest wall, such as ankylosing spondylitis and kyphoscoliosis, will also diminish the effective elasticity of the lungs.

Closing Volume

Before there is any measurable change in FEV_1 or PEFR, those disorders which affect airways resistance may disturb the normal decrease in calibre of the airways during expiration in such a way that some airways, particularly in the dependent parts of the lungs, constrict or even occlude inappropriately early. This can be detected by breathing in, during maximum inhalation, a small volume of inert gas such as argon, and exhaling maximally; a sudden steep rise in argon concentration towards the end of exhalation indicates that exhaled air has suddenly stopped coming from poorly expanded airways, i.e. that they have "closed" prematurely.

Occasionally, bronchitis damages the cartilaginous rings of bronchi and trachea; during attempted expiration the intrathoracic pressure rises and may cause collapse of the damaged intrathoracic airways. In an effort to maintain a high intratracheal pressure, such patients will exhale slowly against a resistance—they will purse their lips and allow air to escape slowly. On the spirograph record of the vital capacity, such airways collapse is seen as a sudden temporary cessation of airflow.

Formal tests of respiratory function do not obviate the need for a careful clinical history, accurate examination and consideration of the chest x-ray. Respiratory function tests enable lung function to be assessed at a single moment in time, but the history is the best way of assessing retrospective progression of the disease.

The chest x-ray may be useful in anticipating which lung function tests are going to be helpful. A large radiotranslucent area surrounded by a thin wall will suggest an underventilated lung cyst, local attenuation of pulmonary arteries will suggest abnormal distribution of blood, and bilateral lower-zone patchy shadowing will suggest interstitial pulmonary fibrosis as a cause of a diffusion defect.

Ventilation-Perfusion Mismatch

The satisfactory transfer of gases between the alveoli and blood depends on the delivery of optimum amounts of each. The delivery of too much blood means insufficient gas exchange, and the delivery of too much air results in wasted ventilation. There are normally homeostatic mechanisms which ensure that underventilation results in local hypoxic vasoconstriction, and interruption of blood supply causes some local bronchiolar narrowing and alveolar collapse, thus attempting to avoid either wasted perfusion or wasted ventilation. Unfortunately these mechanisms are delicate and can easily be overwhelmed by disease, so that in practice ventilation-perfusion mismatch is common.

The concepts involved in calculating and understanding ventilation-perfusion mismatch are not too complicated, but they do involve some fundamental physiology and simple mathematics.

The letters used in calculating ventilation-perfusion mismatch problems have given rise to the "V/Q language" (West, 1977) in which

V is gas volume
Q is blood flow

P is gas pressure
a is arterial gas content
A is alveolar gas content
v is mixed venous gas content
R = respiratory exchange ratio, i.e. CO_2 out/O_2 in

In the normal lungs the blood flow is approximately 5·0 litres per minute and the ventilation about 4·0 litres per minute, giving an overall V/Q ratio of 0·8. However, the V/Q ratio varies surprisingly between the top and bottom of the lungs in the normal individual. The ratio is between 0·6 and 3·0, indicating that the top of the lung is overventilated and the bottom of the lung relatively overperfused. Parts of the lungs which are overventilated (but underperfused) have an increase in the physiological *dead space*, i.e. they contain too much room air, instead of being affected by the normal exchange of respiratory gases which results in reduction of Po_2 and increase in Pco_2. Parts of the lung which are overperfused result in venous blood (containing a low Po_2 and high Pco_2) passing directly to the arterial side—*the venous admixture or shunt effect* (Figure 21).

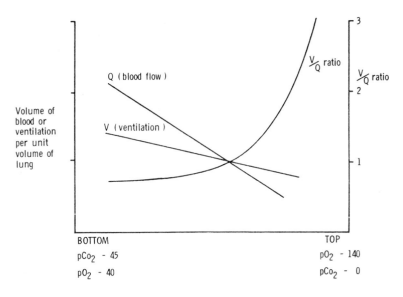

FIG. 21.—The line Q shows the fall in blood flow per unit volume of lung between the bottom and the top of the lungs. The line V shows the smaller fall in ventilation between the bottom and the top of the lungs. It follows that the top of the lungs are relatively overventilated and the bottom relatively overperfused. The curve V/Q shows the ratio between ventilation and perfusion. At one extreme of the V/Q ratio, complete non-perfusion will represent the gases in inspired air, and at the other, complete non-ventilation will represent the blood gases in venous blood.

In the blood there is a relationship between the amount of carbon dioxide and oxygen that can be carried. The relative amounts of each vary because of the Bohr[3] and Haldane[4] effects, which state that the amount of carbon dioxide carried decreases as the oxygen tension rises, and similarly the oxygen carried decreases as the carbon dioxide tension rises. It is important to appreciate that in expired air the relationship between oxygen and carbon dioxide partial pressures is linear since there is no change in the other two components contributing to atmospheric pressure (i.e. P_{H_2O} and P_{N_2}). This follows from Boyle's law, which states that equal volumes of *gas* have the same partial pressure. *Blood* can carry a much greater *volume* of carbon dioxide than oxygen at the same partial pressures of each; this is because carbon dioxide is also given off from bicarbonate, which has to be present in large quantities because it is the principal buffer system in the blood.

It is assumed that alveolar gas is in equilibrium with mixed venous blood. The composition of the following are already known

Inspired air ($P_{O_2} = 140$; $P_{CO_2} = 0$)
Venous blood ($P_{O_2} = 40$; $P_{CO_2} = 45$)
Arterial blood ($P_{O_2} = 100$; $P_{CO_2} = 40$)

The line relating alveolar (or mixed venous) P_{O_2} and P_{CO_2} must therefore pass through these points (Fig. 22).

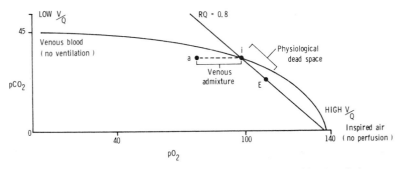

Fig. 22.—This shows the curve relating P_{O_2} and P_{CO_2} in the blood for the whole range of V/Q ratios (from complete non-ventilation, i.e. P_{O_2} and P_{CO_2} as in venous blood, to complete non-perfusion, i.e. P_{O_2} and P_{CO_2} the same as inspired air). This curve is the same as that showing the V/Q ratios in Fig. 21. Point i shows the average V/Q ratio which must exist at an RQ of 0·8 (RQ=ratio of CO_2 out/O_2 in). If the blood gases show a deviation from point i then there must be either overperfusion (shunt or venous admixture) or overventilation (increase in dead space).

This same graph shows all possible ventilation perfusion ratios from pure venous admixture (V/Q=very low) to pure dead space (V/Q=very high). If we know the relative volumes of oxygen and carbon dioxide which are being used (by studying expired air and remembering that equal volumes of gases in equilibrium must always have the same partial pressure) we can superimpose on this graph the ratio of CO_2 given out and O_2 absorbed; it follows that the point where this line cuts the alveolar O_2/CO_2 line must represent the ratio of O_2 to CO_2 in the alveoli which is needed to give rise to the particular ratio of O_2 to CO_2 which the body is known to be using. The particular V/Q ration can be quantified from prior knowledge of the position on the Po_2/Pco_2 line of the V/Q ratios. Furthermore, if a measured sample of arterial blood does not correspond to that predicted from the diagram, there must either be a shunt (venous admixture) or increased dead space. The venous admixture or shunt may be due to V/Q abnormalities *or* a direct anatomical shunt. It is possible to distinguish between these by having the patient breathe 100 per cent oxygen, which will cause the Po_2 to rise if there is V/Q mismatch, because the increased inspired O_2 will increase the Po_2 in previously underventilated but normally perfused alveoli.

Estimation of Pulmonary Causes of Hypoxia

The simplest method of deciding whether peripheral desaturation is due to a shunt effect is to have the patient breathe 100 per cent oxygen. This will increase the oxygen saturation of arterial blood, because even the poorly ventilated alveoli will now be receiving enough oxygen; in contrast, if there is an anatomical shunt, there is almost no rise in arterial Po_2. The same thing occurs when ventilation of normally underventilated lung is increased by exercise. So a rise in oxygen saturation after breathing 100 per cent oxygen improves oxygen saturation in diffusion defects, ventilation/perfusion, inequality, and hypoventilation, but does not raise oxygen saturation due to shunts. Undersaturation of arterial blood due to a diffusion disorder will become rapidly worse after exercise, due to increased tissue utilisation of oxygen which cannot be offset by increasing diffusion of oxygen from alveoli to alveolar capillaries.

CHANGES IN ARTERIAL PO_2 WITH OXYGEN AND EXERCISE IN PULMONARY CONDITIONS CAUSING HYPOXIA

	100% *oxygen*	30% *oxygen*	*Exercise*
Ventilation/Perfusion inequality	improved	unchanged	improved
Shunt	unchanged	unchanged	worse
Diffusion defect	improved	improved	worse
Underventilation	improved	improved	improved

As a rough-and-ready rule, a blood Po_2 of 500 mm can be achieved by breathing 70 per cent oxygen when no significant shunt is present.

With 100% inspired oxygen	Shunt
Blood Po_2–500 mm	15%
Blood Po_2–100 mm	25%
Blood Po_2–50 mm	50%

The Dead-space Effect

Reduction of the Pco_2 below the predicted value usually indicates an increased dead-space effect. This can be quantified if one knows the CO_2 content of expired air. The composition of expired air would be the same as alveolar air if it were not mixed with incoming inspired air. Inspired air which is drawn into the lungs but which does not contain any alveolar air ventilates only dead space; thus expired air contains a mixture of alveolar and dead-space air. The composition of dead-space air is known—hence the size of the dead space can be deduced by finding the amount of CO_2 in expired air. Normally the composition of expired air is given by a point about 30 per cent down from the ideal alveolar air point. Any movement of the expired air point down towards the composition of inspired air must mean the ventilation of dead space. This can be quantified because the distance between the inspired air point and ideal alveolar gas point corresponds to the tidal volume; hence if the ratio of dead space to total volume is known, the size of the dead space can be calculated. The physiological dead space is increased in:

old age	pulmonary embolism
recumbency	emphysema
smoking	anaesthesia.

Increase in the dead space results in wasted ventilation and if this is combined with airways obstruction, serious alveolar hypoventilation may occur. This results in failure to remove carbon dioxide from the alveoli, i.e. in an increase in alveolar Pco_2.

Disorders of the Blood and Red Cell

Each molecule of haemoglobin binds 4 molecules of oxygen; haemoglobin has the remarkable ability of increasing its affinity for oxygen as it takes up oxygen; this property accounts for the steep middle part of the normal oxygen dissociation curve, whereby the saturation of haemoglobin and the *volume* of oxygen carried increases rapidly with only a small change in oxygen partial pressure. The converse of course also applies, so that once haemoglobin starts to give up its oxygen when it reaches the tissues, it does so with increasing ease. The shape of the haemoglobin molecule and the strength of the weak bonds which hold it together (and which must be broken for it to carry oxygen efficiently) are affected by pH, temperature and the amount of carbon dioxide also attached to the haemoglobin molecule. These factors reduce the oxygen-carrying ability of haemoglobin; thus, higher concentrations of CO_2 cause haemoglobin to carry less oxygen whereas, if the ambient Pco_2 is lowered, haemoglobin can transport more oxygen. This phenomenon by which oxygen transport is influenced by Pco_2 is the Bohr effect. The Bohr effect is almost certainly *beneficial* in terms of oxygen delivery to the tissues. Although the total oxygen carried by the haemoglobin is *decreased*, as the Bohr effect shifts the oxygen dissociation curve to the right, it will be seen that the oxygen tension (Po_2) at the tissues is *increased* at a given oxygen saturation. One clinical consequence of this is that in diabetic ketoacidosis, too rapid a correction of the acidosis with bicarbonate, pushing the curve back to the left, may reduce oxygen delivery to the tissues.

2,3 Diphosphoglycerate (DPG)

This organic phosphate is an intermediary in normal carbohydrate metabolism (the glycolytic or Emden Meyerhof pathway). It is present in large quantities in red cells and is known to react with haemoglobin, reducing its oxygen affinity, e.g. low concentrations of DPG cause low tissue tensions of oxygen (because oxygen tends to stay attached to haemoglobin) whereas high levels tend to displace oxygen from haemoglobin. The DPG levels have some clinical relevance; for example, anaemias and hypoxic states are associated with raised (and therefore useful) DPG levels; stored blood has low, and therefore potentially harmful, levels.

The Oxygen and Carbon Dioxide Dissociation Curves

Figure 23 shows the dissociation curves for oxygen and carbon dioxide. Analysis of the curves will show that their shape is predictable, given certain basic data and good planning. The basic data which have to be considered are:

Man has to be able to survive and compete at sea level and up to a reasonable altitude in mountainous parts where the Po_2 is less

Oxygen has to be picked up efficiently and quickly in the lungs by the blood

The pH of the blood has to be kept constant

Carbon dioxide is a waste product of cellular metabolism and therefore has to be removed quickly by the blood

The pH of the blood is kept constant by buffers which are large
quantities of the salt of a weak acid together with the
appropriate weak acid

There are several buffers in the blood, but the main one is the salt
of the acid formed as a result of cell metabolism (that is CO_2
dissolved in water, forming carbonic acid or H_2CO_3; thus, by
eliminating CO_2 the lungs both excrete a waste product and
restore the buffer system

Oxygen must be given up from the blood quickly and easily at the
partial pressure of oxygen at which most cells exist (Po_2 of
around 40 mm). One method is to encourage reduced oxygen
affinity of haemoglobin when the level of carbon dioxide is
raised. This is the situation arising from cell metabolism, which
itself is creating a further requirement for oxygen.

Analysis of the O_2 and CO_2 dissociation curves show that they are
suited to all of these conditions.

At sea level the partial pressure of oxygen is about 140 mm Hg; at
10 000 feet it is only 100 mm Hg. It is therefore desirable for man to
have the same oxygen content (in volumes) in his blood at all levels of
partial pressure down to that at cell level; this explains line A in
Fig. 23. The most desirable line is one which shows no fall in O_2
content as the Po_2 drops to around that at which cellular respiration
occurs. At around Po_2 40–60, the most desirable attribute of haemo-

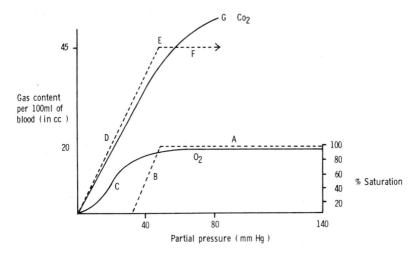

FIG. 23.—This shows on one graph the oxygen and carbon dioxide dissociation curves.
Note that *total* CO_2 carried in the blood is considerably more than the amount of
oxygen which can be carried. The dotted lines are explained in the text; they show how
the dissociation curves can be predicted, given certain biological presuppositions.

globin is that for almost no change in partial pressure it should give up all its oxygen. Line B represents this ideal, while curve C is the compromise linking these ideals and producing the familiar oxygen dissociation curve. How do we explain the altogether different dissociation curve for carbon dioxide? First, remember that carbon dioxide, its acid and the salt (bicarbonate) are going to be the major buffer system, and that there has to be a large quantity of the bicarbonate (from which CO_2 *in vitro* can be extracted). This explains why it is necessary for the total CO_2 content to be so great—it is present in its own buffer. At cell level the most desirable quality of the CO_2 system is that it can accommodate relatively large amounts of CO_2 with very little change in partial pressure, hence line D which shows this idealised state of affairs. However at around point E on this line another requirement is added: in order to encourage the removal of oxygen from haemoglobin there should be a rapid rise in partial pressure of CO_2 for almost no change in CO_2 content (line F represents this ideal). Curve G is the compromise—the CO_2 dissociation curve. (There are slight changes in the slope of the effective part of G according to whether the blood is venous or arterial.)

Acid-Base Balance

The pH of blood is one of the most constant physiological parameters. Tissue metabolism continuously produces acid metabolites which constantly tend to increase the hydrogen ion concentration of the blood. The pH is maintained around 7·4 by the action of buffers, which are the salts of a strong base and a weak acid. The salt is neutral, i.e. has a pH of 7; if more acid is added to a buffer then either more neutral salt is formed, or the base is so much stronger than the added acid that no appreciable change of pH occurs unless vast, unphysiological amounts of acid are added. There are many buffer systems in the body but the most important clinically is the bicarbonate-carbonic acid system. Bicarbonate is the strong base and carbonic acid the weak acid; the concentration of the bicarbonate in the blood is about twenty times that of carbonic acid. The pH of the blood depends on the proportion of base to acid. This is expressed in the infamous Henderson[5]-Hasselbalch[6] equation:

$pH = pK + \log \dfrac{Base}{Acid}$. From a clinical point of view the only thing we have to note is that in order for the pH to remain constant, $\dfrac{Base}{Acid}$ must also remain constant, so that any increase in base should be accompanied by an increase in acid, otherwise, $\dfrac{Base}{Acid}$ would increase.

The weak acid, carbonic acid, readily dissociates into carbon dioxide and water ($H_2CO_3 \rightleftharpoons CO_2 + H_2O$) so that the CO_2 concentration of the blood is an indirect way of measuring the acid component of the most important buffer system in the body.

The CO_2 release from the body is controlled by the lungs; any tendency to alter the CO_2 content of the blood is *respiratory*. Any *primary* increase in CO_2 is a *respiratory* acidosis (as CO_2 is a measure of the carbonic acid) and any primary decrease in CO_2 is a *respiratory* alkalosis.

Any change in one component of the $\frac{Base}{Acid}$ ratio will be compensated for by a similar change in the other component. Thus a respiratory acidosis (elevation of CO_2) will be accompanied by a rise in bicarbonate.

Any *primary* change in bicarbonate is called a *metabolic* change and is accompanied by a similar change in the CO_2 content. Thus, a metabolic acidosis is accompanied by a fall in bicarbonate and then a fall in CO_2. Measurement of the Pco_2 and bicarbonate concentration will usually indicate whether an acidosis or alkalosis is present. The compensatory alteration of either bicarbonate or CO_2 is usually less than the primary abnormality. If the pH is also known it is even simpler to determine whether a patient is suffering from a compensated metabolic or respiratory acidosis or alkalosis. The normal Pco_2 of arterial blood is 40 mm Hg and of venous blood 46 mm Hg. The normal plasma bicarbonate is 23 mmol/l. Example: $Pco_2 = 50$ mm, HCO_3 25 mmol/l—could theoretically be either a respiratory acidosis (raised Pco_2) or a metabolic alkalosis (raised HCO_3). However, the largest change is the elevation of the Pco_2 from the normal of 40 mm to 50 mm so a respiratory acidosis is probably present. When you know that the accompanying pH was 7·32 it will unequivocally be a respiratory acidosis. Similarly a Pco_2 of 20 mm and a bicarbonate of 10 mmol/l (both reduced) could theoretically be a metabolic acidosis or respiratory alkalosis. However, the bicarbonate is very low at 10 mmol/l and as this is probably the primary abnormality a metabolic acidosis is probably present; the accompanying pH of 7·3 makes it a metabolic acidosis for certain. Figure 24 shows the relationship between pH, bicarbonate and Pco_2. At a given pH a rise in Pco_2 will be accompanied by a rise in bicarbonate and vice versa.

The medullary respiratory centre is normally sensitive to changes in arterial Pco_2. An elevated Pco_2 stimulates hyperventilation of the lungs via the respiratory centre and the excess carbon dioxide is rapidly blown off.

Excretion of bicarbonate and hydrogen ion via the renal tubules is a much slower process. There are three mechanisms by which hydrogen ion is secreted into the urine:

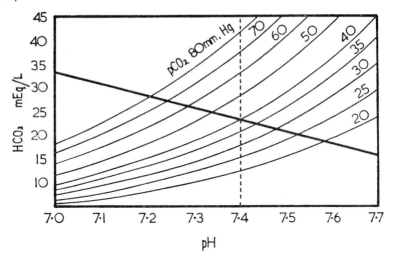

Fig. 24.—The interrelationship between pH, Pco$_2$ and bicarbonate in the plasma. (By courtesy of Dr E. W. O'Brien.)

1. Plasma bicarbonate excreted as carbonic acid

$$HCO_3 + H^+ \rightarrow H_2CO_3$$

2. Excretion of ammonium salts from ammonia manufactured in renal tubules

$$NH_3 + H^+ \rightarrow NH_4^+$$

3. Excretion of sodium dihydrogen phosphate manufactured from disodium hydrogen phosphate

$$Na_2HPO_4 + H^+ \rightarrow NaH_2PO_4$$

The bicarbonate-carbonic acid buffer system is the most important clinically, but there are several other buffer sytems involved in keeping the blood pH constant. Proteins, including haemoglobin and the plasma proteins, act as weak acids and form buffer systems with strong bases such as bicarbonate and phosphate. Oxyhaemoglobin is more acid than reduced haemoglobin, hence, in the tissues where oxy-haemoglobin is reduced to more basic reduced haemoglobin, the acid metabolites are buffered by the reduced haemoglobin. Haemoglobin combines loosely with carbon dioxide, forming "carbamino com-pounds"; when oxyhaemoglobin reaches the tissues where acid metabolites and CO_2 have accumulated it rapidly loses its oxygen at the same time, becoming more avid for carbon dioxide. The process is reversed in the lungs. Reduced haemoglobin, therefore, is important as a buffer against acid metabolites and as a transporter of CO_2.

When blood is collected for estimation of bicarbonate, CO_2 will immediately start to come out of solution unless the blood is collected anaeorobically. Because the buffering properties of blood still remain intact (even though it is in a bottle) the bicarbonate level will also fall. In order to allow for this *in vitro* change in bicarbonate and CO_2 content, the bicarbonate is estimated when the blood has been in contact with a Pco_2 of 40 mm Hg (the Pco_2 of arterial blood); this value is the plasma "standard bicarbonate" concentration.

Causes of Disturbed Acid-Base Balance

Respiratory acidosis (CO_2 retention):
Airways obstruction (asthma and bronchitis)
Failure of bellows function:
 obesity
 ankylosing spondylitis
 poliomyelitis
 chest injuries
 relaxant drugs
Depression of respiratory centre:
 drugs (morphia, barbiturates)
 cerebrovascular accident
 encephalitis
 coma.

Respiratory alkalosis (reduced Pco_2):
Overbreathing:
 hysteria
 diffusion defects
 salicylates (cause stimulation of respiratory centre).

Metabolic acidosis (decrease in bicarbonate):
Ketosis due to diabetes or starvation
Renal failure
Cyclical vomiting in children (causes ketosis)
Severe dehydration
Ingestion of ammonium chloride
Ureterocolic anastomosis
Severe anoxia (lactic acid accumulates).

Metabolic alkalosis (increase in bicarbonate):
Repeated vomiting (pyloric stenosis)
Intestinal fistulae
Milk-alkali syndrome (excessive ingestion of alkalis)
Aldosteronism
Cushing's syndrome
Diuretic therapy.

Treatment

Respiratory acidosis.—The elevated Pco_2 of respiratory failure may be lowered by reversing airways obstruction, stimulating the respiratory centre, or mechanical ventilation.

Respiratory alkalosis.—Rebreathing in a closed circuit will raise the Pco_2 (e.g. hysterics should be made to breathe in and out of a paper bag).

Metabolic alkalosis.—Usually no specific treatment is necessary apart from removal of the cause. Severe alkalosis whether metabolic or respiratory is accompanied by tetany which is due to a reduction in the ionised calcium in the serum. It can be stopped by intravenous calcium chloride (10 ml of 10 per cent solution). Metabolic alkalosis may be caused by hypokalaemia; the cells become depleted of potassium, which is replaced by hydrogen withdrawn from the extracellular fluid, causing an excess of bicarbonate.

Metabolic acidosis.—Diabetic coma should usually be treated with intravenous infusion of bicarbonate (or lactate) as well as rehydration and insulin. Insulin is thought to be less easily utilised in an acid medium (see p. 437 for treatment of diabetic coma).

Standard bicarbonate (BP) is a 1·4 per cent solution and contains 167 mmol/l of bicarbonate and sodium ions. Sixth molar lactate also contains 167 mmol/l of bicarbonate. The 8·4 per cent bicarbonate solution used in the correction of acidosis following cardiac arrest, and in the forced alkaline diuresis treatment of salicylate and barbiturate overdose, contains 1 mmol/ml of bicarbonate.

Replacement of electrolytes, which are found mainly in the extracellular fluid, is based on the fact that the extracellular fluid is about one-fifth of the body weight (usually about 15 litres). In the case of bicarbonate this regime has to be modified, since bicarbonate is also an intracellular ion; it has been found empirically that an assumption that bicarbonate is distributed through fluid equivalent to one-third of the body weight results in adequate replacement of the ion. The plasma is a representative sample of the extracellular fluid; the normal plasma bicarbonate is approximately 25 mmol/l; hence the amount of bicarbonate replacement needed is the plasma deficit per litre multiplied by the number of litres involved, i.e. one-third of the body weight in kilograms (1 litre weighs 1 kilogram).

Example: A 60 kilogram diabetic in diabetic coma has a plasma bicarbonate of 20 mmol/l. He is 5 mmol/l short of bicarbonate, he therefore requires 5×20 mEq $= 100$ mmol.

This is 100 ml of 8·4 per cent bicarbonate (1 mmol per ml) or about ½ litre of 1·4 per cent bicarbonate (167 mmol/l).

CHRONIC BRONCHITIS AND EMPHYSEMA

Chronic bronchitis is a condition characterised by excessive mucus secretion from the bronchial tree, and recurrent cough productive of sputum every day, for three months of the year for at least two successive years. Infection of the bronchi is usually but not invariably present, the commonest infecting organisms being *Haemophilus influenzae* and the pneumococcus; the part played by respiratory viruses in initiating and perpetuating infection is probably much underestimated. Factors which predispose to and aggravate, but probably do not cause, chronic bronchitis are general atmospheric pollution (dust and sulphur dioxide), inhalation of cigarette smoke, damp climate and occupational exposure to harmful dusts and irritant fumes.

The excessive mucus production characteristic of chronic bronchitis is produced by hypertrophied and more numerous mucus-producing goblet cells in the bronchial epithelium, and by dilated mucous glands within the bronchial wall. The severity of the bronchitis can be correlated with the increase in size of the mucous glands. Infection results in thickening of the mucous membrane, micro-abscess formation and viscous, infected sputum. The bronchi are narrowed by the thickened oedematous mucous membrane and viscous, infected mucus which is difficult to expectorate. These changes may be confined to the larger bronchi but more usually the bronchioles are also involved— for this reason the term "obstructive airways disease" is preferable to "chronic bronchitis".

Emphysema is defined as enlargement of the air spaces distal to the respiratory (the most distal) bronchioles, due to dilatation or destruction of the alveolar walls. Emphysema is a frequent accompaniment of chronic bronchitis. It is suggested that if bronchioles as well as bronchi are chronically infected, infection can spread to and destroy alveolar walls leading to loss of functioning lung tissue, fusion of many alveoli and hence to a dilated air space. If the infection is more or less confined to the larger airways, the dominant features will be general narrowing and obstruction to air flow. Emphysema can exist without chronic bronchitis as a precursor, and chronic bronchitis does not invariably cause emphysema.

The late clinical features of chronic bronchitis tend to be different, depending on whether the dominant effect is widespread airways obstruction or destruction of lung tissue (emphysema). In their pure forms these two effects are seen clinically as the "blue bloater" and the "pink puffer". Loss of alveolar wall, as in emphysema, diminishes the area over which diffusion of O_2 and CO_2 can take place; the effect of this is to diminish the P_{O_2} in the blood. The medullary respiratory

centre responds to alteration of the blood CO_2, and the chemoreceptors in the carotid and aortic bodies are sensitive to anoxia. Stimulation
of these chemoreceptors by the anoxia results in an increase in the
depth and rate of breathing which will increase the diffusing surface
available to oxygen, the blood oxygen will rise and the Pco_2 will stay
normal. The oxygen saturation of the blood is only kept normal by
rapid and deeper breathing; in its extreme form this becomes
"dyspnoea". The respiratory centre of "pink puffers" remains sensitive
to a small rise in Pco_2 and their chemoreceptors remain sensitive to a
small fall in Po_2, whereas the respiratory centre of "blue bloaters"
becomes "set" for a higher level of Pco_2 and their chemoreceptors do
not respond to anoxia. The patients who have severe emphysema but
no airways obstruction, therefore, are not cyanosed (i.e. "pink") but
are usually dyspnoeic (i.e. "puffing"). The patients with widespread
airways obstruction are presumed to have a more or less normal ability
to allow gases to diffuse from alveoli to blood, but a diminished ability
to move air in and out of the alveoli through the airways. The high
CO_2 content of the blood causes narrowing of the pulmonary arteries
leading to pulmonary hypertension. Obstruction to the airways results
in collapse of small areas of the lung which are then not ventilated but
may be perfused with blood, which is, therefore, effectively shunted
from pulmonary artery to pulmonary veins. This right-to-left shunting
leads to oxygen desaturation of the arterial blood and cyanosis
("blue"). The pulmonary hypertension results in cor pulmonale, right
heart failure and peripheral oedema ("bloater").

The pulmonary hypertension is due to a combination of several
factors; there is a reduction in the number of capillaries with a
consequent reduction in the cross-sectional area of the blood vessels,
anoxia causes: (i) pulmonary arteriolar vasoconstriction, (ii) increased
pulmonary blood flow, and (iii) increased blood viscosity. Air trapping
within the alveoli increases the intra-alveolar pressure causing compression of capillaries.

"Blue bloaters" tend to be obese and the mechanical work of
moving the heavy chest wall outstrips the oxygen which can be
supplied by the inadequate lungs; there is probably some central
mechanism which reduces the ventilating capacity in obesity.

Normal people respond to a raised Pco_2 by hyperventilating;
however, chronic CO_2 retention does not cause hyperventilation—the
respiratory centre becomes "set" for a higher level of Pco_2. Thus "blue
bloaters" with chronic CO_2 retention lose their compensatory over-
ventilating mechanism. Should this failure of adaptation of the
respiratory centre to a chronically raised Pco_2 not occur, the patient
may be dyspnoeic the whole time in an attempt to blow off CO_2 and
keep the blood Pco_2 normal.

In practice, airways obstruction and emphysema so frequently coexist that differentiation into distinct clinical groups is only rarely possible. While patients with dominant airways obstruction frequently develop secondary polycythaemia, the dominant emphysema patients very rarely do so; there is no satisfactory explanation for this difference.

The only physical signs of uncomplicated chronic bronchitis are those of narrowing of the airways, leading to prolongation of expiration more than inspiration, since the bronchi usually dilate on inspiration and the effect of narrowing will therefore be more marked on expiration. Rhonchi may be heard due to localised areas of bronchial narrowing. When bronchial narrowing becomes widespread, "wheeze" is heard. Crepitations are not a feature of bronchitis; if they occur, they are due to associated left ventricular failure, bronchopneumonia or bronchiectasis. Bronchiectasis is commonly associated with chronic bronchitis. On the plain chest x-ray there are no diagnostic features of bronchitis; the thickened bronchial walls are rarely visible. In fibrocystic disease in children, bronchial thickening and bronchiectasis may be seen as parallel line shadows ("tram-lines"). In the broncho-gram the narrowed bronchi of chronic bronchitis are visible, and the dilated mucous glands fill with lipiodol and are easily seen; the bronchi also end sooner and more abruptly than in normals ("sawn-off tree" appearance).

Antibiotics in Chronic Bronchitis

The two organisms most frequently present in acute attacks of bronchitis are *Strept. pneumoniae* and *H. influenzae*. In the majority of cases *H. influenzae* is the real pathogen. Acute infections are always associated with infection and inflammation within the walls of the bronchi and bronchioles; however, the mucus acts as a reservoir of organisms between acute attacks. Unfortunately, antibiotics can only enter the mucus in *bactericidal* concentration when exudation is present, i.e. when the sputum is purulent. Pathogenic organisms are recoverable from the sputum even when it is mucoid *between* acute attacks. Factors other than infection are likely to be responsible for acute exacerbations of bronchitis. This is supported by the fact that serum precipitins to *H. influenzae* are found in only a quarter of patients with simple bronchitis. For these reasons it is sometimes recommended that antibiotics should only be used in acute exacer-bations if the sputum is purulent, i.e. contains pus. *H. influenzae* is always sensitive to ampicillin and tetracycline; it is, therefore, sug-gested that it is unnecessary to culture the sputum in acute exacer-bations of bronchitis unless:

There is a failure to respond to treatment
Pneumonia is suspected
Bronchiectasis is known to be present.

The quantity of antibiotic in purulent sputum cannot be increased above a certain concentration. In acute exacerbations with purulent sputum, ampicillin or tetracycline 1 g 6-hourly should be given for 5 days, or longer if the sputum remains purulent; in this dose bactericidal concentrations should be reached in the sputum. When the sputum ceases to be purulent, ideally the dose should be reduced to 250–500 mg 6-hourly, at which dose batericidal levels still occur in the tissues. The lowest effective dose of antibiotic should be given because of the danger of superinfection with staphylococci and fungi, and the danger of producing antibiotic-resistant organisms which are possibly a source of danger to the patient and the community. For recurrent attacks of acute bronchitis there are two logical courses: one is to give continuous antibiotics and the other is to give antibiotics immediately an acute exacerbation starts. The orthodox management is to give continuous antibiotics if the sputum remains purulent between attacks. If the sputum is mucoid between acute attacks, antibiotics should not be given continuously, but the patient should have his own supply so that he can start a course as soon as he notices symptoms of an acute exacerbation.

The evidence with regard to prophylactic antibiotics reducing the frequency and/or severity of acute attacks is conflicting. Prophylactic antibiotics probably reduce the duration of acute attacks but not their frequency. There is little evidence that lung damage can be prevented by suppression of bronchial infection.

Physical Signs

The physical signs of "hyperinflation" of the chest are:

Reduced expansion of lower ribs
Diminished breath sounds
Increased resonance on percussion
Reduced cardiac and liver dullness
Use of accessory muscles of respiration
The presence of rhonchi (wheezes)
Filling of the *external* jugular veins during expiration.

Less familiar signs of airways obstruction and hyperinflation are:

Length of the trachea palpable above the sternal notch in expiration. The length of trachea becomes less in hyperinflation because of elevation of the sternum relative to the hilum.

Tracheal descent with inspiration. When there is hyperinflation of the chest the trachea moves downwards during inspiration probably because the diaphragm is lower than in the normal.

Palpable hardening of the sternomastoid and scalene muscles during inspiration, indicating excessive use of the accessory muscles of respiration.

Indrawing of the suprasternal and supraclavicular fossae during inspiration, indicating an excessive fall in intrathoracic pressure during inspiration (in order to try to suck more air through the narrowed airways).

Forced expiration time. During forced expiration with the mouth open *following* maximum inspiration, the time should normally be less than 4 seconds.

The x-ray features of hyperinflation are:

Hypertranslucency of the lung fields

Low and flat diaphragms which, on screening, show diminished excursion

Increase in A-P diameter of the chest

Increase in normal retrosternal translucent area

Splaying out of the pulmonary vessels, whose angles of bifurcation are thereby increased

Rarely, bronchial "tram-lines" may be seen because of the increased "contrast" due to the hyperinflated chest.

Respiratory Failure

The function of the respiratory system is to supply oxygen to the blood and to eliminate carbon dioxide. Failure of the respiratory system will therefore mean a rise in Pco_2 (above 50 mm) and a fall in Po_2 (below 60 mm).

Hypercapnoea.—Elevation of the Pco_2 gives rise to a number of clinical features. The most important are:

Peripheral vasodilatation

Rapid, bounding pulse

Small pupils

Engorged fundal veins

Confusion or drowsiness

Depressed tendon reflexes

Extensor plantar responses

Headache

Papilloedema

Coma.

Elevation of the Pco_2, if compensated, results in a rise in serum bicarbonate. The kidneys compensate by reabsorbing bicarbonate (with sodium) from the tubules—this results in sodium (and water) retention, and peripheral oedema. Peripheral oedema in the absence of heart failure, peripheral vasodilatation and a high cardiac output has given rise to the suggestion that heart failure occurs much less commonly than it is diagnosed in the presence of hypercapnoea. It is important to be aware of this possibility because digoxin dosage may be unnecessarily increased to try and control "heart failure" which is not present. Patients with respiratory acidosis often develop hypo-kalaemia and may not respond to diuretics until potassium supplements have been given.

EMPHYSEMA

Emphysema has already been defined as an increase in the size of the air spaces distal to the respiratory bronchiole, due to dilatation or destruction of the alveolar walls. The lung consists of discrete lobules, or acini, each supplied by several respiratory bronchioles; leaving the respiratory bronchiole are alveolar ducts which lead into individual alveoli. In all types of emphysema (compensatory, focal, bullous, senile or atrophic) there is either dilatation or destruction of the alveolar walls or destruction of the walls of the respiratory bronchioles. Destruction of the walls of the respiratory bronchioles, whether due to bronchitis or deposition of dusts, will lead to several respiratory bronchioles fusing together and forming a large air space in the middle of the lobule, the periphery of the lobule still being composed of normal alveoli. This centrilobular emphysema is the type of focal emphysema seen particularly in dust disease, and sometimes in the early stages of bullous emphysema. If all the alveoli in the lobule (or acinus) are involved in the emphysema, it is said to be panacinar. Panacinar emphysema occurs with dilatation of the air spaces as in compensatory emphysema, when part of the lung enlarges to replace damaged lung, or it occurs if there is destruction of alveolar walls as in bullous emphysema. The mechanisms of alveolar-wall destruction in panacinar (bullous) emphysema are extension from bronchioles, rupture through constant coughing, damage by irritants (cigarette smoke and air pollution) and possibly "avascular necrosis" due to interference with blood supply.

The radiological features of emphysema are those of hyperinflation of the chest, with the addition of dilated proximal pulmonary arteries and attenuated peripheral arteries if there is accompanying pulmonary hypertension.

It should not be forgotten that α_1 antitrypsin deficiency in both heterozygotes and homozygotes may cause primary emphysema, particularly involving the lower zones. The homozygotes almost always have cirrhosis as well, but the heterozygotes may have α_1 antitrypsin levels about 50 per cent of normal. They tend to develop primary emphysema but there is evidence that its onset can be delayed if the patient abstains from smoking.

Cadmium inhalation also causes emphysema and cigarette smoke contains appreciable and measurable amounts of cadmium.

ASTHMA

Asthma is defined as "a disease characterised by variable dyspnoea due to widespread narrowing of intrapulmonary airways which varies over short periods of time either spontaneously or as a result of treatment" (Scadding, 1963).

Note that this definition does not mention allergy, hypersensitivity, or bronchospasm; it emphasises that asthma is dyspnoea due to narrowing of the airways and is to be distinguished sharply from those conditions which cause variable dyspnoea (usually by inhaled allergens) which is due to sudden impairment of diffusion of gases across the alveolar walls (transfer defects). This group of conditions is described on page 158. Their superficial similarity to asthma can lead to unnecessary over-investigation.

The main causes of asthma are:

Allergy to known or unknown allergens. The allergens are usually inhaled, but may be ingested or injected as in the case of an anaphylactic reaction. Asthma of this type is "extrinsic asthma".

Intrinsic asthma, in which there may be some evidence of an allergic origin (e.g. eosinophilia and occasional hypersensitivity to salicylates). However, the natural history of intrinsic asthma differs from extrinsic asthma, in which the evidence for external allergy is more definite although the exact allergen may not have been identified.

Asthma secondary to bronchitis or oedema of the bronchial walls, as in cardiac or renal failure.

In chronic bronchitis there is no dispute that the major airways are narrowed due to thickening of the mucous membrane, while the remainder of the bronchial wall is of a normal thickness; this thickening results from squamous metaplasia and increase in the number of goblet cells. This is such a constant finding in chronic bronchitis that it is one of the ways of assessing chronic bronchitis postmortem; the changes are irreversible. Superimposed on this irreversible airway narrowing there is usually a reversible component.

The reversible component is due to:

Inflammatory or allergic oedema
Plugging of bronchi by exudate and eosinophils
Spasm of bronchial wall smooth muscle.

In simple asthma only the reversible component of airways narrowing is present. There is controversy about the importance of muscle spasm in asthma and the reversible component of airways narrowing in bronchitis.

The main arguments in favour of bronchial mucosal oedema as the most important factor in reversible airways narrowing are:

In some cases the airways narrowing is only slowly reversible when corticosteroids are used

Mucosal oedema and airways narrowing are present postmortem. If the narrowing is mainly due to muscle spasm this should relax after death

Airways narrowing is a feature of pulmonary oedema

The agents which induce asthma, e.g. histamine, are known to produce a sudden allergic oedema in other sites, e.g. the skin and larynx (as in angioneurotic oedema)

The same drugs which can rapidly reverse angioneurotic oedema (e.g. adrenaline, aminophylline and hydrocortisone) can also rapidly relieve asthma.

The main arguments in favour of spasm of the bronchiolar muscles as the most important factor in reversible airways narrowing are:

Hypertrophy of the bronchiolar smooth muscle may be seen at autopsy

The speed of the changes which can occur in asthma are more suggestive of active muscle spasm than oedema analogous to angioneurotic oedema, which is a relatively rare manifestation of an allergic state

Isolated fragments of bronchiolar muscle have been seen to contract actively when they come into contact with allergens to which the patient is sensitive

The pressure generated by bronchial muscle contraction can be measured by balloons in a segmental bronchus.

Extrinsic Asthma

This usually starts in infancy and occurs in atopic subjects. Atopy refers to a type of hypersensitivity unique to man. There is a predisposition to asthma, hay fever, eczema, migraine, rhinitis, urticaria and food allergies. These people become sensitive to many ubiquitous foreign proteins which are not usually antigenic.

The atopic patient has reaginic antibodies (IgE) against the offending allergen. As well as challenge tests to skin, nasal epithelium (in perennial rhinitis) or bronchi, it is possible to demonstrate the presence of allergen-specific IgE antibodies in the serum by means of "radioallergosorbent" tests (RAST). These tests show that four common allergens account for the allergic symptoms in the majority of atopic subjects in the United Kingdom. The four allergens are grass, pollen, house-mite dust and cat epithelium. However, RAST reagents are available for a large number of possible allergens. In a problem case it may be possible to perform RAST testing on nasal or bronchial secretions. Food allergens are a difficult problem because all types of hypersensitivity may be involved, resulting in symptoms 2–36 hours after the offending food is eaten. Diagnosis of food allergy by RAST testing is most likely to be helpful if the symptoms are due to Type 1 (immediate) hypersensitivity.

IgE antibody production sensitises local mast cells and there is a rapid release of histamine, eosinophil mobilising factor and other mediators. This type of sensitivity is called atopy and can be detected by finding a positive skin-prick test, using commonly occurring antigens such as pollens, house dust and aspergillus. The history in asthma is crucial in identifying the likely cause. Subjects who are atopic, i.e. are hypersensitive to common antigens, often have other manifestations such as hay fever, rhinitis and urticaria. The season of maximal symptoms may be relevant to predicting the likely allergen:

February, March, April:	tree pollens
Late June and early July:	grass pollens
Early autumn:	moulds
September to October:	house dust
November to February:	*Aspergillus fumigatus*
Throughout the year:	aspirin and other drugs, tetrazine (the yellow dyes used in orange squashes and the coatings of pills), and foods.

A small group of asthmatics do not have an immediate type reaction and have so-called intermission asthma. This is caused by IgG antibodies and results in a Type III reaction, often causing symptoms 3 to 4 hours after exposure. Intermission asthma may be associated with an allergic alveolitis or eosinophilia. Intermission asthma without either alveolitis or eosinophilia occurs in proteolytic-enzyme-induced asthma (from biological washing powders) or cotton dust (byssinosis).

Aspergillus fumigatus is a ubiquitous fungus and is responsible for a variety of respiratory disorders:

Asthma
Early and intermission asthma (Types I and III allergy) with pulmonary eosinophilia and growth of the fungus in the lungs, leading to bronchopulmonary aspergillosis
Extrinsic allergic alveolitis
Aspergilloma (fungal ball)
Invasive aspergillosis in immunosuppressed patients.

Other Mechanisms of Asthma

Vagal pathways in the mediation of asthma are also sometimes involved. Reflex bronchoconstriction occurs in asthmatics, due to non-immunogenic irritants such as dust and fumes, presumably from stimulation of irritant receptors in larger airways. Aspirin-induced asthma is probably not related to the usual mechanisms of mast-cell damage by IgE reaginic antibodies; it probably causes asthma by stimulating prostaglandin (PgE_2) inhibitor. Exercise-induced asthma is also probably not immunogenic; the asthma comes on usually *after* active exercise, and once it has subsided it cannot usually be reproduced by similar exercise taken some hours later, although by the next day the asthma will again occur with exercise.

Management of Asthma

The severe acute attack is treated with bronchodilators by injection. Status asthmaticus is present if bronchodilators are ineffective in relieving the attack after 24 hours or if the attack is so severe that the patient is unable to speak in sentences. A suitable regime for managing most adult cases of status asthmaticus is:

Parenteral beta 2 agonist

Parenteral hydrocortisone, 100 mg intravenously every 4 hours if the patient has not been on corticosteroids orally or by inhalation. If the patient *has* been on steroids previously, considerably higher doses may be necessary because of previous induction of steroid metabolising enzymes

Beta 2 agonist by nebuliser or positive-pressure respirator using a close-fitting mask

Arterial blood for Pco_2, Po_2, and pH

Chest x-ray (to exclude pneumothorax), and ECG

Oxygen 28–35 per cent by Ventimask

Fluid replacement. Dehydration encourages bronchial-plug formation, and the patient may have been too short of breath to drink adequately. If dehydration is present dextrose 5 per cent, 500 ml every 6 hours should be given

Antibiotics: ampicillin or tetracycline, 500 mg 6-hourly

Consider artificial ventilation and bronchopulmonary lavage if Po_2 is low and/or Pco_2 is elevated.

Beta 2 Agonists

These are selective beta 2 adrenergic stimulators and are preferable in the management of asthma to the older non-selective agonists such as isoprenaline, ephedrine and orciprenaline (Alupent).

Salbutamol (Ventolin) and terbutaline (Bricanyl) are suitable beta 2 agonists and are available in a variety of forms:

	Salbutamol (Ventolin)	Terbutaline (Bricanyl)
Tablets	2, 4 mg	5 mg
Aerosol	100 μg/dose	250 μg/dose
Aerosol powder (Rotacaps)	200 or 400 μg	—
Injection	50 μg/ml 500 μg/ml	500 μg/ml
Infusion	1 mg/ml	500 μg/ml
Solution for ventilator	0·5% solution	10 mg/ml

Atropinic Agents

Some proportion of bronchomotor tone is due to the vagus, and inhibition of this action by the atropine-like drug, ipratropium (Atrovent), as an aerosol, may lead to FEV_1 improvement additional to that achieved by salbutamol. There is a suggestion that this agent preferentially affects the small airways, and that it has a greater effect in chronic bronchitis with asthma than in asthma alone.

Artificial Ventilation

The work of breathing in a severe attack of asthma is considerable, and the oxygen utilisation by the respiratory muscles may account for a large proportion of oxygen transferred from alveoli to pulmonary capillaries. Excessive exhaustion and hypercapnoea are indications for artificial ventilation. Unfortunately, progressive hyperinflation can occur during artificial ventilation, and may result in compression of the heart, causing reduced cardiac output and hypotension. Progressive hyperinflation can be checked by measuring the chest circumference and ensuring that it does not increase by more than one inch after artificial ventilation is started. When a constant-volume ventilator is used, progressive elevation of the inflation pressure after a prolonged expiratory phase means that exhalation is incomplete. It is important that peak inspiratory inflation pressure is adjusted to allow for some prolongation of the expiratory phase, but that inflation does not occur too quickly, otherwise excessive pressures are generated and may result in rupture of alveoli not protected by very narrow airways. Airways resistance is high in asthma and pulmonary compliance is low; this is because tidal ventilation is occurring near total lung capacity.

Recently it has been appreciated that the small airways, after about 15 divisions, do not constitute a high resistance to air flow. One of the earliest manifestations of damage to the small airways is collapse, and loss of lung volume and vital capacity, and it may also lead to V/Q abnormalities in the absence of any measurable change in airways resistance.

The changes in blood gases and FEV_1/FVC following bronchodilators may be complex because bronchodilators may improve VC if they act predominantly on the smaller airways rather than the larger airways. In this case there will be an apparent deterioration in FEV_1/FVC ratio despite clinical improvement. A similar explanation probably accounts for occasional paradoxes between PEFR and FEV, as indicators of improvement after treatment of asthma.

At low lung volume, e.g. when the functional residual capacity (FRC) is reduced, the small airways close completely. This happens in normals at the lung bases at the end of full expiration. The volume of lung at which the small airways close is known as the "closing volume". The volume of lung at which the small airways close tends to rise with age and smoking; the small airways may close even during normal tidal breathing. The same effect occurs in heart failure, obesity and anaesthesia. The FRC is reduced in the supine position, and even if there is no change in closing volume the same airways still close during tidal breathing. This effect can be overcome by increasing the FRC by increasing the positive end-expiratory pressure (PEEP). This prevents collapse of small airways during expiration, i.e. it *reduces* the closing volume below the tidal range (Branthwaite, 1978).

Other Facets of Severe Asthma

Hypoxia occurs because of disturbed ventilation/perfusion relationships in the lungs; the Po_2 may not return to normal despite an improvement in FEV_1. Furthermore the Po_2 may remain at dangerously low levels despite marked symptomatic improvement. Before discharging a patient with severe asthma from hospital, therefore, it is wise to check that the Po_2 has returned to normal. Practical experience suggests that patients admitted with status asthmaticus who are discharged early from hospital are often readmitted with another attack within a few days of returning home. In the early stages of status asthmaticus there is an inverse relationship between the arterial oxygen pressure and the pulse rate. If other causes of tachycardia can be excluded a pulse rate above 130/min is suggestive of an arterial oxygen pressure below 50 mm. Hypoxaemia, when severe, may lead to a metabolic acidosis superimposed on a respiratory acidosis if the Pco_2 is raised; treatment with bicarbonate is sometimes indicated. The level of the Pco_2 is not always a reliable guide because severe asthma may result in hyperventilation and a low Pco_2; an elevated Pco_2 always indicates a severe attack.

The FEV_1 and PFR are not always reliable guides—sometimes the patient improves symptomatically and the Po_2 rises despite the fact that the FEV_1 remains unchanged. The vital capacity may be a more useful monitor of progress. The reason for this is that airways narrowing results in trapping air within the lungs, increasing the functional residual capacity (FRC), causing stretching of the lungs. The work needed to move the tidal volume in and out of these stretched lungs is much more than the work needed to move the same tidal volume out of lungs which are not stretched. The FEV_1 measures airways narrowing; the airways may remain the same size but the work needed to move the tidal volume in and out is less if the lungs are not stretched. Clinical improvement in asthma may occur because the FRC is reduced and not because the FEV_1 has improved.

Other physiological disturbances may occur:

Transient right ventricular hypertrophy on ECG
Transient hypokalaemia possibly caused by steroids and overventilation
Transient elevation of blood urea.

Corticosteroids used to treat the acute attack can be stopped as soon as the attack is over. Some airways obstruction occasionally persists between acute attacks, particularly in intrinsic asthma. It may then be reasonable to give long-term corticosteroids. These should be given if they can be shown to improve significantly the FEV_1. When being considered for long-term steroid treatment the patient should be admitted to hospital and daily FEV_1 measurements recorded for 4–5 days *before* starting on steroids, and then for 5–7 days afterwards. It sometimes takes seven days for steroids to produce an improvement, however; if, after this, the mean FEV_1 readings are the same as before steroids they should not be given continuously in extrinsic asthma. The situation is not quite so clear-cut in intrinsic asthma; the poor prognosis of this condition may justify continuous steroids on the grounds that they *may* reduce the frequency of acute attacks even if they do not improve airways obstruction between attacks.

Long-term Management of Asthma

Regular use of peak flow meter by patient to detect presymptomatic relapse
Disodium cromoglycate
Antibiotics as soon as there is any evidence of a chest infection
Regular breathing exercises (*J. roy. Soc. Med.*, 1978)
RAST testing and possible desensitisation
Corticosteroids, either by inhalation or by inhalation and by mouth.

Occupational Asthma

A number of biological, chemical, industrial and household substances can cause asthma which may be difficult to identify if it is of the intermission type. Examples are:

Biological enzyme detergents
Flour
Wood resins
Solder flux (asthma in electronic workers)
Isocyanates (printer's asthma).

Intrinsic Asthma

Most chronic asthmatics are in this group. The disease is much commoner in women over the age of 40; there is no previous history of allergy or evidence of atopy. There is often higher blood eosinophilia than in extrinsic asthma. The prognosis is poor, and early continuous corticosteroids may be justified. It is particularly in this group of asthmatics that the disease may lead to chronic bronchitis, exacerbations of which in turn aggravate the asthma.

In this group it is always worth trying an atropinic aerosol such as ipratropium (Atrovent) since one pathogenic mechanism may be disturbance of bronchomotor tone due to vagal action.

Bronchitis and Associated Asthma

Chronic bronchitis causes permanent airways narrowing; in some patients this is accompanied by additional narrowing of the airways which may vary over short periods of time, either spontaneously or as a result of treatment; therefore, by definition, these patients have asthma as well. In some patients with chronic bronchitis acute exacerbations are dominated by this asthmatic component, in others further infection and inflammatory oedema are dominant in the acute exacerbation. Chronic bronchitics in whom the asthmatic component is predominant may have eosinophils in blood and sputum in the same way as other asthmatics; similarly, the acute exacerbation may respond to treatment of the asthmatic component more than to treatment of the infection. In these patients the question always arises whether the asthmatic component is due to the infecting organisms acting as allergens. This is a difficult thing to prove; attempts to do so have not been entirely successful; however, such a reasonable hypothesis should not be lightly discarded.

Extrinsic Allergic Alveolitis

This is a disease of non-atopic subjects, due to inhalation of organic dust of about 2 μm in size, which can enter alveoli. Re-exposure usually causes symptoms of malaise and dyspnoea, particularly in farmers' lung and pigeon-fanciers' lung, in which a large antigen dose is received intermittently. Where exposure is less intermittent to a smaller dose of antigen (e.g. when a single budgerigar is the antigen source) the symptoms may be much more insidious and difficult to elicit.

The disorder is caused by Type III (immune complex) disorder. The immune complexes activate complement and produce tissue damage; however, some features of the disorder also involves Type IV hypersensitivity (i.e. cell-mediated immunity), causing granuloma formation and possible transfer of reactivity by sensitised lymphocytes. Occasionally complement activation can occur with organic dusts without the intermediary of immune complex formation.

Extrinsic allergic asthma is associated with narrowing of the airways which is a response of Type I (immediate) hypersensitivity reactions. Another type of hypersensitivity reaction is the Type III (Arthus) reaction. Following repeated exposure to antigen, circulating antibodies develop. On re-exposure to the antigen an antibody-antigen reaction takes place which differs from the immediate one of Type I allergy: it takes 3–6 hours to develop and is associated with vascular damage and local oedema. This reaction occurs at the site of exposure to the antigen, which in the respiratory system is the alveoli. Unlike Type I reactions the severity of this reaction is related to the dose of antigens. Extrinsic allergic alveolitis describes the conditions caused by these Type III hypersensitivity reactions. All the conditions have a number of features in common as a result of their common type of hypersensitivity:

Symptoms begin suddenly 3–6 hours *after* exposure

Repeated exposure at short intervals will result in a chronic disease

The acute symptoms are caused by alveolar-wall oedema, which causes sudden dyspnoea and cough. There is also a systemic reaction which generally consists of pyrexia, shivering, malaise and myalgia. There is *no* evidence of airways obstruction

The chronic disease is caused by organising fibrosis of the alveolar oedema and results in restrictive lung-function tests (impaired ventilation tests) as well as diffusion abnormalities

Circulating precipitating (IgG) antibodies are present in the serum, although they may be transient.

The known diseases causing extrinsic allergic alveolitis are:

Farmers' lung	Maple bark disease
Bird breeders' lung	Wheat weevil (flour) disease
Bagassosis	Suberosis
Weavers' cough	Malt weevil lung
Pituitary snuff-takers' lung	Thatchers' lung
Smallpox handlers' lung	Cheese washers' lung
Mushroom pickers' lung	Paprika splitters' lung.

A number of additional causes of extrinsic alveolitis have been identified and include:

Humidifier lung, due to immune reactions to amoebae contaminating the water
Ventilation pneumonitis, due to *Micropolyspora faeni* growth in large ventilation systems.

Long-standing cases of extrinsic allergic alveolitis often develop fibrosis of the interstitial tissues of the lung. Similar fibrosis may develop in the absence of any of the known predisposing causes; this idiopathic type of pulmonary fibrosis used to be called diffuse interstitial pulmonary fibrosis, but is now called cryptogenic (idiopathic) fibrosing alveolitis.

Fibrosing alveolitis is a disease characterised by an inflammatory processs in the lungs beyond the terminal bronchioles having as its essential features a cellular thickening of the alveolar walls, and large mononuclear cells, presumably of alveolar origin within the alveolar spacies, as well as interstitial granuloma formation.

Clinically, fibrosing alveolitis is characterised by dyspnoea, dry cough, crepitations, particularly over the lower zones, and finger clubbing. In extrinsic allergic alveolitis clubbing is less common and the disease tends to affect the upper lobes. Corticosteroids are more useful when there are a large number of mononuclear cells present. They are unlikely to be of value if there is thickening of the alveolar walls. There is no constant relationship between the biopsy appearances and length of survival. Spontaneous remissions occur.

PNEUMONIAS

Pneumonia usually implies infection of alveoli, although there are exceptions to this, such as lipoid and aspiration pneumonias.

Classical lobar pneumonia is due to *Streptococcus pneumoniae*. Complications are minimal with prompt antibiotic treatment by penicillin. Among the complications which may occur are sterile pleural effusion, empyema (infection in the pleural space), lung abscess, pericardial involvement and septicaemia leading to meningitis and endocarditis.

Staphylococcal pneumonia frequently complicates other pneumonias such as influenza and aspiration pneumonias, as well as complicating staphylococcal septicaemia. In children staphylococcal pneumonia may occur as a primary infection and is common in cystic fibrosis. Characteristically it causes multiple, cavitated, ill-defined, round opacities on the chest x-ray. Hospital-acquired infection will be due to a coagulase-positive (virulent), penicillinase-producing organism.

Frequent blood cultures should be taken, as staphylococcal septicaemia is a frequent complication. Pyopneumothorax is also a common complication in children.

Recurrent Pneumonia

In a patient who has had several attacks of pneumonia, always consider if one of the following are present:

Lowered resistance to infection (leucopenia or hypogammaglobulinaemia)
Diabetes mellitus
Aspiration
Bronchial obstruction (adenoma, carcinoma, foreign body, external compression of the bronchus)
Bronchiectasis of the bronchus of the infected lobe. (Note: bronchiectasis may be secondary to fibrosis caused by old tuberculosis; in these cases the recurrent pneumonia is often in the upper lobes.)
Recurrent pulmonary infarcts.

Aspiration Pneumonia

A second attack of pneumonia within six months, or a second attack in the same lobe as a previous attack at any time, should alert to the probability that aspiration is occurring. There may be a clear history of dysphagia or possible inhalation of a foreign body (e.g. following the party trick of throwing up nuts and catching them in the open mouth, or a bout of coughing following a dental extraction). However aspiration pneumonia may occur when sinusitis is present and pus may be aspirated at night while the patient is asleep. Liquid paraffin taken for constipation is sometimes aspirated during sleep, and nose drops with an oil base may be accidentally aspirated. Microscopic globules of oil may be coughed up in the sputum if aspiration of any oil has occurred. In cases of recurrent pneumonia it is always worth having the sputum examined for oil droplets. Pneumonia may recur in lobes with normal bronchi if pus is aspirated from bronchi which are bronchiectatic.

Friedländer's[7] Pneumonia

This is usually a severe pneumonia, in which the patient coughs up odourless, thick, gelatinous, reddish-green sputum (due to blood staining of the green pus characteristic of Friedländer's bacillus). The upper lobes are more frequently affected than the lower and abscess formation is very common. The pneumonia may be followed by fibrosis or bronchiectasis.

Viral Pneumonia

Mycoplasma pneumonia is associated with a sudden onset of cough and fever accompanied by headache and myalgia. Dyspnoea may be marked, in the absence of physical signs in the lungs. The chest x-ray may show extensive bilateral patchy or nodular shadows, sometimes of lobar distribution. About 60 per cent of patients develop a rising titre of cold agglutinins (antibodies which will agglutinate group O red cells at 4°C). They appear in the blood one to four weeks after infection, and may remain for several months. Confirmatory evidence of primary atypical pneumonia is the demonstration in the serum of complement-fixing antibody to *M. pneumoniae* and isolation of *M. pneumoniae* from the sputum or throat swab. The organism is slow growing and the sputum cultures may take several weeks to become positive. The organism is sensitive to tetracycline. The complications of primary atypical pneumonia are central nervous system involvement (headaches, photophobia and meningism), haemolysis, and peripheral venous thrombosis due to a high titre of circulating cold agglutinins. Rarely, arthralgia, pleural effusions and skin lesions resembling erythema multiforme occur. A useful diagnostic feature is the high ESR and normal white-cell count. A normal white-cell count makes bacterial pneumonia unlikely.

In epidemics of influenza, the B virus may cause a fulminating rapidly fatal viral pneumonia; between epidemics the pneumonia is much milder. Psittacosis (ornithosis) is an acute respiratory illness due to a virus acquired from the excreta of birds which are usually ill. The birds are not necessarily psittacine birds such as parrots and budgerigars; chickens and pigeons may also be responsible. Systemic features such as splenomegaly and meningo-encephalitis occur. The disease is modified by tetracycline and chloramphenicol. Other virus illnesses such as chickenpox, measles and cytomegalic inclusion disease may cause a specific pneumonia.

Legionnaires' Disease

Legionnaires' disease was first described in 1976, and is due to infection with a bacillus, *Legionella pneumophila*. The organism inhabits large ventilation systems, although it may also be water borne; this disease usually occurs in epidemics although there are occasionally sporadic cases. The commonest features are:

fever, dry cough, chest pain
confusion
haematuria and gastro-intestinal bleeding
hyponatraemia
abnormal liver function tests
lobar consolidation of the lungs which is slow to resolve.

The diagnosis is confirmed by blood or sputum culture and serological tests. Treatment is with penicillin and erythromycin, with the addition of rifampicin if there is no improvement.

MEDICAL COMPLICATIONS IN SURGICAL PATIENTS

The major medical conditions associated with surgery are:

Pulmonary complications
Myocardial infarction
Thrombo-embolism.

Pulmonary Complications

The major pulmonary complications relate to alveolar collapse and pulmonary oedema, although infection and aspiration are also frequent. Alveolar collapse occurs because of:

Shallow breathing
Airways obstruction
Absorption atelectasis if the inspired oxygen concentration is too high
Pulmonary oedema.

Shallow breathing, because of pain or chest "splinting" as a result of recumbency, results in a fall in functional residual capacity (FRC). This means two things: one is that tidal breathing occurs in conditions of reduced compliance, and therefore involves more work, and the other is that tidal breathing occurs at lung volumes at which the closing volume of the small airways coincides with the range of tidal breathing; this results in more small airways closing and a worsening of already disturbed V/Q ratios.

Pulmonary oedema occurs in post-operative patients for a variety of reasons headed by left ventricular failure and overtransfusion. Nonetheless, other factors are also involved, such as capillary leak due to damage by circulating endotoxins and inflammatory products. Neurogenic pulmonary oedema may occur if there is damage to the central nervous system by hypoxia. Excessive inspired oxygen can also result in pulmonary oedema.

Cardiac Complications

It is now recognised that the risk of developing a myocardial infarction in the post-operative period is much greater if a patient has had a previous infarct. Further, the mortality from myocardial infarction in the post-operative period is around 50 per cent. The risk of developing an infarct are about 5 per cent if the infarction was more than 6 months previously, 15 per cent if between 3 and 6 months previously and 40 per cent if less than 3 months previously.

Pulmonary Embolism and Deep Venous Thrombosis

The incidence of post-operative venous thrombosis is known from a large number of series to be at least 20 per cent. The incidence of deep venous thrombosis shown by ascending venography or labelled fibrinogen scan is considerably higher than that detected by clinical signs.

PREDICTION AND PREVENTION

Pulmonary Complications

Apart from the clinical history and examination, the most reliable predictors of pulmonary complications are:

> Blood gases (cyanosis does not occur until Po_2 falls to 70 mm Hg); a raised Pco_2 alerts to unsuspected obstructive airways disease
> Vital capacity
> Maximum breathing capacity
> Peak flow rate (which can be correlated with ability to cough).

The chest x-ray appears to contribute surprisingly little of predictive value, although a pre-operative chest x-ray is useful from the point of view of comparative changes post-operatively. Other than attention to anaesthetic details, cessation of smoking and pretreatment of bronchitis with antibiotics, pre- and post-operative physiotherapy have been shown to reduce mortality and to produce objective improvement in FVC, FEV_1, and PEFR. In the United States considerable use is made of "incentive spirometers" to encourage patients to improve their respiratory function.

Cardiac Complications

Many attempts have been made to devise an index of risk factors. One acceptable index is that of Goldman *et al.* 1977:

> Myocardial infarct in previous 6 months
> Gallop rhythm or distended jugular veins
> Dysrhythmia
> More than 5 premature ventricular contractions per minute
> Emergency operation
> Po_2 less than 60 mm Hg.

The presence of a previous myocardial infarction, the physical features found on examination (raised venous pressure or gallop rhythm), and any rhythm disturbance on the ECG account for about half the significant predictor risk factors.

Deep-vein Thrombosis (Rose, 1979)

There are many trials of various prophylactic measures to reduce the incidence of post-operative thromboembolic complications.

Oral anticoagulation.—There is little dispute that oral anticoagulation with warfarin is effective, particularly in high-risk patients. The risk of haemorrhage is greater, but probably not as much as is supposed. Despite the incontrovertible evidence of the prophylactic value of oral anticoagulation in the management of fractures of the femoral neck, only about 3 per cent of surgeons routinely anticoagulate such patients.

Early ambulation and leg elevation.—Probably of no real benefit.

Intermittent external pneumatic leg compression.—Nearly all the studies show reduction of venous thrombosis comparable with low-dose heparin. The compression has to be continued for several weeks post-operatively.

Aspirin.—There is some evidence that aspirin reduces the incidence of pulmonary embolism without affecting the frequency of deep-vein thrombosis.

Dextran.—Dextran is a polymer of glucose which acts as a plasma expander and also affects platelet stickiness and other coagulation factors. It undoubtedly reduces thromboembolic complications, but it has to be continued for the duration of the risk, and complications resulting from bleeding, renal failure and fluid overload probably preclude its use.

Low-dose subcutaneous heparin.—The evidence is now good that subcutaneous heparin is valuable and associated with few complications. However, the largest multicentre trial did not show a reduction in overall mortality, although there was a reduction in thromboembolic complications.

Identifying Patients at Risk of Developing Deep-vein Thrombosis Post-operatively

Because of the logistic problems involved in giving subcutaneous heparin to surgical patients, attempts have been made to identify patients at special risk. High-risk patients can be identified by five factors (Crandon *et al*, 1980):

1. Increased euglobulin lysis time (a measure of the ability to dissolve any small clots that may form)
2. Level of fibrin-related antigen (i.e. an indication of the amount of fibrin present)
3. Age

4. Percentage overweight
5. Presence or absence of varicose veins.

Shock Lung (Adult respiratory distress syndrome)

The condition is characterised by pulmonary oedema in the absence of left atrial hypertension. It is important to remember the other causes of pulmonary oedema without cardiac enlargement on the chest x-ray, these include:

Inhalation
Virus pneumonia
Mitral stenosis
Constrictive pericarditis
Pulmonary embolism
Fat embolism
Inhalation pneumonia.

The cardinal features of shock lung are tachypnoea, hypoxia, and pulmonary oedema on chest x-ray following surgery, major trauma or septicaemia. The condition affects predominantly alveoli, causing endothelial proliferation and fibrinous exudation. It has a mortality of 50 per cent; at post-mortem there is high incidence of thrombotic lesions.

Probable pathogenic mechanisms are:

Spasm of pulmonary veins
Increased capillary permeability due to cerebral hypoxia; this is supported by the fact that denervation of lung prevents shock lung syndrome in animals. Humoral factors such as serotonin derived from platelets or damaged tissue, and endotoxin from Gram-negative organisms are also implicated in increasing capillary permeability. In this situation there are obvious dangers in using dextrans.

The physiological effects of shock lung are V/Q mismatch resulting in shunting of blood, and gas diffusion defects. The magnitude of the shunt may increase with high inspired oxygen. Measurement of shunts may be important prognostically, and also the inspired oxygen tensions can be chosen rationally, so that inspired oxygen concentration do not exceed those necessary to maximally oxygenate the blood, given the level of pulmonary shunting (see p. 137).

Prevention of Shock Lung

Avoidance of overtransfusion
Filtration of blood through millipore filters
Early positive-pressure ventilation

Raised end-expiratory pressure to ensure tidal volume is on
   compliant part of curve
Judicious oxygen.

It is probably better not to use steroids. There may be long-term
lung damage in survivors.

PULMONARY EMBOLISM AND INFARCTION

Experimental and clinical work has suggested that the mechanical
obstruction effects of a clot lodging in the pulmonary circulation are
the most important factors leading to death from pulmonary embolism.
Small pulmonary emboli can be lysed and disappear. In a patient with
no previous heart or respiratory disease, over half the pulmonary
circulation must be occluded before death occurs, although patients
with emphysema, mitral stenosis or previous left ventricular failure
are unable to tolerate emboli of this size. The purely mechanical
effects of a pulmonary embolus have been underemphasised; however,
it is also probable that other factors are involved. Following pulmonary
embolism there is tachypnoea; this does not occur when the pulmonary
artery is experimentally occluded, suggesting a *reflex* nervous mechanism; hypoxia frequently occurs, but theoretically this should not
happen if the circulation to one lung alone is obstructed, suggesting
that *reflex* bronchial constriction also occurs.
   Clinically tachypnoea and slight cyanosis may be the earliest or only
signs of pulmonary embolism. Emboli which occlude so much of the
pulmonary arteries that the circulation through the lungs virtually
ceases cause hypotension, hypoxia, shock and cardiac arrest. Pulmonary embolism occasionally causes chest pain which is indistinguishable
from the pain of myocardial ischaemia. In fact the chest pain of a
large embolus is probably due to a sudden reduction of blood flow to
the coronary arteries.
   Pulmonary emboli which do not cause sudden death or are not soon
dispersed usually produce signs of right ventricular strain. A rare
physical sign is a transient murmur over the affected pulmonary artery
due to blood passing the obstruction. In the plain chest x-ray there
are only three signs of pulmonary embolism:

1. Enlarged pulmonary arteries
2. Abrupt ending of a pulmonary artery
3. Hypertranslucency of part of the lung fields due to absent blood
   flow.

Pulmonary Infarction

If the thrombo-emboli are small enough to block the small pulmonary arteries, infarction of part of the lung may occur. Infarction caused by small pulmonary artery occlusion occurs much more readily if pulmonary vein function is also disturbed. Infarction of the part of the lung generally occurs in a cone, with the base of the cone on one of pleural surfaces—it may, therefore, be on one of the *interlobar fissures*. In effect this means that the shape of the resulting shadow on x-ray can be anything from triangular or round to linear. Sometimes the only x-ray sign is the resulting pleural effusion, which is usually bloodstained but can be serous; elevation of the diaphragm is occasionally the only x-ray sign. The intrapulmonary shadowing following a pulmonary infarct may not appear for up to 24 hours after pleuritic chest pain; haemoptysis or pyrexia suggest that infarction has occurred. The electrocardiogram in both pulmonary infarction and pulmonary embolism may be normal or may show a dysrhythmia, right ventricular hypertrophy pattern, or features of posterior myocardial infarction due either to unidentified pulmonary-coronary reflexes or reduced blood flow.

A normal lung scan and chest x-ray virtually excludes significant pulmonary embolism. However, the reverse is not necessarily true, and filling defects in the lung scan may be due to pathologies other than pulmonary embolism; for example, asthma or bronchitis may result in small areas of collapse which are not perfused. This can be overcome by combining perfusion lung scanning, using labelled macro-aggregated albumin with a labelled xenon ventilation scan. This requires a gamma camera, which is not widely available. It is disconcerting that 25–30 per cent of all patients undergoing surgery develop evidence of deep vein thrombosis as judged by the labelled fibrinogen uptake test, and that about 20 per cent of patients have evidence of pulmonary embolism as judged by combined ventilation and perfusion scanning. The figures correspond to those obtained from autopsy material.

Management.—In a case of suspected pulmonary embolism two additional investigations may be mandatory, namely, lung scanning and pulmonary arteriograms. The pulmonary arteriograms can be performed after some practice in any x-ray department; the catheter should be placed if possible in the pulmonary artery so that contrast in the right ventricle does not obscure the view of the lower pulmonary arteries. It is not essential to make pressure recordings in the cardiac chambers.

Emergency pulmonary arteriography is a comparatively safe procedure.

Treatment of Pulmonary Embolism and Infarction

Prevention of further thrombosis: heparin
Lysis or removal of established pulmonary emboli
Attention to the source of the emboli (see page 82)
Prevention of thrombo-embolic pulmonary hypertension.

As a general rule, pulmonary infarcts which are judged to be small, in that the embolus which caused them has not produced any haemodynamic disturbance, should not be overinvestigated or treated by thrombolysis. If on clinical, electrocardiographic and radiological evidence a pulmonary embolus is judged to be large then pulmonary angiography should be performed and the embolus located or the extent of occlusion of pulmonary arteries demonstrated. If it is then decided to institute thrombolytic treatment, the catheter is left in the appropriate pulmonary artery and streptokinase and hydrocortisone infused for 24 hours in the same dose as for deep vein thrombosis. Further pulmonary arteriograms should then be obtained.

It has been shown that thrombolytic therapy can dissolve large pulmonary emboli. It should be considered in the relatively uncommon occurrence of pulmonary embolism in which death is not immediate and in which there is evidence of persisting haemodynamic disturbances due to the embolus, or when x-rays reveal persisting obstruction of one or more of the major pulmonary arteries.

Pulmonary embolectomy (Trendelenburg's[8] operation) is considered if the patient is unlikely to survive long enough for thrombolytic therapy to have time to work, or if there is no evidence of clot lysis or improvement after 24 hours.

The evidence of the Urokinase Pulmonary Embolism Trial Study Group indicates that the patients who will benefit most from thrombolytic therapy are those who are critically ill from massive pulmonary embolism. There is no evidence that thrombolytic therapy in the early stage of embolism will reduce the incidence of late complications. Further deterioration with heparin or thrombolytic therapy would be an indication for pulmonary embolectomy.

There are numerous references to the long-term dangers following either pulmonary embolism or deep vein thrombosis. As a general rule all cases of deep vein thrombosis and pulmonary embolism or infarction should receive oral anticoagulants for at least 6 months. The risk and importance of repeated thrombo-embolism are so great that anticoagulants for this length of time are essential. The common practice of discontinuing oral anticoagulants when a patient is mobile or after an empirical period of 6 weeks after a deep vein thrombosis is difficult to justify.

There are particular dangers of thrombo-embolism in women on oestrogen-containing oral contraceptives. It is wise to consider giving prophylactic anticoagulants to any woman who is to have an operation and who is taking or who has taken them within the previous two months.

TUBERCULOSIS

Pulmonary tuberculosis is acquired by droplet infection with human *Mycobacterium tuberculosis* (Koch's[9] bacillus). The first infection of the lung produces an acute inflammatory response at alveolar level which soon forms a typical tubercle consisting of fibrous tissue, lymphocytes and Langhans[10] giant cells (Ghon[11] focus). The lung is very rich in lymphatics, and living tubercle bacilli disseminate by lymph spread to the hilar lymph glands; here the disease may be contained. The combination of initial tuberculous infection of the lung together with lymphatic spread to the hilar lymph glands is known as the primary complex. Lymphatic spread of the bacilli in the primary infection may be responsible for infection of pleura and vertebrae. Live tubercle bacilli may be disseminated from the original infected alveoli to other parts of the lung by the airways, or an infected lymph gland may rupture into a blood vessel, causing haematogenous spread. By far the commonest occurrence is complete healing of the primary focus and its associated primary complex.

About 4–6 weeks after the first tuberculous infection all the cells in the body become sensitised to the presence of tubercle bacilli or protein products derived from them. As a result of this hypersensitivity, further contact with tubercle bacilli produces an extremely vigorous inflammatory response. This inflammation is accompanied by caseation and fibrosis. Within such a fibrocaseous mass, tubercle bacilli may either become walled off and harmless or, less commonly, liquefaction may occur and tubercle bacilli multiply and spread (fibrocaseous or post-primary tuberculosis).

Primary Tuberculosis

For the first four weeks after infection there are no abnormal signs; after this the patient develops signs of tuberculin sensitivity: erythema nodosum, phlyctenular conjunctivitis and a positive tuberculin skin test. After eight to twelve weeks the primary lung focus may be seen in the chest x-ray. It may be accompanied by hilar lymphadenopathy which, if severe, causes bronchial obstruction leading to consolidation and collapse. At this stage haematogenous (miliary) and lymphatic spread to pleura and bone may occur.

Primary tuberculosis may occur at any age; the frequency of complications depends upon the age group:

Ages 0–7 years: High incidence of miliary spread particularly 3–6 months after infection. Pleural effusions and cavitation are unusual.

Age 7–12 years: Relatively few complications

Age 13–20 years: Pleural effusions 3–6 months after infection are common. Progress of the intrapulmonary primary focus to cavitated fibrocaseous tuberculosis is common.

Meningitis tends to occur about a year after primary infection, bone and kidney involvement later. Pleural effusion tends to occur after about 5 months and erosion of bronchial walls at about 9 months.

Management.—Clinical evidence of tuberculous infection at any age is always treated, whether it be pleural effusions or change of tuberculin skin test from negative to positive. Treatment is continued for at least two years with at least two antituberculous drugs to which the bacilli are fully sensitive. Pleural effusions are treated with repeated aspirations as well as antituberculous chemotherapy. If the effusion persistently recurs, intrapleural hydrocortisone is used. Tuberculin testing is done with old tuberculin (OT), which is a heat-sterilised protein derivative of human *Myobacterium tuberculosis*. The Mantoux test involves the intradermal injection of 0·1 ml 1 in 10 000 (1 unit) of old tuberculin, the test is read in 2–4 days, and the size of both the erythema and the accompanying induration should be recorded. Induration with a diameter of more than 0·5 cm is a positive reaction. If the reaction is negative the test should be repeated, using 0·1 ml of 1 in 1000 OT (10 units).

The Heaf[12] test involves intradermal injection to a depth of 1 mm of a concentrated solution of Purified Protein Derivative (PPD) by means of a mechanical gun with 6 pointed prongs which project for 1 mm when the gun is actuated. A positive Heaf test corresponds to a positive Mantoux test at a dilution of OT of approximately 1 in 1000. PPD is a purer form of the antigen from tubercle bacilli than old tuberculin. Certain factors may depress the skin reaction in a patient who should have a positive tuberculin test:

Inactive old tuberculin
Old age
Healed childhood tuberculosis
Sarcoidosis
Miliary tuberculosis
Corticosteroid administration
Malignant lymphomas
Exanthemata
Severe febrile illness.

Following a primary tuberculous infection the patient becomes tuberculin positive and this gives some natural immunity if the patient is again infected. Artificial immunity can be given by vaccination with BCG vaccine (Bacille Calmette[13] -Guérin[14]), which is an attenuated strain of bovine tubercle bacilli. It is given intradermally to people who are known to be tuberculin negative. Usually a small primary lesion develops at the site of injection six weeks later, and the patient becomes tuberculin positive. Occasionally BCG vaccination is accompanied by ulceration, induration and regional lymphadenopathy, particularly if given accidentally to a tuberculin-positive patient. This may require antituberculous chemotherapy. In this country it is usual to offer BCG to:

> All school children at the age of 13–14 who are not already tuberculin positive
> All tuberculin-negative contacts of cases of tuberculosis
> People at special risk such as doctors and nurses
> The newborn children of tuberculous mothers.

Post-primary (Adult) Tuberculosis

Following primary tuberculosis, living tubercle bacilli may remain dormant in the healed primary complex. Post-primary tuberculosis arising from infection by these organisms is "endogenous reinfection"; this is probably unusual. Another method of reinfection is by inhalation of a fresh dose of tubercle bacilli from outside—"exogenous reinfection". These external bacilli may be immediately involved in an intense inflammatory reaction which prevents their multiplying further. However, the inflammatory reaction may be insufficient to contain them, and the organisms and inflammatory reaction may continue to "fight it out". The inflammation heals by caseation and fibrosis, if caseation occurs into a bronchiole the patient will cough up live tubercle bacilli and cavitation is said to have occurred. The evidence of exogenous reinfection is:

> Coinciding with a fall in open cases of tuberculosis in the population there has been a parallel decrease in notifications of new cases of tuberculosis.
> People who had primary tuberculosis before the advent of antituberculous chemotherapy occasionally develop post-primary (adult) tuberculosis due to *drug-resistant* organisms.
> Post-primary tuberculosis due to ordinary *M. tuberculosis* occasionally develops in people who have previously had BCG; if endogenous reinfection had occurred then their tuberculosis should be due to the organisms given in the BCG.
> Occasionally cluster cases of tuberculosis occur in close contacts, suggesting case-to-case transmission of organisms.

However, despite this evidence favouring exogenous reinfection, many tuberculosis experts feel that endogenous reinfection is commoner.

The patient who coughs up live tubercle bacilli is said to be sputum positive or an open case. Haemoptysis will occur if cavitation involves a blood vessel. Fibrosis may lead to contraction of the part of the lung involved, together with distortion of neighbouring structures such as trachea, pleura, chest wall and interlobar fissures; it may also lead to dilatation of neighbouring bronchi, bronchiectasis and secondary infection. Common methods of presentation of adult tuberculosis are weight loss, night sweats, haemoptysis, cough and sputum. The chest x-ray may show evidence of old primary tuberculosis: ill-defined, patchy shadowing usually in one upper zone, which may be cavitated or calcified and accompanied by evidence of fibrosis. Post-primary tuberculosis generally involves the apical segment of the upper lobes, and the primary focus the peripheral part of the middle or lower zones—the reason for the difference in distribution is not known. Tomography is often necessary to confirm cavitation or calcification.

The annual number of deaths from tuberculosis in England and Wales is still over 1300. This number far exceeds the death rate from any other notifiable infectious disease. It is salutary to note that 20 per cent of cases dying from tuberculosis are diagnosed only after death. In other words, every District General Hospital in the country should expect to have at least one patient a year dying of unsuspected tuberculosis. Asian immigrants are more than 20 times as liable to have tuberculosis as the indigenous population. They are also more likely to have a non-respiratory manifestation of the disease. The most common forms of presentation of pulmonary tuberculosis are:

Middle-aged smokers with persistent cough
Unresolved pneumonia
Discovered by Mass Miniature Radiography. This has now been abandoned routinely because the yield was less than one active case per 1000. However, the equipment remains available for certain categories in which the yield remains high, e.g. contacts, immigrants, prisons and mental hospitals
Deterioration in general health, and weight loss
Ill health in immigrants
Haemoptysis
Patients on steroids; diabetics and post-gastrectomy patients.

Non-respiratory Tuberculosis

It is important to note that, in the elderly, tuberculosis may present as a wasting illness with fever and without pulmonary manifestations. Antemortem diagnosis may depend on marrow, lymph-node or liver biopsy. In cases of doubt a therapeutic trial with PAS and isoniazid is justified.

In immigrants non-respiratory tuberculosis is the rule and the features may include fever, generalised cervical or hilar lymphadeno-pathy, hepatosplenomegaly, as well as bone or genito-urinary involvement.

Treatment of Tuberculosis

Primary chemotherapy refers to treatment for patients who have never previously had any antituberculous chemotherapy. In Britain about 4 per cent of newly diagnosed patients have infection with organisms which are resistant to at least one of the main primary drugs, and in order to prevent the emergence of resistant strains of organisms at least two of the drugs must be given. In practice this means starting initial intensive therapy with three drugs in case the patient happens to be one of the 4 per cent whose organisms are resistant to one drug. The result of tubercle bacillus sensitivity to chemotherapy will not be known for at least 6 weeks after treatment.

In Britain streptomycin and isoniazid are always included in the initial stage of primary therapy and the third drug may be PAS, ethambutol or rifampicin. In developing countries thiocetazone may be used because of its cheapness. Initial therapy is continued for at least 6 weeks, but the exact duration depends on the site and extent of the disease.

Continuation therapy is with two drugs to which the organism is known to be sensitive. Continuation therapy is continued for at least 1 year for non-cavitated disease and for 1½–2 years for cavitated disease. All combinations of drugs used in continuation therapy contain isoniazid. The second drugs in the various regimes are PAS, ethambutol, rifampicin and thiocetazone.

Retreatment of relapsed tuberculosis and drug-resistant organisms.—If the organisms are still sensitive to the primary drugs, these drugs may again be used. If the organisms have developed resistance, rifampicin and ethambutol are the most useful drugs, provided they have not been used previously, because the incidence of side-effects is lower with these than with the other reserve antituberculous drugs. Abroad (particularly in India and East Africa), successful treatment of tuberculosis has been obtained both with carefully controlled intermittent chemotherapy and short-course regimes, but these are not used in this country.

Examination of contacts.—Adult contacts who are tuberculin negative six weeks after the patient has been in hospital should be given BCG and regular chest x-rays (BCG is given if the contact is tuberculin negative after a delay of six weeks after the patient's admission, as the contact may already be in the process of developing a positive tuberculin test as a result of his last contact with the patient). Adult contacts who are tuberculin positive should receive regular chest x-rays and tuberculin tests. All the children who are tuberculin negative six weeks after the patient has been admitted should be given BCG. Children who have not previously had BCG and are tuberculin positive should receive two years antituberculous chemotherapy if they are between the ages of 0 and 7, and 12 and 20. Opinion is divided about tuberculin-positive children between the ages of 7 and 12. Some would advocate regular check-ups and no antituberculous chemotherapy unless further evidence of tuberculosis develops; others would give antituberculous chemotherapy on the grounds that most children at this age are tuberculin negative, and that a child who is tuberculin positive has evidence of tuberculous infection which has probably recently been acquired from the newly discovered hospital case. The reason why 7 to 12 years is a special age group is that the complications of primary tuberculosis at this age are less than in infants and adolescents.

The principal side-effects of the antituberculous drugs in *reverse* order of frequency of incidence are:

Isoniazid: Peripheral neuropathy. This is commoner in patients who inactivate isoniazid slowly (slow inactivators). It can be prevented by giving pyridoxine at the same time. There is no evidence that the rate of healing of tuberculosis is different in slow and fast inactivators of isoniazid on the same dose of the drug. Psychosis, intellectual impairment, insomnia and epilepsy occur rarely with isoniazid. There have also been reports of a possible carcinogenic effect.

Streptomycin: Vestibular disturbances (nystagmus, ataxia, vertigo), fever, skin rash and very rarely, deafness. It is a wise precaution for everyone having steptomycin to have caloric and audiometry tests before starting on the drug. When the drug is stopped the vestibular disturbances are usually reversible. Deafness is usually not reversible.

PAS: Gastro-intestinal disturbances, goitres, hypothyroidism, hypokalaemia, liver damage and a glandular-fever-like syndrome.

Ethambutol: The only major toxic effect so far is a reversible form of optic neuritis which presents as blurring of vision. A unique form of red-green colour blindness and an arcuate central scotoma may be associated. Visual function should be tested before the drug is given. The drug is mainly excreted via the kidneys, hence renal failure may cause accumulation.

Rifampicin: No serious toxic effects have yet been reported. Mild gastro-intestinal disturbance, and liver impairment have occurred. The drug causes a red colour of urine and sputum. It also interferes with colour reaction for bilirubin in the serum giving false high bilirubin readings.

Capreomycin: The side-effects are similar to although less frequent than those of kanamycin; the most important are nephrotoxicity and ototoxicity.

Pyrazinamide: Liver damage (therefore fortnightly transaminase estimations for the duration of treatment), gout, fever and photosensitivity.

Cycloserine: Severe depression, epilepsy and confusion.

Prothionamide: Gastro-intestinal disturbances, liver damage, peripheral neuropathy, gynaecomastia and possibly teratogenic effects (hence, to be avoided in pregnancy).

Other Mycobacteria

Mycobacteria are acid- and alcohol-fast bacilli of which *M. tuberculosis* and *M. leprae* are two types. Most of the others occur as opportunists in man and rarely can cause disease. *Histologically* the disease they cause is identical to that caused by *M. tuberculosis* but *clinically* the diseases are very different. These opportunist mycobacteria were called "atypical" or "anonymous". For practical clinical purposes there are three important opportunist mycobacteria in this country:

1. *M. kansasii*
2. *M. avium (Battey bacillus)*
3. *M. marinum (M. balnei).*

The opportunist mycobacteria are classified into groups according to certain biochemical, cultural and morphologic differences. They grow rather more rapidly than *M. tuberculosis*, therefore a culture report back in four weeks instead of the usual six should alert one to the possibility that opportunist mycobacteria are present.

Some of the opportunist mycobacteria are saprophytes and are normally found in soil and water; they are occasionally found in association with *M. tuberculosis*. They should only be assumed to be causing the disease if they are repeatedly isolated. Infection by individual opportunist mycobacteria can be tested for by Mantoux testing using antigen prepared from the organism. The incidence of infection with opportunist mycobacteria varies in different parts of the world from 10 per cent of all tuberculosis in some parts of the United States to about 1·5 per cent in this country. Some of the opportunist mycobacteria are partially sensitive to the first-line antituberculous drugs.

1. *M. kansasii* can cause a pulmonary disease virtually identical to that caused by *M. tuberculosis*. Certain differentiating chest x-ray appearances have been claimed, namely more cavitation and less fibrosis. Infection with *M. kansasii* is much commoner among urban

dwellers and coal miners with pneumoconiosis. It is virtually confined to adult men, some of whom have had previous tuberculosis due to *M. tuberculosis*; there is no evidence of spread of the disease in close contacts; *M. kansasii* does *not* exist in the soil or water.

2. *M. avium* (*Battey bacillus*). This causes cervical adenitis particularly in children and is now the commonest cause of "tuberculous" adenitis.

3. *M. marinum* (*M. balnei*). This rarely causes outbreaks of skin granulomas (swimming-bath granulomas).

SARCOIDOSIS

Sarcoidosis is characterised by involvement of various organs with non-caseating granulomas. Similar granulomas occur in foreign-body reactions, tuberculosis, fungus infections and in lymph glands draining a carcinoma. The relationship of sarcoidosis to tuberculosis is still not clear, most cases have a negative tuberculin test but the incidence of tuberculosis in patients with sarcoidosis is 10 per cent. The clinical course of the disease is variable; an acute form with a duration of three to four weeks is more common in young women under the age of 30. They develop erythema nodosum and hilar lymphadenopathy, and only occasionally involvement of other organs. The chronic form develops insidiously and often begins with fever, cough and dyspnoea. The pulmonary manifestations are hilar lymphadenopathy and infiltration by fibrous tissue; on the chest x-ray this is seen as soft, irregular, nodular shadows and linear streaks often radiating from the hilum. The acute form commonly has a good prognosis and the chronic form a poor one. In the chronic form pulmonary function tests usually show a diffusion defect, but the impairment of diffusion bears no relationship to the severity of the x-ray shadowing. A diffusion defect is sometimes found even when the chest x-ray is normal. Other organs frequently involved are lymph nodes, eyes (uveitis and keratoconjunctivitis sicca), skin (erythema nodosum), spleen, liver, bone, salivary glands and nervous system. Bone cysts occur in the terminal phalanges of the hands, they do not occur unless there is skin involvement. Nervous-system involvement has been recorded in the absence of any other signs. Neurosarcoid is more common with the acute variety; response to corticosteroids is usually poor. Hypercalcaemia, which may cause nephrocalcinosis, is probably due to hypersensitivity to vitamin D, resulting in excessive gastro-intestinal absorption of calcium; hypercalcuria may occur in the absence of hypercalcaemia. Increased gamma globulins also occur. Serum alkaline phosphatase is normal, unlike many of the other causes of hypercalcaemia.

The diagnosis is confirmed by a negative tuberculin test, a positive

Kveim[15] test and histological evidence. The most usual sites for biopsy are liver, scalene node and conjunctiva. Rarely it may be necessary to obtain a paratracheal gland by mediastinoscopy or a bronchial biopsy by bronchoscopy. The Kveim test is almost always positive in acute sarcoid although it may be negative in chronic sarcoid. Occasional false positive Kveim tests occur—their frequency depends on the antigen used. The diagnosis may also be confirmed by studying the lymphocytes obtained from bronchial washings.

Corticosteroids are used for the treatment of the hypercalcaemia, involvement of eyes and nervous system, disfiguring skin lesions, diffusion defects and intrapulmonary shadowing which remains unchanged for three months. Progressive dyspnoea, particularly in the early stages, is an indication for high doses of steroids which should be reduced when there is clinical improvement but should probably be continued in smaller doses for at least three months. In younger patients enlarged hilar lymph glands usually disappear within a year. They are more likely to remain in older patients, when they may calcify. Pleural effusions do not occur in sarcoidosis.

DRUG-INDUCED LUNG DISEASE

A large number of drugs have adverse reactions involving the respiratory system. The lungs and airways may be involved in a generalised reaction caused by the drug (e.g. drugs causing a syndrome resembling systemic lupus erythematosus or asthma as part of an anaphylactic reaction). Involvement of the lungs may be the only adverse reaction produced (e.g. pulmonary eosinophilia). The drug-induced lung diseases are:

Asthma

Penicillin	Vitamin K
Tetracycline	Bromsulphthalein
Erythromycin	Iron dextran
Streptomycin	Suxamethonium
Griseofulvin	Antisera
Cephaloridine	Vaccines
Ethionamide	Aspirin
Monoamine oxidase inhibitors	Indomethacin
Organic iodides	Pituitary snuff
Local anaesthetics	

Pulmonary eosinophilia

Nitrofurantoin	Sulphonamides
PAS	Imipramine
Penicillin	

Systemic lupus erythematosus

Penicillin
Tetracycline
Gold
Sulphonamides
Phenylbutazone
Griseofulvin
Hydralazine
Isoniazid

Phenytoin
Streptomycin
Procainamide
PAS
Thiouracil
Troxidone
Methyldopa
Carbamazepine

Polyarteritis

Iodides
Hydantoins
Penicillin
Gold salts

Thiouracil
Phenothiazines
Sulphonamides

Lipoid pneumonia

Liquid paraffin
Ephedrine nose drops

Cod-liver oil

Intra-alveolar oedema and fibrosis

Busulphan

Hexamethonium and other
ganglion-blocking drugs

Local atelectasis and alveolar oedema

Oxygen—when administration of high concentrations is prolonged.

Local pleural fibrosis

Methysergide

Mediastinal and generalised lymphadenopathy

Phenylbutazone ⎫
PAS ⎬
Hydantoins ⎭

Histology of glands in these conditions may
resemble sarcoidosis, glandular fever and
lymphoma respectively

Pulmonary infarcts

Oral contraceptives

BRONCHIAL CARCINOMA

The evidence implicating cigarette smoking as a cause of bronchial
carcinoma is now overwhelming. The carcinogen in cigarette smoke
thought to be responsible is 3-4-benzpyrene. Atmospheric pollution

probably plays a minor role in causation but the evidence is conflicting; the incidence of bronchial carcinoma is lower in coal miners even though their smoking habits are the same. It is suggested that pneumoconiosis results in obstruction of lung lymphatics, limiting lymphatic spread of carcinoma. Certain mining and industrial processes are associated with a high incidence of bronchial carcinoma in exposed workers, e.g. asbestos, nickel, chromate, arsenic workers, and pitchblende and uranium miners.

Carcinoma of the bronchus is responsible for over one-third of cancers in men, and is responsible for nearly 10 per cent of all deaths in men. Despite widespread publicity of its dangers, the amount of tobacco consumed in this country has not declined, nor has the incidence of bronchial carcinoma. It is interesting that the incidence of death from bronchial carcinoma is now constant in men below the age of 60, but the incidence in younger women, and in men over this age, is still increasing. This corresponds to the two periods when cigarette smoking became widespread in this country—among men during the First World War and among women during the Second World War.

The main pathological types are:

Squamous cell (or epidermoid—because the cells resemble the epithelium of the bronchi).—These tend to occur in the main bronchi.

Anaplastic, a common variety of which is the oat-cell carcinoma. This is the most common type associated with non-metastatic endocrine abnormalities. This type is highly malignant and is often associated with massive involvement of the mediastinum.

Adenocarcinoma.—This tends to occur in the periphery of the lung; it is the commonest bronchial carcinoma in women and is not associated with smoking. It accounts for less than 5 per cent of bronchial carcinoma in men and is mainly responsible for the uncommon occurrence of bronchial carcinoma in non-smokers. It is the commonest histological type associated with asbestosis.

Alveolar-cell carcinomata.—These are uncommon and are usually widespread throughout the lung; they may arise from several foci or spread by aspiration metastasis. Histologically they resemble adenocarcinoma. Rarely they may be responsible for defects of diffusion; on x-ray alveolar-cell carcinoma is seen as diffuse, small, ill-defined nodules.

Histological proof of the diagnosis of carcinoma is desirable and is obtained by bronchoscopy, sputum cytology, pleural biopsy, pleural aspiration or lymph-node biopsy. For ten days following bronchoscopy, cells indistinguishable from carcinoma cells may appear in the sputum even when no carcinoma is present; if the patient is suffering from tuberculosis or chronic bronchitis, the sputum may contain cells which are similar to neoplastic cells. Cells derived from a pleural effusion due to pulmonary infarction may resemble adenocarcinoma cells. Approximately 10 per cent of bronchial carcinomas present with evidence of central nervous system involvement.

Treatment

The two main forms of treatment are surgery or radiotherapy. Apart from differences in the tumour histology there are a number of factors which exclude surgery:

Severe coincidental lung disease; chronic bronchitis severe enough to cause an FEV_1 less than 60 per cent of the predicted normal for age and weight

Severe coincidental disease in other systems

Old age. The operative mortality of most series increases over the age of 65.

Mediastinal involvement with evidence of widening of the carina on bronchoscopy, or paratracheal gland involvement

Pleural effusion which recurs after aspiration, provided infection distal to bronchial obstruction is not responsible for the persisting effusion

Paralysed diaphragm, recurrent laryngeal palsy or Horner's syndrome

Extension to the chest wall

Metastases—very occasionally exceptions are made when there is a solitary cerebral metastasis.

The current orthodox policy is to advise surgery for cases of squamous and adenocarcinoma deemed operable, and radiotherapy for anaplastic and oat-cell carcinomas. There has now been a 5-year M.R.C. follow-up of cases of anaplastic carcinoma treated by surgery and radiotherapy; results indicate that radiotherapy is marginally better than surgery for oat-cell and small-cell anaplastic tumours (Medical Research Council, 1969).

The question of earlier diagnosis of lung cancer in people at risk (smokers over the age of 40) is important. It seems that earlier detection of cases by regular six-monthly chest x-rays does improve the 5-year survival in operable cases.

Inoperable and anaplastic tumours are treated with radiotherapy; sometimes this is combined with cyclophosphamide or nitrogen mustard. Recurrent pleural effusions are treated with radioactive gold, nitrogen mustard or pleurodesis.

Bronchial carcinoma of whatever type carries a worse prognosis in women than in men.

NON-METASTATIC EXTRAPULMONARY COMPLICATIONS OF BRONCHIAL CARCINOMA

Endocrine

Cushing's syndrome. This is due to formation by the tumour of a peptide resembling ACTH. Often the first manifestation of Cushing's syndrome is a severe hypokalaemic alkalosis which is extremely resistant to treatment with potassium infusion and spironolactone. Most cases of Cushing's syndrome arise in young women. The occurrence of the disease in a middle-aged man should arouse the suspicion that a bronchial neoplasm is responsible. This is the commonest endocrine manifestation of carcinoma of the bronchus. Severe muscle weakness and pigmentation are usually present.

Hypercalcaemia. This is caused by a parathormone-like substance elaborated by the tumour. The hypercalcaemia may cause thirst, polyuria, fits and mental confusion, muscle weakness and constipation. The level of serum calcium can be brought down with steroids and the syndrome usually improves when the tumour is treated either surgically or with radiotherapy.

Inappropriate secretion of ADH. This results in a dilutional hyponatraemia; symptoms do not occur unless the serum sodium drops below 120 mmol/l. Paradoxically there may be sodium in the urine. There may also be a renal tubular defect resulting in glycosuria, aminoaciduria and potassium loss. The condition can be improved with fludrocortisone.

Carcinoid syndrome. This syndrome can occur with bronchial carcinomas as well as adenomas.

Hypo- and hyperglycaemia.

Thyrotoxicosis.

Acromegaly.

Gynaecomastia.

Red-cell aplasia.

Polycythaemia.

Other tumours associated with polycythaemia are:

Renal carcinoma
Benign renal tumours
Cerebellar haemangiomas
Fibroids
Adrenal carcinoma or hyperplasia
Ovarian tumours
Hepatomas
Phaeochromocytoma.

Neurological Complications

All parts of the nervous system may be affected.

Encephalopathy with dementia, cerebral degeneration or leuco-
dystrophy
Cerebellar degeneration
Extrapyramidal syndromes
Myelopathy
Neuropathy (motor and sensory)
Myasthenia
Motor neurone disease.

Other Non-metastatic Manifestations:

Dermatomyositis
Pulmonary osteoarthropathy
Enteropathy resulting in malabsorption
Thrombophlebitis
Haemolytic anaemia, bleeding diatheses due to excess fibrinolysins,
megaloblastic anaemia due to the tumour utilising all available
folic acid
Skin disorders.

The course of these syndromes is very variable; in some patients
they remit if the primary tumour is treated, in others they progress
despite "adequate" treatment of the primary. Some, particularly the
neuropathies, fluctuate regardless of treatment of the primary. The
syndromes may antedate the appearance of the bronchial carcinoma
by several years.

PULMONARY FIBROSIS

Pulmonary fibrosis is the end result of many lung diseases, including
extrinsic allergic alveolitis, pneumonia and tuberculosis. The main
causes are:

Chronic infections
Pneumonia
Fibrocystic disease
Bronchiectasis

Cardiovascular disorders
Chronic pulmonary oedema
Haemosiderosis

Dust diseases
Silicosis
Pneumoconiosis
Asbestosis and berylliosis

Unknown causes
  Sarcoidosis
  Intrinsic fibrosing alveolitis

Lung involvement in systemic diseases
  Rheumatoid disease
  Systemic sclerosis
  Scleroderma
  Wegener's granulomatosis
  Histiocytosis X
  Polyarteritis

Neoplasms
  Alveolar-cell carcinoma
  Lymphangitis carcinomatosa
  Leukaemia

Miscellaneous
  Irradiation
  Goodpasture's[16] syndrome
  Alveolar proteinosis
  Alveolar microlithiasis
  Loeffler's[17] syndrome

Intrinsic (Cryptogenic) Fibrosing Alveolitis

The condition is characterised by fibrosis of the alveolar walls and cellular exudation into the alveoli, which causes dyspnoea, crepitations and lower-zone fibrosis. Clubbing is common, and no cause of the disorder is identifiable. The disease may occur in an acute or chronic form and progression is usually not associated with spontaneous remissions.

The spectrum of the disease blends into those disorders which are also associated with pulmonary changes, for example:

  Rheumatoid disease
  Systemic lupus erythematosus
  Dermatomyositis
  Chronic active hepatitis
  Ulcerative colitis
  Systemic sclerosis

In cryptogenic alveolitis antibodies found in the autoimmune diseases also occur frequently, for example:

  IgM Rheumatoid factor
  Antinuclear factor
  Anti DNA antibodies (usually single-stranded DNA).

Treatment

The only treatment is corticosteroids, which should be started in a moderate dose (20 mg/day) and increase gradually if there is no response. If a response occurs the dose can be cut back *gradually*. If high doses of steroids produce no improvement they should be gradually withdrawn.

Miscellaneous Causes of Lung Fibrosis

Goodpasture's syndrome consists of multiple haemorrhages into the lungs in association with glomerulonephritis, and is a variant of polyarteritis nodosa. In pulmonary haemosiderosis there are also multiple haemorrhages into the lungs, but this disease is much more chronic and not associated with nephritis; it may be idiopathic or secondary to chronic pulmonary venous congestion, as in mitral valve disease. Alveolar proteinosis and microlithiasis are very rare diseases in which a protein substance and numerous minute calcified particles respectively are deposited in the alveoli.

INDUSTRIAL DUST DISEASE

Silicosis

Silicosis is due to inhalation of particles of silica in exposed workers. Small amounts of silica dust can be disposed of by the ordinary processes of phagocytosis, inhalation of larger amounts result in silica particles remaining in the substance of the lung, and this provokes an intense inflammatory reaction—the silicotic nodule. With continued exposure these nodules will appear throughout both lungs and in the lymphatics and lympth glands. The silicotic nodules enlarge and coalesce; this may be avoided if the patient is removed from exposure. The conglomeration is greatest in the upper zones and is possibly associated with tuberculosis; distortion of the lung by fibrosis results in bullous emphysema. Cor pulmonale and pneumothorax are frequent complications.

On x-ray the first appearance is of well-defined, dense nodules throughout both lung fields; later, the nodules enlarge and become ill-defined. Conglomeration of nodules is seen particularly in the upper zones; the hilar lymph glands are enlarged and frequently calcified. Later, when emphysema supervenes, the masses are even easier to see; they tend to move medially and finally may become continuous with the enlarged lymph glands of the mediastinum.

Coal-miners' Pneumoconiosis

This may develop in workers exposed to pure coal dust (e.g. stokers and trimmers aboard coal-burning ships) as well as in coal-miners. In miners, pneumoconiosis is often accompanied by silicosis. The x-ray appearances in the first instance are similar to those of silicosis, with progression to coarse nodules. Unlike silicosis, these nodules are less well-defined and are not associated with bullous emphysema or lymph-gland enlargement. Clearing of the dust particles is slower from alveoli which are relatively fixed, i.e. those in the centre of the lung lobules and those immediately underlying pleura and lung septa. This results in emphysema which is characteristically "focal"—this is the stage of simple pneumoconiosis. Complicated pneumoconiosis is said to have occurred when the nodules in the upper zone coalesce, a process called progressive massive fibrosis (PMF); tubercle bacilli are fre-quently isolated from the fibrotic areas at postmortem, but clinical tuberculosis is uncommon in coal-miners' pneumoconiosis. Treatment prophylactically with antituberculous drugs has no effect on the development of PMF. The lesions of PMF frequently cavitate and calcify; they result in compression and distortion of neighbouring lung tissue and frequently cause bronchiectasis and thrombosis of arteries and veins. Obstruction of lymphatics in the dust diseases results in inefficient clearing of any fluid; hence, pulmonary oedema tends to occur more readily than when lymph drainage from the lungs is normal. Patients with coal-miners' pneumoconiosis are more breath-less than those with pure silicosis who have a similar amount of shadowing. Cor pulmonale is more common in coal-miners' pneumo-coniosis, clinical tuberculosis more common in silicosis.

There is an international classification of radiological opacities in the lung fields provoked by inhalation of mineral dusts. Categories numbered 1 to 3 indicate the "profusion" of the opacities (extent and density of distribution). Category 1 indicates that the opacities occupy an area of one-third of both lung fields, Category 2 that most of both lung fields are involved, and Category 3 that the opacities are very numerous. The size of the opacities is indicated by letters: p (punctiform) indicates nodules up to 1·5 mm, m (micronodular) indicates nodules 1·5–3 mm and n (nodular) nodules 3–10 mm in size. The letters A, B and C indicate the extent of massive fibrosis; the letter D denotes distortion of any thoracic structure (mediastinum, lung fissures, diaphragm, trachea or pleura) by the fibrosis of compli-cated pneumoconiosis (Pneumoconiosis and Allied Occupational Chest Diseases, 1967). Compensation for pneumoconiosis is possible from Category 2 onwards; at this stage PMF may develop even if the miner is removed from exposure. The presence of pneumoconiosis does not always mean that a miner has to leave mining; further compensation is not affected by the fact that he continues to work in the mines and later develops more severe pneumoconiosis. In men who have or are destined to have rheumatoid disease the radiological appearances of pneumoconiosis are atypical (Caplan's syndrome).

Usually on a background of Category 1 or 2 pneumoconiosis, well-defined round opacities may appear suddenly in the periphery of any part of the lungs. They may come and go in crops, may calcify, or may disappear leaving thin-walled cavities. The opacities can be very large and result in surprisingly little functional impairment.

Asbestosis

This is due to inhalation of dust containing the silicates of magnesium and iron in workers and miners who handle asbestos and mica. Characteristically there is fine mottling and streaky diffuse shadows, particularly in the lower zones. The pleura and pericardium are thickened and shaggy in outline. Clubbing is common and there is probably no predisposition to tuberculosis. Minimum exposure is necessary to develop the disease; people exposed to asbestos dust cough up "asbestos bodies" in the sputum but these do not necessarily mean that the person has lung fibrosis due to asbestos, they merely indicate previous exposure to asbestos.

Exposure to asbestos dust leads to a predisposition to develop mesotheliomata, which are malignant tumours of serous membranes such as pleura, pericardium and peritoneum. Mesotheliomata are much commoner in exposure to blue or Cape asbestos (crocidolite); they appear to be commoner in people exposed to asbestos dust but who have not worked with asbestos, e.g. the wives of asbestos workers, and local populations near asbestos mines. The relationship between pleural plaques and mesothelioma has not yet been established. There is also a predisposition to develop bronchial carcinoma, particularly peripheral adenocarcinoma.

REFERENCES

BRANTHWAITE, M. A. (1978) *Management of Medical Emergencies*, ed. H. Baderman, p. 48. London: Pitmans.

CRANDON, A. J., PEEL, K. R., ANDERSON, J. A., THOMPSON, V. & McNICOL, G. P. (1980) *Brit. med. J.*, **2**, 345.

CROFTON, J. (1978) *Clin. Radiol.*, **29**, 353.

GOLDMAN, L., CALDERA, D. L. & NUSSBAUM, S. R. (1977) *New Engl. J. Med.*, **297**, 845.

FORGACS, P. (1978) *Lung Sounds*. London: Baillière Tindall.

JOURNAL OF THE ROYAL SOCIETY OF MEDICINE (1978) Symposium on Assessment and Treatment of the Respiratory Cripple, **71**, 55.

MEDICAL RESEARCH COUNCIL REPORT (1969) *Lancet*, **2**, 501.

PNEUMOCONIOSIS and ALLIED OCCUPATIONAL CHEST DISEASES (1967) London: H. M. Stationery Office.

ROSE, S. D. (1979) *Medical Clinics of North America*, **63**, 1205.

SCADDING, J. G. (1963) *Brit. med. J.*, **2**, 1428.

SIMON, G. (1978) *Principles of Chest X-ray Diagnosis*. London: Butterworth.

WEST, J. B. (1977) *Ventilation/Blood Flow and Gas Exchange*. Third edit. Oxford: Blackwell Scientific Publications.

General References

CUMMING, G. & SEMPLE, S. J. (1980) *Disorders of the Respiratory System*. Second edit. Oxford: Blackwell Scientific Publications.

NUNN, J. F. (1977) *Applied Respiratory Physiology*. Second Edit. London: Butterworth.

EPONYMS

1. René Théophile Hyacinthe Laënnec (1781–1826)

Laënnec, born in Quimper in Brittany, was brought up by an uncle who was a physician in Nantes. Laënnec eventually went to Paris and studied with Baron Corvisart (Napoleon's physician), who had just translated Auenbrugger's *Inventum Novum* into French. Laënnec discovered his "auscultation mediate" in 1818; the *immediate* method being impractical by virtue of the sex of his buxom patient, he hit upon the "mediate" (or intermediate) method of listening to the chest through a rolled-up tube of paper. Unlike Auenbrugger's discovery of percussion, the value of Laënnec's stethoscope was immediately recognised. Laënnec succeeded Corvisart as Professor of Medicine at the College de France. The ruthless Dupuytren was a contemporary.

2. Thomas Hodgkin (1798–1866)

While a student in Guy's Hospital he visited Laënnec and was largely responsible for introducing the stethoscope to London. Like his contemporaries, Addison and Bright, he received some of his medical education in Edinburgh. Guy's and St Thomas' Hospitals then existed as a partnership which was subsequently dissolved. Hodgkin transferred from Guy's to St Thomas' at this time. He died of cholera in Palestine while on a trip to the Holy Land and is buried at Jaffa in Israel.

3. Christian Bohr (1855–1911)

Professor of Physiology in Copenhagen. Father of Niels Bohr the atomic physicist.

4. John Scott Haldane (1860–1936)

Haldane was born and qualified in Edinburgh; in 1887 he went to work for his uncle John Burdon-Sanderson, at Oxford; his son, John Burdon-Sanderson Haldane, was also a physiologist, and mapped out the X chromosome and designed the midget submarines used in the Second World War. J. S. Haldane discovered the affinity of haemoglobin for carbon monoxide; he developed the Haldane gas analyser and did important work on the effect of altitude on respiration.

5. Lawrence Joseph Henderson (1878–1942)

Henderson was educated at Harvard; he trained first in physical chemistry, then medicine. He was interested in the mathematical relationship between body chemicals, and invented the nomogram. He introduced the concept of "systems" or complicated relationships, between physiocochemical and biological variables. He wrote an influential essay, *The Order of Nature*, and was an exponent of the biochemical equivalent of "gestalt," that is to say, that the whole is greater than the sum of its parts. When the Harvard Business School opened, he established the Harvard Fatigue Laboratory, believing that "systems" exist even in complicated social interrelationships.

6. Karl Hasselbalch (1874–1962)

Hasselbalch was a Danish biochemist who later added certain mathematical refinements to Henderson's original formula.

7. Carl Friedländer (1847–1887)

Friedländer died of tuberculosis, having been compelled to give up his post as a pathologist. He had worked with Virchow, von Recklinghausen and Volkmann (of the contracture), and had been drafted into the Prussian Army for the Franco-Prussian war of 1870.

8. FRIEDRICH TRENDELENBURG (1844–1924)
Trendelenburg qualified in Berlin and spent a year in Glasgow, eventually becoming
Professor of Surgery in Leipzig. He performed the first pulmonary embolectomy
(unsuccessfully) in 1908. The first successful embolectomy was performed in 1924 by
Trendelenburg's pupil Kirschner on Trendelenburg's 80th birthday.

9. ROBERT KOCH (1843–1910)
Koch received the Nobel Prize for Medicine in 1905. He qualified in Göttingen, worked
in Berlin with Virchow, then entered general practice, and in his amateur laboratory he
proved that anthrax, which was prevalent in the area, was due to a transmitted bacillus;
he perfected many microbiological techniques. Ten years later in 1882 he discovered
the tubercle bacillus and in the next year the cholera vibrio. (Koch did not prove that
tuberculosis was an infectious disease; this was already widely known as a result of the
work of a French army surgeon, Jean Antoine Villemin, who had succeeded in
transmitting tuberculosis from one animal to another.) In 1885 Koch became Professor
of Hygiene in Berlin and had a whole succession of eponymous workers including
Ehrlich, von Behring, Loeffler, Neisser and Klebs. He described "old" and "new"
tuberculin, but came under a scientific cloud because of his misplaced belief that
tuberculin could cure tuberculosis; as a result large numbers of patients flocked to
Berlin and Koch was widely criticised for his unsubstantiated (but long awaited)
announcement of the "cure". Wordly pressures forced Koch to claim he had discovered
the "cure"; the public and the profession were expectant and the Kaiser pressed Koch
to make the announcement. In 1893 at the age of 50 he was divorced and within two
months married Fraulein Freiburg (21). He became *persona non grata* in many circles,
and this and the tuberculin debacle accounted for his later willingness to travel widely.
He subsequently investigated a large number of infectious diseases in India and Africa.

10. THEODOR LANGHANS (1839–1915)
Langhans studied under Henle and then under Virchow and von Recklinghausen. He
succeeded Edwin Klebs as Professor of Pathology in Berne, where he, Kocher (of the
incision) and Sahli (haemoglobinometer) were a formidable contemporary trio.

11. ANTON GHON (1866–1936)
Ghon became Professor of Pathology in Prague. In 1920 be described the primary
tuberculous focus in children.

12. FREDERICK ROWLAND GEORGE HEAF (1894–1973)
British physician.

13. LÉON CHARLES ALBERT CALMETTE (1863–1933)
Calmette worked with Pasteur and opened the first overseas Pasteur Institute, in
Saigon. Later he founded a dispensary in Lille for treating tuberculosis and remained
there during the First World War. He had pigeons in the laboratory, which aroused the
suspicions of the Germans that he was sending messages to the Allies; because of this
his wife was interned and Calmette himself humiliated. When Metchnikoff died,
Calmette became deputy director of the Pasteur Institute in Paris. In 1924 BCG was
given to doctors free of charge until the Lubeck disaster in 1930 in which 150 children
died because of improper preparation of BCG by German workers.

14. JEAN MARIE CAMILLE GUÉRIN (1872–1961)
He was born in Poitiers and trained as a vet. He eventually became head of the
Tuberculosis department of the Pasteur Institute in Lille, and received many honours
for his work with Calmette.

15. MORTEN ANSGAR KVEIM (1892–1966)
Kveim at first studied humanities, but then qualified in medicine in Oslo and became a general practitioner. However, in 1936 he developed an interest in dermatology, and in 1940 devised his skin test for sarcoidosis.

16. ERNEST WILLIAM GOODPASTURE (1886–1960)   .
Goodpasture qualified in Johns Hopkins University, Baltimore; he went on to become Professor of Pathology at Vanderbilt Medical School, Tennessee.

17. WILHELM LOEFFLER (1887–1972)
Basle and Zurich physician.

3

GASTRO-ENTEROLOGY

EXAMINATION OF THE ALIMENTARY SYSTEM

The external and remote clues of disorders of the alimentary tract are often as informative as the detailed examination of the abdomen itself. It is, therefore, mandatory to look carefully for circumstantial evidence of alimentary disease and one of the most frequently overlooked pointers is an abnormality at the beginning of the alimentary tract, namely, in the mucosa of the mouth and tongue.

The examination of the alimentary system should begin at the finger tips. Clubbing of the nails occurs in cirrhosis, Crohn's[1] disease and chronic diarrhoeas, whereas koilonychia occurs in severe iron deficiency anaemia and is a feature of the Plummer[2]-Vinson[3] syndrome (dysphagia, iron deficiency anaemia and koilonychia). White crescents in the nails, or leukonychia, are said to be a feature of alcoholic cirrhosis; pigmentation of the nails occurs with excessive use of phenolphthalein as a purgative.

The hands may show palmar erythema involving the finger tips, thenar and hypothenar eminences; the condition occurs in cirrhosis but is also seen in pregnancy, following oestrogen ingestion and in patients with rheumatoid arthritis. Tylosis palmaris or hyperkeratosis of the palms occurs in carcinoma of the oesophagus. The skin creases should be inspected for pallor and pigmentation; pigmentation of the skin creases is highly suggestive of Addison's disease.

The hair should be observed—there may be changes due to pernicious anaemia (premature greying) or kwashiorkor (reddening of the hair). The hair and skin may be involved in vitamin deficiencies such as scurvy and pellagra. The skin should be carefully inspected for spider naevi as evidence of liver disease; they are often diagnostic but may occur in pregnancy, weather-beaten facies and following oestrogen ingestion. The skin may also show jaundice with scratch marks and bruising as evidence of liver disease.

Careful inspection of the mouth is essential before proceeding to the abdomen. Carious teeth and abnormally shaped teeth should be noted. Hutchinson's[4] teeth occur in congenital syphilis but only the permanent teeth are affected: they are abnormally widely spaced and the incisors are notched and pointed. The gums are swollen and often bleed if there is gingivitis, scurvy, primary amyloid or hypertrophy due to anticonvulsant drugs. The gums may be stained in fluorosis or with tetracyline administration at an early age. The gums may become swollen and necrotic with chronic mercury poisoning.

The mucous membranes of the mouth may be involved in systemic skin disorders such as scleroderma, pemphigus and lichen planus. They are also involved as part of the Stevens[5]-Johnson[6] syndrome, Behçet's[7] disease, generalised allergic reactions and vitamin deficiencies.

Loss of the filiform papillae of the tongue occurs in iron deficiency and pernicious anaemia, as well as riboflavin deficiency, which may cause angular stomatitis in addition. The mucosae may be involved in any bleeding diathesis; the ones most relevant to the alimentary system are Henoch-Schönlein purpura, liver disease and hereditary telangiectasia. The mucosae may be pigmented in Addison's disease; circumoral pigmentation occurs in the Peutz[8]-Jeghers[9] syndrome (circumoral pigmentation and small-intestinal polyposis). Circumoral purpura are a feature of scleroderma associated with acrosclerosis and calcification of the soft tissues of the fingers (Thibierge[10]-Weissenbach syndrome). The lymph drainage of the stomach is ultimately into the left supraclavicular glands; these glands frequently become the seat of metastases from carcinoma of the stomach. A large number of eponyms have been given to these glands when they are enlarged; the most macabre is that of Troisier[11] who noted the ominous physical sign in himself.

The abdomen itself is then inspected: its general shape, movement with respiration and distension are observed. The presence of operation scars, abnormal peristalsis, dilated veins, and hernias should be noted. The abdomen should be palpated with the patient lying flat. Before starting to palpate, it is essential to ask the patient if there is any local tenderness. After inspecting the abdomen carefully, palpation should only be performed while looking at the patient's face, in order to catch the first sign that palpation is causing pain. The abdomen is conventionally divided into nine segments: right and left hypochondrium, right and left lumbar region, right and left iliac fossae, epigastrium, umbilical region and hypogastrium. Each segment should be palpated twice, the first time lightly and the second time more firmly.

The liver may be enlarged, tender or shrunken. Regeneration nodules may be palpable; the presence of umbilicated nodules is pathognomonic of secondary carcinoma. In amyloidosis, the liver is often very large but there is seldom any evidence of hepatocellular failure or portal hypertension. The liver may be smaller than normal due to fibrosis, the small liver can only be detected by percussing the upper border which should lie at the level of the fifth rib in the midclavicular line in the normal. A Riedel's[12] lobe may extend down into the right lumbar region; this is a normal variant and is more often seen in women.

The characteristics of a splenic enlargement are:

Well-defined medial border which is notched
It is impossible to get above the swelling
A groove is felt between the swelling posteriorly and the erector spinae, whereas no such groove occurs with renal swellings
The swelling is dull to percussion.

The normal spleen can be percussed; percussion should begin posteriorly and extend along the 10th rib towards the mid-line. The limit of dullness of the normal spleen is the mid-axillary line.

The gall bladder, if palpable, is generally felt as a smooth rounded swelling projected below the edge of the liver. Enlargement of the liver displaces it downwards. If the liver is not enlarged the surface markings of the gall bladder are either the intersection of the right costal margin and a line drawn from left superior iliac spine through the umbilicus or the angle between the costal margin and the lateral border of the right rectus abdominis muscle.

Renal swelling is characterised by being felt in the loin, by being able to get the exploring finger above the swelling, by movement with respiration, and by a band of resonance extending over it anteriorly, due to gas in the colon.

ABDOMINAL PAIN

There is a very useful and sometimes life-saving dictum—"Any abdominal pain lasting more than six hours is likely to be surgical."
These are some tips which may be useful:

Digoxin causes vomiting and diarrhoea *but do not assume* in a patient who is on digoxin that vomiting is due to digoxin *until* you have *examined* the abdomen.
In all cases of abdominal pain always *examine carefully all* the hernial orifices.
Strangulation of part of the gut wall can occur in a hernia which *later* reduces itself (Richter's hernia).
Intestinal obstruction may *not* cause vomiting until very late.
Localised perforation, and peritonitis going on later to generalised peritonitis, can occur when the bowel sounds and abdominal x-rays remain *absolutely normal.*
Any cause of severe abdominal pain, e.g. acute cholecystitis or pyelitis, may cause a reflex paralytic ileus—the abdominal x-ray may show multiple fluid levels but the gut is *not* usually distended.

Ileus may be caused by drugs and electrolyte disturbances.

Feel the femoral pulses and listen for bruits—abdominal aortic aneurysms can cause abdominal pain, as can a mesenteric embolus.

In a coloured patient, remember sickle-cell anaemia—the abdominal pain is usually due to infarcts in the mesentery or anterior abdominal wall—the gut sounds are often normal in the presence of quite severe pain.

Diabetic ketosis and porphyria may cause severe abdominal pain.

Always test the serum amylase—pancreatitis is surprisingly common *but* as a rule any cause of local or general peritonitis can cause a rise in the serum amylase to levels which are claimed to be diagnostic of pancreatitis. Pancreatitis does not always cause pain in the back.

Don't forget the rectal examination. Tenderness PR is *not* normal. If the patient is tender PR, peritonitis either localised or generalised is probably present.

Ask for a second opinion sooner rather than later.

Radiology of the Alimentary System

Chest X-ray

A dilated oesophagus is seen as a well-demarcated opacity continuous with the right upper mediastinum; in the lower chest it may cause a double outline to the right border of the heart. Within the dilated oesophagus there may be particles of food and fluid levels. Associated with a dilated oesophagus there may be evidence of aspiration pneumonia or consolidation in aspiration segments. Scleroderma may cause oesophageal narrowing with dilatation above as well as abnormal lung shadowing which is usually bilateral and which may progress to "honeycomb" lung.

A rolling hiatus hernia may cause an abnormal shadow with fluid levels behind the heart, a lateral film shows that the shadow is situated posteriorly. Rare types of diaphragmatic hernia may be seen in the chest x-ray: one is herniation through the foramen of Morgagni,[13] which is situated anteriorly and is an area of weakness at the attachment of the diaphragm to the sternum; it occurs much more commonly on the right side; another is herniation through a patent foramen of Bochdalek,[14] which represents the embryonic pleuroperitoneal canals; it is usually left-sided and is frequently filled with loops of small intestine or colon. Also sometimes to be seen in the chest film are enlargement of liver or spleen, free gas under the diaphragm or absent or distorted gastric gas shadow due to hiatus hernia, large spleen or a tumour of the stomach.

Plain X-ray of the Abdomen

Certain structures should be routinely inspected as in the examination of the chest x-ray. The most important are the size of the liver, spleen, kidneys and psoas shadows (which become indistinct if there is fluid in the peritoneum). The plain x-ray allows the lumbar spine, pelvis, sacro-iliac joints and sometimes the hip joints to be assessed. The presence of calcification should be noted, particularly in relation to gall bladder, kidneys, pancreas, aorta and arteries: phleboliths and calcified lymph glands may be present. Care should be taken not to confuse swallowed radio-opaque pills, particularly those which contain iron or calcium, with pathological calcification. In the pelvis calcification may be seen in large uterine fibroids, ovarian dermoid cysts, vesical calculi, prostate and the bladder wall in schistosomiasis.

The plain abdominal x-ray is most frequently required to assist in the diagnosis of an acute abdomen. Apart from the routine inspection of any x-ray, the following should be borne in mind with regard to the presence and diagnosis of an acute abdomen:

Fluid in the peritoneal cavity (ascites or peritonitis).—Fluid in the peritoneal cavity results in a general loss of definition of the shadows seen in the x-ray particularly of gas-filled bowel and psoas shadows. In the erect film the gas-filled bowel floats upwards and occupies a position under the diaphragm, and in the supine film the gas shadows usually appear more in the centre of the abdomen. Gas-filled loops of the bowel may be separated by a greater distance than normal.

Gas in the peritoneal cavity.—This is usually seen as a radio-translucent crescent under the diaphragm. As well as perforation, gas will be found in the peritoneal cavity following laparotomy, pneumoperitoneum and paracentesis abdominis.

Distension of part of the gut with or without fluid levels.—The radiological signs of obstruction are excessive dilatation with accumulation of fluids in the dilated loops of bowel. Fluid levels will be seen in x-rays taken in erect or lateral positions but not in the supine position. The gas that accumulates in obstructed bowel is probably due to swallowed air. In general, paralytic ileus involves much of the alimentary tract and fluid levels are numerous.

Abnormal calcification.—This may be helpful in the case of cholecystitis, impacted gall-stone causing intestinal obstruction, or ureteric calculus as the cause of the abdominal pain.

Enlarged viscus or intra-abdominal mass.—If seen on the plain film an intra-abdominal mass may be the clue to the diagnosis.

Two conditions give rise to localised paralytic ileus manifested by local dilatation of loops of bowel, these are arterial occlusion to part of the gut, and localised peritonitis, e.g. following acute appendicitis, cholecystitis, pancreatitis, salpingitis or ruptured ectopic pregnancy.

The approximate site of intestinal obstruction can sometimes be determined from the plain film. Large-bowel obstruction produces gas-filled loops of bowel around the edge of the x-ray although, of course, later, the changes of small-intestinal obstruction will become superimposed as the effects of the obstruction alter function higher in the intestines. The ileum generally occupies the central portion of the abdomen, and the jejunum the upper left quadrant. In ileal obstruction there are likely to be more dilated loops than in jejunal obstruction. The appearances of the gas-filled bowel may give an indication of the site of the obstruction. The jejunal mucosal folds lie very close together at right-angles to the long axis, and are easily seen when the jejunum is filled with gas. In the ileum the mucosal folds are sparse and flat and may not be seen.

Fibreoptic Endoscopy

The rapid improvement and increasing robustness of fibreoptic endoscopes has led to their rapid introduction into routine gastro-enterological practice. There can be little doubt that their use is now mandatory for the correct management of many gastro-intestinal conditions. Their very usefulness and the relative ease and comfort with which they can be passed poses logistic problems. The orthodox routine indications for endoscopy are still controversial, but it is generally accepted that about 30 per cent of patients with negative barium meals may have a significant lesion discovered by endoscopy. The available evidence suggests that endoscopy is generally unnecessary in patients who have a radiologically confirmed duodenal ulcer, but all patients with a gastric ulcer should have an endoscopic biopsy in case the ulcer is malignant.

Endoscopy should now be considered with radiology as an essential investigation in patients with acute gastro-intestinal bleeding and anastomotic ulcer symptoms. Radiology is unable to detect acute gastric erosions and about half of all anastomotic ulcers escape detection.

Gallium Scanning

There is now evidence that malignant tumours of the colon and rectum take up labelled gallium much more than normal tissue and ^{67}Gallium scans may be of value in identifying malignant, large-bowel tumours.

Faecal Occult Blood Tests

Three tests are used:

Haematest.—This is probably too sensitive, having a 70 per cent false positive ratio.

Occultest.—This is insensitive. At least 2 ml of blood are required to give a positive result.

Fecatest.—This has a sensitivity midway between Haematest and Occultest. To be sure that occult blood is not present, three negative stools should be obtained. If one of the three is positive, it may be worth re-examining the stool with the patient on a temporary meat-free diet. If in doubt a radioactive chromium-labelled red-cell test can be used to detect occult bleeding.

Peptic Ulcer

Incidence and Pathogenesis

The incidence of hospital admission for, and probably the total incidence of, duodenal ulceration is declining. Both duodenal and gastric ulcers are now commoner in social classes 4 and 5.

In duodenal ulcers there is evidence of an increase in gastrin production which increases acid production from the gastric parietal cells; there is also failure of the normal mechanism inhibiting gastrin secretion. Somatostatin is a hormone that occurs in the wall of the stomach, inhibiting the release of many hormones, including growth hormone, glucagon, insulin and gastrin. Gastrin is a generic name for several polypeptides of different sizes and activities. One variety of gastrin is more effective in promoting the secretion of intrinsic factor. Gastrin secretion is stimulated both by food in the stomach and by vagal action.

In addition, in duodenal ulcer there is evidence of an increase in the number and sensitivity of parietal acid-producing cells.

Race: in every country where studies have been made the incidence of duodenal ulcer is always higher than gastric ulcer. However, in some countries the incidence of gastric ulcer is higher than in this country, e.g. Japan, parts of India and Finland. Chronic peptic ulcers are almost unknown in the South African Bantus.

Known aetiological factors:

Zollinger-Ellison syndrome
Cushing's syndrome
Hyperparathyroidism
Cirrhosis—portal and biliary
Severe burns
Septicaemia
Coma.

There is also increased incidence in other diseases, e.g. emphysema, chronic bronchitis, pulmonary tuberculosis, rheumatoid arthritis and atherosclerosis.

Heredity: there is often a strong family history in cases of peptic ulceration. Ulceration in the same site is common in the same and succeeding generations. Blood group O, plus non-secretion of blood group substances in the exocrine secretions, is associated with a higher incidence of duodenal ulceration; this applies particularly to anastomotic ulcers following partial gastrectomy, or vagotomy plus drainage. Carcinoma of the stomach is associated with non-secretion in blood group A people.

Smoking: the incidence of peptic ulcers is lower in non-smokers.

Personality: the incidence of duodenal ulcers is higher in anxiety-prone personalities and in people with responsible jobs.

Drugs: Many drugs produce dyspepsia and an increased incidence of gastric bleeding; the same drugs may exacerbate an already present peptic ulcer, but there is little evidence that in normal doses drugs cause ulcers. Aspirin in *high* doses taken *continuously* in women may cause gastric ulcer.

Drugs which may produce dyspepsia and bleeding are:

Aspirin
Steroids
Phenylbutazone
Indomethacin
Non-steroidal, anti-inflammatory drugs.

Gastric ulcers are associated with a lower-than-normal acid secretion; they are more common if there is chronic gastritis and are *much* commoner if there is a coexisting duodenal ulcer. This may be because the duodenal ulcer delays gastric emptying, promoting stasis and damage to the gastric epithelium resulting in gastric atrophy and loss of mucosal resistance. Distortion of the pylorus by the duodenal ulcer may also lead to reflux of bile into the stomach which can also damage the gastric mucosa. Because duodenal ulcers promote gastric stasis which may lead to reflux oesophagitis, symptoms of reflux oesophagitis are common with a chronic duodenal ulcer.

Treatment of Peptic Ulceration

H_2 **receptor antagonists.**—These drugs reduce the effect of gastrin and pentagastrin (a synthetic analogue of gastrin) on the acid-producing parietal cells. Because of the failure of the older antihistamines to affect gastric acidity, Black postulated the existence of two types of histamine receptors: those blocked by older antihistamines and those blocked by cimetidine. Cimetidine is undoubtedly beneficial in healing duodenal ulcers, but there is evidence of a high relapse rate when the drug is stopped, and it may have to be given continuously; there are also doubts about its long-term side-effects, particularly hepatocellular damage, impotence, drowsiness, confusion and gynaecomastia. All gastric ulcers should be checked by repeat barium meal and endoscopy for complete healing; this does not apply to duodenal ulcers: chronic scarring of the duodenal cap means that no ulcer crater, oedema or fresh scarring can usually be demonstrated on a barium meal in an acute exacerbation of duodenal ulcer symptoms.

No medical measures have been shown to prevent relapse of peptic ulceration; medical treatment is directed towards symptomatic relief and promotion of healing. The main forms of medical treatment are:

Bed rest.—Symptoms of both gastric and duodenal origin disappear more rapidly with bed rest; however, only gastric ulcers have been shown to heal more rapidly with bed rest and there is no evidence that duodenal ulcers are affected.

Smoking.—There is some evidence that stopping smoking promotes the healing of gastric ulcers. There is no evidence with regard to duodenal ulcer or whether stopping smoking prevents relapse of ulcers.

Diet.—The evidence is that milk and milk products are no more beneficial than a diet of the patient's own choosing. Maximum acidity occurs when meals are taken at hourly or four-hourly intervals; the optimum interval between meals is about two hours. These findings have been confirmed.

Antacids.—Most of the effective antacids only reduce the acidity of the stomach for about twenty minutes, although they usually relieve the pain of peptic ulceration for much longer. Sodium bicarbonate is the most effective alkali—its main disadvantage is that it is absorbed from the stomach and may give rise to alkalosis. Calcium carbonate does not cause systemic alkalosis but may cause hypercalcaemia and the milk-alkali syndrome. Magnesium oxide is the third most effective antacid but magnesium salts produce diarrhoea; this can be counteracted by giving calcium salts, which tend to constipate, at the same time. Other antacids are much less effective; magnesium trisilicate is about one-tenth as effective as sodium bicarbonate and 300 ml of aluminium hydroxide gel is equivalent to about 5 g of sodium bicarbonate.

Prolonged medical treatment of peptic ulcers with high doses of alkalis and milk (which contains large amounts of calcium) may lead to renal damage with retention of calcium, albuminuria and a raised blood urea, which are the hallmarks of the milk-alkali syndrome. There is usually nephrocalcinosis and sometimes nephrolithiasis; polyuria may occur due to the raised calcium and blood urea. Associated nausea and vomiting with ulcer pain may suggest an exacerbation of the peptic ulcer.

Anticholinergic drugs.—These drugs are atropine-like in their activity and act on the stomach by reducing its motility and preventing vagal-induced acid secretion. They often effectively relieve ulcer symptoms but do not accelerate healing. There are three absolute contra-indications to the use of anticholinergic drugs, namely, a history of acute glaucoma, prostatism and pyloric stenosis. Side-effects are those of atropine, i.e. blurred vision, dry mouth, tachycardia and paralytic ileus.

Carbenoxolone (Biogastrone).—This has been shown to be effective in the healing of gastric ulcers. It usually causes fluid retention and potassium depletion, which should be treated with a thiazide diuretic and liberal potassium supplements. It is generally agreed that a gain in weight of over 4 lb in six weeks is an indication for diuretic treatment. The drug should not be used in the presence of renal disease, hypertension or cardiac failure. A specially coated form of carbenoxolone is available for the treatment of duodenal ulcers.

Complications of peptic ulcers include:

Haematemesis and melaena	Penetration and fistulae
Perforation	Malignant change
Pyloric stenosis	Milk-alkali syndrome.

Management of Haematemesis and Melaena

About a quarter of peptic ulcers are complicated by haemorrhage. The tendency to bleed is greatest in the first year after an ulcer develops; thereafter, the likelihood of haemorrhage is the same throughout the disease. The mortality from haemorrhage is higher in chronic than acute ulcers and is much higher over the age of 50. Over 95 per cent of bleeding from the upper gastro-intestinal tract is due to peptic ulceration; however, most of the problems of management involve the exclusion of causes other than chronic ulceration.

The bleeding which follows salicylate ingestion is due to acute gastric erosion. The chance of bleeding with salicylates is no greater in patients with a peptic ulcer or a previous history of dyspepsia. Some haemorrhage is said to occur in 50–70 per cent of patients taking aspirin. Bleeding is much less with enteric-coated tablets but absorption is delayed so that they are only useful for long-term treatment—they will not relieve pain quickly, which is the commonest reason for taking aspirin. The treatment of haemorrhage due to salicylates includes the administration of vitamin K, because salicylates lower the blood level of prothrombin as well as reducing platelet aggregation. There is little evidence that cimetidine influences the outcome when bleeding is due to oesophageal varices, gastric erosions or peptic ulceration.

The main diagnostic difficulty in the management of haematemesis is the exclusion of oesophageal varices. The history is sometimes helpful; apart from a history of alcoholism or recurrent liver failure, exposure to many industrial chemicals results in liver damage and portal hypertension. A previous history of chronic dyspepsia is important in helping to decide the site of bleeding; however, the incidence of peptic ulcers in cirrhotics is higher than in the general population. The finding of splenomegaly or other signs of portal hypertension is the most useful pointer to bleeding varices; associated signs of hepatocellular failure should always be looked for. A barium meal should be performed as early as practicable following an upper gastro-intestinal haemorrhage. Ideally, endoscopy should be performed as soon as possible to establish the site of the haemorrhage. There is no evidence that an emergency barium meal predisposes to further haemorrhage. Oesophageal varices are demonstrated in about 70 per cent of cases in which they are present. In about a quarter of cases in which bleeding is due to a peptic ulcer, a barium meal does not reveal an ulcer crater. If this negative barium meal is accompanied by a short or absent history of previous dyspepsia in a patient under the age of 50, than it is very likely that the bleeding is due to acute ulceration, which is accompanied by a low mortality when treated conservatively.

Long-standing peptic ulcers (particularly chronic gastric ulcers) are associated with a higher mortality when treated conservatively. The treatment of severe haemorrhage, whatever the cause, is immediate blood transfusion, sedation, bed rest and feeding small, frequent meals after a period of 24 hours after bleeding has stopped. If haemorrhage from the stomach is continuous or repeated it may be helpful to pass a Ryle's tube. Occasionally bleeding continues because the stomach is distended with clot. This should be evacuated with ice-cold water. Rarely, in a desperate situation, adrenaline and thrombin in methyl cellulose instilled into the stomach may stop bleeding.

If bleeding has been severe it is wise to set up a central venous pressure line; a fall in CVP may be the first sign that a second bleed has occurred.

The problems of transfusion of large amounts of blood should be borne in mind, namely:

> Circulatory overload
> Potassium intoxication
> Hypocalcaemia (due to citrate anticoagulant in the blood chelating the calcium in the body)
> Hypercoagulation states
> Serum hepatitis and other infections
> Air embolism
> Allergic and febrile reactions
> Mismatched blood

Surgical Treatment

Acute bleeding ulcers in patients under the age of 50 are usually treated conservatively. In patients over the age of 50 who have chronic ulcers, and recurrent or sustained bleeding, emergency laparotomy is performed. The procedure carried out at laparotomy varies; all the procedures involve oversewing a small ulcer or removing or oversewing a large ulcer. The three forms of treatment currently in vogue for both bleeding duodenal and gastric ulcers are:

1. Partial gastrectomy
2. Vagotomy and antrectomy (to remove the gastrin-secreting portion of the stomach and pylorus)
3. Vagotomy and pyloroplasty.

If at operation no ulcer or single bleeding point is seen or palpated, the stomach and duodenum are inspected internally, either by performing a gastrostomy or by inserting a sigmoidoscope and inflating the stomach. If the bleeding is due to acute erosions and is not life-threatening no further operation is performed; if no bleeding points are seen partial gastrectomy is usually carried out.

Perforation.—There are three phases of the clinical picture following perforation. The first is the dramatically sudden onset of intense abdominal pain accompanied by rigidity and guarding; the pulse rate and blood pressure are normal and bowel sounds are absent. The second stage or stage of delusion develops when abdominal pain subsides and the patient seems to be improving—but the abdomen remains rigid. The third stage is that of generalised peritonitis. Two factors modify the clinical picture, the first is a small perforation which becomes localised by omentum or adhesions; the second is perforation in the elderly, in whom the clinical picture may be less severe in the early stages. Once the diagnosis has been made, laparotomy should be performed without delay. If the perforation is small it can be sutured; if large, a partial gastrectomy is usually performed. Careful conservative treatment of acute perforation in highly selected cases is occasionally used; with correct selection of patients the mortality is much the same as for emergency laparotomy.

Pyloric stenosis.—Pyloric stenosis is almost invariably due to scarring secondary to a duodenal ulcer or to a carcinoma of the stomach; only rarely does a gastric prepyloric ulcer lead to pyloric stenosis. Benign gastric ulcers usually occur on the lesser curve of the stomach, hence an ulcer in the prepyloric region should be presumed to be malignant until proved to be benign (by gastroscopy, repeat negative barium meal, or intragastric photography).

With the development of pyloric stenosis the symptoms of duodenal ulcer usually change. The delay in gastric emptying leads to secondary ulceration of the stomach, and the increased intragastric pressure may lead to reflux oesophagitis. The symptoms of gastric ulcer and peptic oesophagitis often become superimposed on those of the duodenal ulcer. Repeated vomiting leads to gastric distension and electrolyte changes. The narrowing of the pylorus is due to fibrosis or oedema in relation to the nearby ulcer; in addition, spasm of the muscle of the pyloric canal probably occurs as well. The diagnosis is suggested by the history of changed symptoms, vomiting, recent weight loss and constipation. Physical signs include visible gastric peristalsis and distension, succussion splash, dehydration and alkalosis. The alkalosis may be aggravated by the administration of antacids, and may cause a lowering of the ionised calcium in the serum and cause either latent or overt tetany which may be accompanied by a positive Chvostek's[15] or Trousseau's[16] sign. Tetany may also be caused by potassium loss due to the repeated vomiting. The alkalosis that occurs is due to loss of hydrogen ion in the vomit; secondary uraemia may occur due to dehydration, or potassium or sodium depletion damaging the kidneys. Despite the alkalosis the urine may be acid if hydrogen ion is excreted in order to conserve potassium. Anticholinergic drugs are definitely contra-indicated, as they reduce gastric motility and hence further impair gastric emptying.

In the management of pyloric stenosis, gastric aspiration is performed intermittently or continuously—this reduces the friability of the stomach should operation be necessary. If the volume of juice aspirated after an overnight fast exceeds 500 ml the diagnosis is confirmed.

If most of the pyloric obstruction is due to inflammatory oedema the symptoms should subside in 2–3 days. Operation is indicated if: (i) the vomiting persists more than three days, (ii) more than 500 ml is repeatedly aspirated from the stomach after overnight fasting, (iii) the barium meal reveals a distended stomach with narrowing of the pyloric canal so that the lumen is less than 3 mm.

Occasionally, long-standing pyloric stenosis presents in unusual ways:

> Diarrhoea probably due to multiplication of organisms in the poorly emptying stomach
> Nephrocalcinosis and tubular damage due to prolonged alkalosis, hypokalaemia and hyponatraemia
> Mental changes due to hyponatraemia.

Penetration.—Chronic peptic ulcers may penetrate any adjacent organ; however, the commonest is the pancreas, and the ulcer is usually situated on the posterior wall of the stomach or duodenum. Perforation should be suspected if the ulcer symptoms become severe and continuous. There is usually evidence of pancreatic inflammation (continuous back pain and raised serum amylase). Barium meal may show barium in the penetrating ulcer or fistula.

Malignant change.—This does not occur with duodenal ulcers but occurs occasionally in long-standing gastric ulcers. It is important to note that carcinoma may undergo peptic ulceration and it is frequently impossible to say which came first.

Elective Operation for Peptic Ulceration

The main factors influencing a decision for elective operation for peptic ulcer are:

The presence of complications of peptic ulceration weighs heavily in favour of surgery. Following haemorrhage, operation is advisable over the age of 50; below this age it is acceptable to wait to see if bleeding recurs. Perforated ulcers which have been sutured require elective surgery if there is recurrence of ulcer symptoms. Organic pyloric stenosis and a long ulcer history are strong indications for surgery.

Failed medical treatment.—Recurrence of symptoms after a prolonged course of medical treatment, no further relief of pain with alkalis, interruption of sleep, frequent time off work, or a long history of frequent relapse favour surgery.

Chronic gastric ulcers, particularly if there is doubt as to whether they are benign or malignant.

There is considerable variation as to what operation should be performed to promote healing and prevent recurrence of ulcers. Duodenal ulcers are associated with a high output of hydrochloric acid which is controlled by gastrin secretion from the antrum of the stomach and by the vagi. If the acid output by the stomach is very high, both section of the vagi (vagotomy) and removal of the gastrin-producing part of the stomach (antrectomy) are necessary. Lesser degrees of hyperchlorhydria can be treated by vagotomy alone; however, section of the vagi reduces the motility of the stomach and the operation must be accompanied by some form of "drainage procedure". The drainage may be by enlarging the pyloric canal (pyloroplasty) or a side-to-side anastomosis between the stomach and the jejunum (gastro-jejunostomy). The advantage of pyloroplasty or antrectomy over gastro-jejunostomy is that there is no "blind loop", although it is not always possible to perform a pyloroplasty or antrectomy if there is severe scarring, and they are less suitable procedures than gastro-jejunostomy for very sick patients. The recurrence rate of duodenal ulcer following any vagotomy and drainage procedure is higher than with partial gastrectomy; in addition there are ill effects from sectioning the vagi, viz., diarrhoea, which is usually but not always temporary, and disturbances of the motility of stomach and oesophagus which leads to a feeling of fullness, belching and dysphagia in some patients.

Which Vagotomy?

There are three types of vagotomy:

1. Truncal
2. Selective (i.e. branches supplying the stomach are cut)
3. Proximal gastric (i.e. only fibres supplying the acid-secreting mucosa are cut).

The proximal gastric vagotomy is more difficult and time-consuming to perform, but because innervation of the remainder of the stomach is kept intact the operation need not be accompanied by a drainage procedure. Recurrent ulceration may be more frequent with this type of operation but postoperative diarrhoea and metabolic disturbances appear to be less frequent.

Some surgeons still prefer to perform a Pólya[17] partial gastrectomy for duodenal ulcer, in which the gastric stump is sutured to a jejunostomy and there is a blind loop through which bile can drain. The difference between a Pólya partial gastrectomy and a gastro-jejunostomy is that in the gastro-jejunostomy a side-to-side anastomosis is performed but the pylorus and duodenum are left intact, so that stomach contents can either pass through the duodenum or straight from the stomach to jejunum. In the Pólya gastrectomy the first part of the duodenum together with the distal stomach is removed and the remainder of the stomach is anastomosed to jejunum; the duodenum is closed proximal to the ampulla of Vater[18] so that bile can still reach the intestines. Resection of part of the stomach and the blind loop have their own problems, but the rate of recurrence of duodenal ulceration is much less; the duodenal ulcer itself is resected and vagotomy can always be performed later if necessary.

For gastric ulcers a Billroth[19] I partial gastrectomy is favoured by most surgeons. The first part of the duodenum, pylorus and antrum are removed and a gastro-duodenal anastomosis performed. Anastomotic or recurrent ulcers do not usually occur after partial gastrectomy for gastric ulcer, but are more likely after partial gastrectomy for duodenal ulcer—the incidence is 1–2 per cent.

Complications of Partial Gastrectomy

The immediate complications are those of any abdominal operation. Within a few weeks of the operation other complications may occur.

Early dumping syndrome.—After a meal there is a sensation of epigastric fullness and nausea, accompanied by faintness, sweating and palpitations. Many mechanisms have been held responsible for these symptoms. The main ones are:

Rapid distension of the jejunum;

Hypovolaemia caused by rapid flow of water from the extracellular fluid as a result of rapid transit of gastric contents with a high osmotic pressure into the jejunum. Attempts have been made to infuse fluid intravenously at the time fluid is being lost into the jejunum, in order to maintain the blood volume. Also insulin (or tolbutamide) has been give before the meal to lower the blood sugar and encourage more rapid absorption of carbohydrate from the jejunum, thus preventing the outpouring of fluid into the jejunum.

Failure of peripheral arterioles to constrict in response to rapid diversion of blood flow to splanchnic areas.

Late dumping syndrome.—This is due to hypoglycaemia. Soon after food reaches the jejunum there is rapid absorption of carbohydrates leading to an increase in blood sugar which stimulates insulin secretion. If too much insulin is secreted there will be an overswing and hypoglycaemia will occur. The attacks usually occur 2–4 hours after a meal but may appear much earlier. They generally diminish in severity in the course of time.

Afferent or blind-loop syndrome.—This consists of a feeling of fullness and nausea, relieved by vomiting almost pure bile. It is suggested that there is transient obstruction of the blind loop into which the bile and pancreatic ducts open. The obstruction is due to mechanical distortion and is relieved when vomiting of the contents of the blind loop occurs. Sometimes the dumping syndrome is superimposed on the blind-loop syndrome. The treatment is surgical and usually consists in converting the operation to a Billroth I type gastrectomy and adding a vagotomy.

Stomal (anastomotic) ulceration.—The incidence varies from 1 to 15 per cent in different series, and depends on the type of partial gastrectomy. It is much less with a Pólya than with a Billroth I partial gastrectomy. The presenting features are pain induced by food, haematemesis and melaena or iron deficiency anaemia, with persistently positive occult blood in the stools. Sometimes pain is entirely absent. It is usually difficult to demonstrate an ulcer crater on the barium meal, although gastroscopy occasionally helps. The stoma may be more rigid than normal due to local scarring; diagnosis is often very difficult if pain is absent or slight and the barium meal reveals no abnormality. The finding of persistent occult blood is highly suggestive. Anastomotic ulcers do not usually heal by medical means; operation is technically much more difficult than the original partial gastrectomy. The operation usually consists of vagotomy, with or without attention to the stoma. When anastomotic ulceration recurs following vagotomy the completeness of the vagotomy can be tested by the insulin test. Measurement of the gastric acid also helps—if the acid output is high anastomotic ulceration is more likely.

Weight loss.—Most patients lose weight following a partial gastrectomy. It is more marked following a Pólya partial gastrectomy and vagotomy with drainage than following a Billroth I partial gastrectomy. The most important cause is probably a diminished intake of food. Because of the reduced size of the stomach the patient feels full after only a small meal; the dumping syndrome may make the patient afraid to eat. Chronic iron deficiency anaemia and superficial gastritis following partial gastrectomy both reduce the appetite. Occasionally malnutrition of protein leading to a kwashiorkor-like state may dominate the clinical picture.

Malabsorption and steatorrhoea.—The main causes for malabsorption of fat following partial gastrectomy are:

> Imperfect mixing of pancreatic juice with contents of jejunum
> Too rapid a delivery of food to the small intestine with too rapid transit
> Reduced pancreatic and biliary flow
> Bypassing of upper duodenum (in the case of a Pólya partial gastrectomy)
> Stagnant-loop syndrome. Several strains of the bacteroides group of bacteria which may colonise a stagnant loop can deconjugate bile salts. Deconjugated bile salts are less efficient at emulsifying fats and they are also toxic to the mucosa of the small bowel.

Iron deficiency.—Over 50 per cent of patients develop iron deficiency anaemia following partial gastrectomy; this is usually preceded by a low serum iron and a raised iron-binding capacity. There are several reasons why iron deficiency occurs: pre-operative haemorrhages deplete the iron stores, intermittent blood loss may continue after operation, the upper duodenum is the main site of iron absorption and this may be bypassed. Achlorhydria is associated with diminished absorption of iron, but this may be reversed by ascorbic acid and other reducing substances.

Vitamin B$_{12}$ deficiency.—The incidence of megaloblastic anaemia following partial gastrectomy is about 7 per cent, and incidence of a low serum B$_{12}$ about 15 per cent. Occasionally, subacute combined degeneration occurs in the absence of anaemia or megaloblastic changes in the bone marrow. The usual cause of B$_{12}$ deficiency is failure of absorption of B$_{12}$ due to lack of intrinsic factor because of atrophy of the remaining part of the stomach; occasionally it is due to a stagnant loop. Very rarely, the diet is deficient in vitamin B$_{12}$.

Patients who have a low serum B_{12}, or megaloblastic bone marrow without anaemia, should be given regular B_{12} because there may be an improved sense of well-being and a gain in weight as well as a reversal of the megaloblastic marrow abnormality.

Folic acid deficiency.—This is much rarer than iron deficiency and B_{12} deficiency following partial gastrectomy; it is probably due to inadequate intake of folate. This may improve if the appetite is increased with iron and B_{12}.

Bone disease.—Osteomalacia is commoner than osteoporosis and occurs in 1–3 per cent of patients following a partial gastrectomy. The distinction between osteoporosis and osteomalacia is difficult, particularly as the two frequently coexist. Pseudo-fractures only occur in osteomalacia, as do biochemical disturbances; so that diminished calcium and phosphorus levels in the serum (with a raised urinary excretion of phosphorus if there is secondary hyperparathyroidism) and an elevated serum alkaline phosphatase, indicate osteomalacia; however, osteomalacia can be present even if the blood biochemistry is normal. In addition bone biopsy may show widening of the osteoid seams.

Osteoporosis should only by diagnosed on x-ray—a lateral x-ray of the lumbar spine is by far the most useful. Osteoporosis may follow a long-continued negative calcium balance. The main causes of post-gastrectomy bone disease are:

Decreased intake of calcium, vitamin D and protein
Steatorrhoea
Altered pH of duodenum—calcium absorption is favoured by an acid pH.

Treatment consists of prophylaxis with calcium and vitamin D, and yearly check-ups at a post-gastrectomy clinic. Treatment of the established condition is with calcium, vitamin D and anabolic steroids. A satisfactory way of dealing with post-gastrectomy problems is for all patients to be seen yearly at a post-gastrectomy clinic and to be given courses of iron, vitamin D, folic acid and vitamin B_{12} for one month every year (the most suitable month is the one in which the patient's birthday falls).

GASTRITIS

The two most important forms of gastritis clinically are acute gastritis due to ingested irritants, and atrophic or chronic gastritis. Two rare forms of gastritis are "acute infective" due to invasion of the stomach walls by organisms, and "giant rugal hypertrophy" (Ménétrier's disease). One condition which frequently gives rise to confusion is "hypertophic gastritis"; this term is usually given to a radiological appearance in which the mucosal folds of the stomach appear prominent, and it is usually associated with the presence of a duodenal ulcer. Histologically the abnormally large mucosal folds are normal, although occasionally such coarse folds are seen in patients suffering from dyspepsia, in whom no ulcer is found.

Acute Gastritis

This consists of rapid exfoliation of surface epthelial cells, and infiltration with inflammatory cells. It is not usually accompanied by bleeding as in the case of alcoholic gastritis. Similar changes occur in the gastric mucosa in some febrile illness and in staphylococcal gastro-enteritis. Acute gastritis may be accompanied by haemorrhage when it is due to aspirin ingestion.

Atrophic (Chronic) Gastritis

In its most severe form this is seen in pernicious anaemia. It is also common in people over 40, particularly cigarette smokers, in people who drink hot fluids, in association with heavy alcohol consumption, and in gastric carcinoma. The incidence of gastric ulcer is higher in patients with atrophic gastritis than in the normal population. The exact relationship between atrophic gastritis and iron deficiency anaemia is not settled. The incidence of iron deficiency in patients with atrophic gastritis is higher than normal, but patients with atrophic gastritis are more liable to bleed. In a few patients with atrophic gastritis, achlorhydria and iron deficiency anaemia, correction of the anaemia results in return of the gastric mucosa to normal and normal secretion of acid. It is now generally accepted that atrophic gastritis probably predisposes to iron deficiency anaemia.

The radiological appearences of atrophic gastritis are:

> Tubular stomach with the greater and lesser curves roughly parallel
> "Bald" fundus with absent mucosal folds
> Thin mucosal folds on the greater curvature
> Active peristalsis
> Normal duodenal cap.

Megaloblastic Anaemia

Megaloblastic anaemias are almost always due to a deficiency of either vitamin B_{12} or folic acid. The ultimate cause of the megaloblastic blood picture in B_{12} and folate deficiency is reduced DNA synthesis in the cells of the bone marrow; vitamin B_{12} is necessary for the metabolism of folic acid, the end result of which is essential for normal DNA synthesis. B_{12} is also an essential coenzyme in transmethylation reactions. The accumulation of methyl tetrahydrofolic acid in B_{12} deficiency is referred to as the "methyl folate trap". B_{12} deficiency may result in folate deficiency because of the amount of methyl folate lost in the urine (Fig. 25).

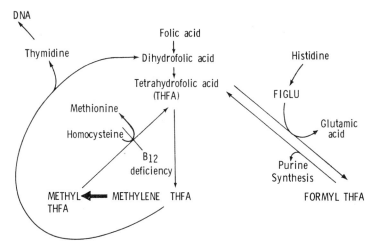

Fig. 25.—This shows the metabolism of folic acid and shows the mechanism of B_{12} deficiency causing an accumulation of methyl tetrahydrofolic acid (the "methyl folate" trap). Folic acid is necessary for the conversion of FIGLU to glutamic acid. Deficiency of folic acid leads to FIGLU accumulation.

The beneficial effect of vitamin B_{12} on subacute combined degeneration is due to actions other than its effect on folate metabolism or transmethylation. Folate is required for the metabolism of L histidine through formimino glutamic acid (FIGLU) to glutamic acid. Folate deficiency leads to an accumulation of FIGLU; this can be enhanced by giving the patient increased amounts of histidine. Increased excretion of FIGLU in the urine is used as a test of folate deficiency. In addition to its involvement in transmethylation in the folate metabolic pathway, vitamin B_{12} analogues are also involved in other transmethylation reactions, e.g. the B_{12} analogue coenzyme B_{12} is involved in the conversion of methyl malonyl coenzyme A to succinyl coenzyme A (Fig. 26) Another B_{12} analogue, known as methyl B_{12}, is involved in homocystein methylation to methionine, as well as the methylation of transfer RNA. Because of their involvement in DNA synthesis, deficiency of B_{12} or folate affects all dividing cells in the body, particularly those which are dividing the fastest, i.e. marrow, epithelial and intestinal cells. The effects of deficiencies on these cells are the cause of many of the observed manifestations of B_{12} and folate deficiency like atrophic gastritis and reversible small-intestinal malabsorption such as occurs in tropical sprue and pernicious anaemia.

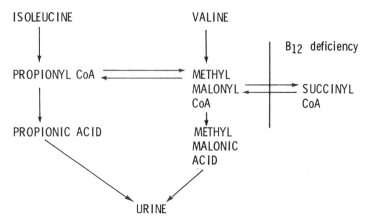

FIG. 26.—This shows the effect of vitamin B_{12} deficiency which leads to excess methyl malonic and propionic acid in the urine.

Physiology of Vitamin B_{12}

Vitamin B_{12} is present in most animal tissues but has to be synthesised by micro-organisms. Vitamin B_{12} is absorbed attached to intrinsic factor, a glycoprotein secreted by the parietal cells of the gastric mucosa. The complex is absorbed into the ileal mucosal cells and the B_{12} is then detached from intrinsic factor and reattached to a circulating transport globulin, transcobalamin II, which transports about 20 per cent of circulating B_{12}; it has a rapid turnover and is the transport protein which allows B_{12} to pass through the cell walls. In the systemic circulation B_{12} is also transported on transcobalamin I which is an alphaglobulin that binds B_{12} more firmly and releases it more slowly than transcobalamin II, and probably acts as a storage for B_{12}.

Transcobalamin I itself may be abnormal and bind B_{12} excessively, resulting in effective B_{12} deficiency but with normal circulating levels of B_{12}. Transcobalamin I is produced by the white cells and is present in excess in leukaemia and hepatomas.

Abnormalities of transcobalamin II also occur. B_{12} deficiency may also occur in the presence of normal amounts of circulating B_{12} because of failure to produce methyl B_{12}, which is the analogue essential for folate metabolism, while the level of hydroxycobalamin remains normal.

Pernicious Anaemia

Pernicious anaemia is due to a malabsorption of vitamin B_{12} because of a deficiency of intrinsic factor due almost invariably to gastric atrophy associated with circulating antibodies to intrinsic factor.

These IgG antibodies to intrinsic factor are of two types; *blocking* antibody, which prevents intrinsic factor combining with B_{12}, and *binding* antibody, which prevents the binding of intrinsic factor + B_{12} to the ileal absorption sites. The blocking antibody is present in about 60 per cent of patients, while both antibodies are present in about a third of patients. The stomach of patients with pernicious anaemia contains a third intrinsic factor antibody, which is an IgA. Intrinsic factor antibodies are also found in some patients with Graves' disease, and diabetes, and in relatives of patients with pernicious anaemia. Patients with pernicious anaemia also have raised titres of antibody to gastric parietal cells, and often antibodies to thyroid cytoplasm and thyroglobulin.

Clinical Features of Pernicious Anaemia

Vitamin B_{12} deficiency affects every system; the non-specific features such as malaise and anorexia usually respond dramatically to treatment with B_{12}, even before there is any improvement in haemoglobin concentration. Pernicious anaemia is not rare and shows striking geographical and regional variation. In the UK for example it is much commoner in Scotland than in South East England. It is important to appreciate that the symptoms may be very varied, e.g.:

Soreness of the tongue	Pyrexia
Diarrhoea	Yellowness of the skin
Dyspepsia	Weight loss
Paraesthesia	Oedema.

The physical signs are usually those of anaemia, often accompanied by slight hepatosplenomegaly. The signs of subacute combined degeneration are due to a mixture of peripheral neuropathy and posterior-column and pyramidal loss. The commonest features being numbness, paraesthesiae, mild ataxia, irritability, memory loss often with positive Rombergism, and posterior column loss. The reflex changes are variable and depend on which part of the nervous system is predominantly affected. A number of other diseases are sometimes associated with pernicious anaemia:

Carcinoma of the stomach (especially likely in men)
Iron deficiency
Diabetes mellitus
Vitiligo
Graves' disease
Rheumatoid arthritis
Addison's disease and hypoparathyroidism
Myasthenia gravis.

Diagnosis of B_{12} Deficiency

Blood picture.—There is increased size of erythrocytes (90 fl) which contain an *increased* amount of haemoglobin (32 pg) and fragmentation of cells resulting in poikilocytosis (pear shaped cells). There is also leucopenia with increased lobulation of granulocyte nuclei as well as inclusion bodies such as Howell-Jolly bodies.

Bone marrow.—Erythropoiesis is megaloblastic, which leads to increased reticulocytes and macrocytic erythrocytes. It is important to be aware that iron deficiency can completely mask the presence of megaloblastic erythropoiesis.

Serum B_{12}—This is now measured by saturation analysis in which the sample is mixed with a known amount of radioactive B_{12}; a B_{12} binder then picks up labelled and unlabelled (sample) B_{12} in the proportions they are present in the mixture. The higher the sample B_{12} the less labelled B_{12} will be picked up by the binder. There is considerable daily variation in B_{12} levels. Low B_{12} levels occur in pregnancy, folate deficiency and iron deficiency.

Coenzyme B_{12}—This is the coenzyme for conversion of methyl malonyl coenzyme A to succinyl coenzyme A. Deficiency of B_{12} will therefore lead to accumulation of methyl malonic acid. Valine can be used as a loading test to increase methyl malonic acid excretion. Other organic acids further back in methyl malonyl coenzyme A production may also accumulate in pernicious anaemia and be excreted in the urine (e.g. propionic and succinic acid).

Schilling test.—An oral dose of radioactive labelled vitamin B_{12} is given with a large dose of parenteral unlabelled B_{12}. If the oral dose has been absorbed, some will be excreted in the urine provided the patient is not already B_{12}-depleted; the purpose of the large, unlabelled dose of B_{12} is to ensure that the plasma-binding sites are all saturated with B_{12} so that the labelled B_{12} is free in the plasma (if absorbed) and will be excreted in the urine. The test can be repeated giving intrinsic factor with the oral labelled B_{12} if the patient has pernicious anaemia. This will improve absorption, and therefore excretion, of labelled B_{12}. If oral absorption of B_{12} is due to disease of the terminal ileum, intrinsic factor added to oral B_{12} will not increase absorption.

HIATUS HERNIA

These are of three types:

1. Sliding: the whole oesophago-gastric junction moves up into the chest. The symptoms are those of reflux oesophagitis and the size of the hernia is no guide to the severity of the symptoms.

2. Para-oesophageal: the fundus of the stomach herniates into the

chest alongside the gastro-oesophageal junction, which remains in the normal position. The main symptom is dysphagia.

3. Mixed sliding and para-oesophageal: this is commoner than the pure para-oesophageal. The symptoms are those of reflux oesophagitis and dysphagia.

The pain of hiatus hernia usually comes on when the patient is lying flat or bending forwards. It is almost invariably made worse by drinking hot fluids and this has been used as the basis of a clinical test for the presence of hiatus hernia—"the hot tea test". Relief of the pain with liquid alkalis is an important diagnostic feature. Like cardiac pain there may be relief with trinitrin. A large para-oesophageal hernia may displace the heart and give rise to ECG changes.

Complications include stricture formation, aspiration pneumonia, gastric ulceration within the hernia, and oesophageal ulceration. Bleeding from the hiatus hernia may be chronic and insidious or profuse. The indications for surgical treatment of hiatus hernia are:

> No systematic relief of the symptoms of oesophagitis after six months conservative treatment. The size of the hernia is of no importance
>
> Development of a gastric ulcer in a hernia after six months' treatment
>
> Development of a stricture
>
> Recurrent bleeding in a young person; in an old person conservative management of recurrent bleeding is usually satisfactory
>
> Occurrence of aspiration pneumonia
>
> Incarceration or strangulation of the hernia.

DYSPEPTIC SYMPTOMS

As with pain arising from any other site, certain specific points should be noted with abdominal pain or discomfort:

> Site
> Intensity
> Duration
> Character
> Constancy (whether continuous or colicky)
> Radiation
> Relieving factors
> Precipitating factors
> Periodicity (exacerbation and remissions)
> Associated features.

Oesophageal reflux is suggested by heartburn, burning pain on drinking hot fluids or dysphagia. A variety of symptoms has been described in duodenal ulcers, gastric ulcers and non-ulcer dyspepsia. The majority of patients with non-ulcer dyspepsia have either atrophic gastritis or a normal mucosa.

Salicylates

Several series show that 60–70 per cent of normal people have gastro-intestinal bleeding when they take salicylates. The available evidence suggests that this blood loss is much the same for all types of salicylate preparation, except that it may be less with enteric-coated aspirin. There is, of course, considerable delay between taking enteric-coated aspirin and absorption, hence they are not suitable for rapid relief of pain (the purpose for which most people take an aspirin). Furthermore, absorption is variable; enteric-coated salicylates are usually suitable for patients on long-term salicylates, provided that the degree of absorption is checked by a blood salicylate level at an appropriate time. There is no doubt that acute erosions can occur where particles of salicylate come into contact with the gastric mucosa, that the incidence of gastric ulcers is higher in women who habitually take salicylates and that the incidence of perforation of ulcers is higher in patients who take salicylates. It is also likely that patients who have a severe gastric haemorrhage after taking a small dose of salicylates have a hypersensitivity to them. Bleeding may occur from a large area of the gastric mucosa and is probably not always caused by simple erosions due to direct contact of particles of salicylate.

The amount and frequency of bleeding following ingestion of salicylates is not greater in patients who have an established peptic ulcer. Salicylates can produce gastro-intestinal bleeding when given parenterally. They can also cause thrombocytopenia and hypoprothrombinaemia. Vitamin K should always be given to patients whose gastric haemorrhage is assumed to be due to salicylates.

Corticosteroids

There is a widespread clinical belief that patients on long-term corticosteroids have a higher-than-usual incidence of gastro-intestinal haemorrhage and gastric perforation. However, many careful clinical surveys have failed to confirm these views, although it is agreed that patients with rheumatoid arthritis on steroids (and other ulcerogenic drugs) have a higher incidence of gastro-intestinal haemorrhage. The surveys also agree that although gastric perforation is no commoner than in normal people, the symptoms and signs of perforation are masked by steroids and this may lead to dangerous delay in making the diagnosis.

Gastro-enteritis and Infective Diarrhoea in Adults in the U.K.

The most important infective causes of diarrhoea in adults are:

Salmonella
Shigella[20] (bacillary dysentery)
Virus infections—probably the commonest cause of outbreaks of infective diarrhoea from which bacteria are not isolated
Amoebic dysentery
Pathogenic strains of *E. coli*—these are virtually confined to children under the age of 1 year
Rarities such as cholera
Bacterial contamination of food, e.g. staphylococcal and *Cl. botulinus* toxins. One common trap is to assume that a sudden onset of diarrhoea is infective in origin—remember, diarrhoea may be "spurious"—small amounts of liquid stool may be passed in a patient (not necessarily elderly) suffering from chronic constipation.

Other important causes of diarrhoea are:

Purgative abuse
Ulcerative colitis (or proctocolitis)
Crohn's disease
Diverticulitis
Spastic colon
Carcinoma

Management of Diarrhoea

Before starting symptomatic or specific treatment it is essential to try to establish the definitive cause or try to exclude certain possible causes if the precise cause cannot be found. This means that every case of sporadic diarrhoea of sudden onset for which no cause is known should have stools examined for ova, cysts and amoebae, and the stools cultured. In the majority of cases sigmoidoscopy should be performed particularly if the patient has lived abroad—amoebic dysentery is notorious as a cause of episodic attacks of diarrhoea. The amoebae may be excreted in the stool when the patient has no diarrhoea or the amoebae may not be seen although diarrhoea is severe. Sigmoidoscopy will often show the characteristic shallow ulcers in the colon.

Symptomatic Treatment of Diarrhoea

Absorbents—claimed to absorb the "toxins" in the bowel lumen, examples kaolin or pectin

Opiates—reduce peristalsis in the colon, examples codeine phosphate, morphia

Anticholinergic drugs—also reduce peristalsis in the colon.

The most suitable drugs for symptomatic treatment of diarrhoea are:

Kaolin and morph. BPC 15–30 ml 6-hourly

Codeine phosphate 15–30 mg 6-hourly.

There is no convincing evidence that proprietary drugs such as Lomotil have any advantage over the older and simpler remedies.

Specific Treatment

The most frequent clinical problems are patients with diarrhoea who have:

1. A stool culture which grows a *Salmonella* ("enteric fever") or a *Shigella* (bacillary dysentery) without evidence of systemic spread (fever, malaise, leucocytosis, elevated ESR), or complications such as severe dehydration.

2. Negative stool culture.

There is now general agreement, that, except for *Salmonella typhi*, *Shigella shigae* and *Sh. flexneri*, whatever organism is grown from the stool the patient should not receive antibiotics *unless there is evidence of systemic spread*. Antibiotics are potentially dangerous—they do not usually control the infection, they prolong the carrier state and they increase the chance of a subsequent relapse. The use of proprietary antibiotic-containing remedies such as Neovax, Neo Sulfazon and Entero-vioform is usually no more effective than symptomatic treatment, and these preparations may be potentially dangerous.

Systemic infection with *any* of the Salmonella organisms including *S. typhi*, *S. paratyphi*, *S. typhimurium*, etc. should be treated with chloramphenicol or ampicillin.

Systemic infection with any of the Shigella organisms should be treated with sulphonamides (sulphadimidine 2 g followed by 1 g 6-hourly) if the organism is sensitive (in the U.K. most strains of Shigella are now resistant to the sulphonamides). Other useful drugs are streptomycin, neomycin, nalidixic acid and the tetracyclines.

Diarrhoea may be severe enough to produce dehydration and electrolyte deficiencies; these should be treated with adequate replacement therapy.

The decision not to treat Shigella or Salmonella enteritis with antibiotics may be modified in the case of severely debilitated and old patients or in infection with rare virulent forms of Salmonella to Shigella.

In the event of an outbreak of infective diarrhoea (usually due to Shigella) scrupulous cleanliness is the most effective prophylactic treatment. There is nothing to be gained by giving prophylactic antibiotics to uninfected neighbouring patients.

Conclusion.—When diarrhoea persists or recurs following an acute attack of gastro-enteritis, consider the possibility of persisting infection or acquired disaccharide intolerance. Post-dysenteric diarrhoea is very common. Patients who have had proven amoebic dysentery in the past or who have lived in areas where it is endemic and who develop persistent diarrhoea for which no other cause can be found can justifiably be given a therapeutic trial of emetine if symptomatic treatment is not working. Infective diarrhoea should be treated symptomatically. Antibiotics should not be given, if infection is localised to the gastro-intestinal tract, for the majority of infections with Salmonella or Shigella organisms.

Diagnostic Difficulties with Diarrhoea

A proportion of patients with diarrhoea who have had routine gastro-enterological studies have no apparent cause established. The problem should be looked at again with the following points in mind:

> It is important to confirm the diarrhoea—a daily stool weight over 200 g per day on a normal diet indicates some malabsorption. This simple investigation is under-used; the unpleasantness of stool weighing can be mitigated by placing a polythene sheet in the lavatory bowl before defaecation, sealing and then weighing the bag.
>
> Have another careful look for abdominal scars indicating previous bowel surgery and possible fistula formation.
>
> *Acquired disaccharidase deficiency.* This may occur following an infective cause of gastro-enteritis. Usually symptoms only occur if the patient consumes more than 2 pints of milk a day. The diagnosis of lactase deficiency can be tested by showing a rise in blood sugar with 25 g of glucose and galactose separately (the two monosaccharides in the disaccharide lactose) but no rise with 50 g of lactose.
>
> *Purgative abuse.* Phenolphthalein derivatives can be detected by adding alkali to the stool and noting a pink colour, and senna derivatives by finding anthraquinone products in the urine.
>
> *Villous papilloma of the rectum.* These produce hypochloraemia and hypokalaemia.
>
> *Acute viral enteritis.* In adults this is due to rotavirus infection. It is usually a self-limiting disease, although world-wide it is

responsible for a considerable mortality. The diagnosis is made by finding the virus in the stool.

Pseudomembranous colitis. In this condition diarrhoea occurs 2–3 weeks after antibiotics are stopped and is due to infection with *Clostridium difficile*. Like all clostridia, *Cl. difficile* produces an exotoxin; this causes the ulcers. The commonest causative antibiotic is clindamycin but the infection can occur following other antibiotics such as ampicillin and the cephalosporins. The diagnosis is made by finding the characteristic ulcers on rectal biopsy. Treatment is with antibiotics to which the organism is sensitive (usually vancomycin, metronidazole or tetracycline).

Campylobacter enteritis. This organism is a relatively common cause of diarrhoea particularly in children. It is a difficult organism to culture unless a specific medium is used. It is common in those who work closely with animals. The presenting features are usually bloody diarrhoea and severe abdominal pain usually following a prodromal influenza-like illness. It is usually a self-limiting disease but should always be treated to prevent septicaemia and excretion of the organisms. The treatment of choice is erythromycin.

Whipple's[21]-disease (intestinal lipodystrophy). This is a rare condition due to an infecting organism which has not yet been clearly identified. The lymphatics of the wall of the small bowel are filled with foamy macrophages. The condition is characterised by generalised as well as gastro-intestinal features. In addition to diarrhoea and steatorrhoea there may be pigmentation, lymphadenopathy, non-erosive arthritis, pericarditis, pleural effusion and cerebral damage (it is a rare cause of treatable dementia). The diagnosis is made on the basis of the small-bowel histological appearances.

INTESTINAL MALABSORPTION

This is one of the conditions where a high index of suspicion is essential. Steatorrhoea is not a *sine qua non* of malabsorption—only the more severe cases have any alteration in frequency or consistency of the stool or an increased excretion of faecal fat. Deficient absorption of single substances may lead to isolated symptoms, and for this reason intestinal malabsorption should be suspected in any of the following:

> Iron deficiency anaemia particularly if it is unresponsive to iron therapy
> Loss of weight

Hypoproteinaemia
Raised alkaline phosphatase
Recurrent aphthous ulceration or soreness of the tongue
Osteoporosis, osteomalacia or tetany
Macrocytic anaemia
Diarrhoea and abdominal discomfort
Hypokalaemia
Following partial gastrectomy

Two screening tests used most frequently to exclude malabsorption are the xylose excretion test and the estimation of faecal fat excretion. Following a 25 g oral dose of d-xylose at least 5 g should be excreted in the urine in the next five hours. In malabsorption usually less than 2 g is excreted; the test is of less value if there is delay in gastric emptying, renal impairment or if there is severe diarrhoea and a very rapid transit time through the small intestine. It is not valid in people over the age of 65. In a few patients the 25 g dose gives rise to diarrhoea so that a 5 g dose is sometimes advocated. Xylose is not digested in the gut and is absorbed by passive diffusion, there is no active phosphorylation and it is not absorbed across a concentration gradient.

A normal person on a normal diet rarely excretes more than 6 g of fat per day in the stools. For this reason the daily faecal fat excretion in the stools collected for a 3-day period on a ward diet is a reasonably reliable indication as to the presence of steatorrhoea. The use of continuous markers such as cuprous thiocyanate is common in metabolic wards. The principle is that the patient takes a known amount of marker per day and once a steady excretion rate of marker is obtained the fat content and marker content of a faecal sample can be related to daily fat excretion. These are the most acceptable screening tests although other investigations may be necessary to confirm the diagnosis:

Barium meal follow-through.—The main features in steatorrhoea are a delayed transit time, dilatation of loops in the small bowel (calibre of jejunum more than 3·0 cm is abnormal); in later films the barium flocculates.

Flocculation, clumping and scattering are due to excessive amounts of mucus in the small intestine. The purpose of using non-flocculating barium is because similar appearances may be seen in normal people if ordinary barium is used.

Peroral jejunal biopsy.—Abnormal appearances are:

(i) *Subtotal villous atrophy* in which there is almost total loss of villi and all that remains is the crypts between the villi.

(ii) *Partial villous atrophy* is intermediate between subtotal villous atrophy and normals.

There is often *no* correlation between the severity of the mucosal lesion as judged histologically and the degree of malabsorption. It is important that other histological features suggesting malabsorption should be present before implicating reduced villous height as evidence of malabsorption. These are:

>Increased mucosal thickness
>Decreased epithelial surface cell height
>Inflammatory cell infiltration of mucosa and submucosa.

Other investigations are necessary to establish the extent to which different substances are not being absorbed and the general nutritional status of the patient. The most important ones are:

>Serum levels of iron, vitamin B_{12} and folic acid
>Tests of ability to absorb vitamin B_{12} (Schilling test), and folic acid (FIGLU test). Folic acid is almost always reduced in steatorrhoea, particularly gluten-sensitive enteropathy and tropical sprue.
>Serum level of bone alkaline phosphatase, calcium and phosphate. X-ray of bones to find evidence of osteoporosis or osteomalacia. Tetany may occur if the level of ionised calcium falls critically
>Serum proteins
>Serum electrolytes, of which potassium is the most important. Rarely, hypokalaemia may lead to secondary paralytic ileus
>Glucose tolerance test. The curve is flat in intestinal malabsorption; it is very occasionally of diabetic type if malabsorption is due to pancreatic failure and loss of islet cells
>Prothrombin time, to detect malabsorption of vitamin K
>Vitamin A absorption is almost always impaired in steatorrhoea and vitamin A absorption tests can be used to confirm the diagnosis. Serum carotene levels are also low in fat malabsorption.

Causes of Malabsorption

Loss of Functional Epithelium (Villous Atrophy)

Gluten sensitive enteropathy
Idiopathic steatorrhoea
Disaccharide intolerance
Stagnant loop syndrome
Coeliac syndrome
Infestations which destroy the mucosa, e.g. *Giardia lamblia* and *ankylostoma duodenale*
Drug damage: phenindione, neomycin and other antibiotics, phenolphthalein, colchicine, PAS, folic acid antagonists and irradiation.

Infiltration of the Wall of the Small Intestine

Crohn's disease
Scleroderma
Amyloid disease
Whipple's disease
Reticulosis.

Damage to Vascular Supply or Disturbance of Motility

Superior mesenteric artery occlusion
Polyarteritis nodosa
SLE
Diabetes
Congestive heart failure
Constrictive pericarditis.

Short-circuiting of Small Intestine

Gastrocolic fistula.

Resection of Small Intestine

Diminished Splitting of Food due to Lack of Digestive Juice

Pancreatic insufficiency
Obstructive jaundice or liver failure.

Diminished Splitting of Food due to Inadequate Mixing with Digestive Juices

Partial gastrectomy.

Diminished Splitting of Food due to Inactivation of Digestive Juice

Zollinger-Ellison syndrome.

Disaccharide Intolerance

Deficiency of enzymes which split disaccharides into their constituent monosaccharides may occur as an inborn error of metabolism. The disaccharide most frequently involved is lactose, whose constituent monosaccharides are glucose and galactose. Disaccharides cannot be absorbed unless they are split into monosaccharides. The undigested disaccharides are fermented by intestinal bacteria producing irritant organic acids; these, together with the osmotic effect of the sugar leads to diarrhoea which is very acidic. The symptoms are diarrhoea with a high content of lactic acid, abdominal distension and colic. Disaccharide intolerance in children does not usually heal spontaneously.

The diagnosis is made by a lactose tolerance test, in which the rise in blood sugar (glucose) is compared after an oral dose of 100 g of lactose and 50 g glucose; the rise in blood sugar should be the same following each. The pH of the stools is tested. The amount of disaccharidase in the jejunal mucosa can be measured in specimens obtained at peroral biopsy. It is essential to know the site of the biopsy if the mucosal cell content of disaccharidase is used to confirm the diagnosis, because the disaccharidase content of cells varies according to their position. It is lower in surface cells of the jejunum than of the ileum. Flocculation and clumping may be seen in the barium meal follow-through if lactose is mixed with the barium. This may be compared with the normal appearance of the follow-through when the barium is given without lactose in a lactase-deficient patient.

Lactase deficiency may be a common cause of functional diarrhoea. Lactase deficiency may also be acquired as a result of other gastro-intestinal conditions, e.g. partial gastrectomy, gastro-enteritis, coeliac disease, malnutrition and ulcerative colitis. The lactase deficiency may improve as the associated condition improves; furthermore some of the symptoms of the primary condition may be alleviated if lactose is excluded from the diet. Lactose is the main sugar in milk so that exclusion of milk from the diet may be beneficial. In ulcerative colitis the situation is even more complex as there is evidence that the proteins in milk may also aggravate the condition. About one in four patients with ulcerative colitis may be helped by a milk-free diet. Other disaccharidase deficiencies occur but are very rare.

Acquired lactose intolerance is a possible explanation for the chronic diarrhoea which may follow treated bacterial or viral gastro-enteritis.

The Coeliac Syndrome

It is now widely accepted that the coeliac syndrome can be premalignant. The commonest malignancy is a lymphoma of the small intestine or draining mesenteric glands, the next commonest carcinoma of the oesophagus, and thirdly carcinoma or lymphoma elsewhere. Nearly all patients who develop a malignancy after the coeliac syndrome have had malabsorption for more than 10 years. Features which should alert one to the possibility that the coeliac syndrome is complicated by a malignancy are a long history, profound sudden weight loss, abdominal pain and anorexia. The coeliac syndrome may occur with skin disorders, particular psoriasis, rosacea and dermatitis herpetiformis. The skin condition as well as the malabsorption may respond to a gluten-free diet. Before deciding that a patient is not responding to gluten withdrawal it is essential to wait at least 6 months and to ensure that the patient is not occasionally taking gluten-containing foods. In older patients chronic pancreatitis is a relatively common cause of malabsorption.

Coeliac Disease

In coeliac disease, in which there is sensitivity to gluten in the diet, there may be an immunological hypersensitivity or damage to the mucosa by toxic polypeptides. There are usually high antibody titres to gluten antigens, and often to milk antigens as well. Steatorrhoea is not always present. There may only be specific defects in absorption (e.g. iron or folic acid). The subtotal villous atrophy may be patchy, although there is nearly always some lymphocyte infiltration. There is a poor correlation between the biopsy appearances and the severity of malabsorption. The condition can present at any age, even in the late seventies. The presentation may be:

Diarrhoea	Abdominal pain
Anorexia	Persistent glossitis
Weight-loss	Skin disorders
Obscure deficiency syndrome	Clubbing.

Stagnant Loop Syndrome

The upper small intestine is normally sterile; the presence of large numbers of coliform and bacteroides organisms may lead to malabsorption. Excessive numbers of bacteria may be present if there is any slowing of transit through the small intestines, e.g. in the presence of a stricture or Crohn's disease; excess bacteria may be present if they are allowed to multiply excessively, e.g. in a diverticulum or blind loop following a partial gastrectomy. Excessive numbers of coliform organisms cause malabsorption by splitting bile salts into substances which are ineffective in the splitting of fat and which are toxic to the mucosa of the small intestine. The organisms also utilise vitamin B_{12} in competition with the host. The number of organisms is related to gut mobility, accounting for the overproduction of micro-organisms which occurs when a blind loop is present. The type of organism is also dependent on diet, particularly the protein intake. In the large bowel, anaerobic organisms predominate and the pseudomembranous colitis due to altered bacterial flora is due to invasion by *Clostridium difficile*. Whipple's disease, which affects the small bowel, is also due to local invasion by micro-organisms. Some of the breakdown products of micro-organisms are carcinogenic. The presence of micro-organisms in the gut also affects absorption of carbohydrates, a lower number of micro-organisms allowing more efficient absorption.

The diagnosis can be made by performing bacterial counts on the contents of the jejunum; this is obtained by a special capsule which avoids contamination with any other part of the gut. The coliform organisms break down tryptophane to indole and then indican; this is absorbed and excreted in the urine. The urinary indican level is high if there are excessive numbers of coliform and bacteroides organisms in the jejunum. The absorption of vitamin B_{12} will also be abnormal in the stagnant-loop syndrome. The diagnosis can be clinched by demonstrating a reduction in jejunal organisms, a decrease in urinary indican, diminished faecal fats, and an improvement in vitamin B_{12} absorption following treatment with broad-spectrum oral antibiotics. The serum folate is often abnormally high in the stagnant-loop syndrome because the organisms are able to manufacture folate, which is then absorbed.

A test for excessive overgrowth of intestinal bacteria is the labelled carbon-glycocholic acid breath test. The bile acids, cholic and cheno-deoxycholic acids, are linked by an amide bond to their glycine or taurine conjugates and this bond may be broken down only by the action of bacterial enzymes. In the test C^{14}-labelled glycocholic acid is given by mouth. Bacterial deconjugation of the C^{14} glycine from the cholic acid caused by excessive bacteria (or by the normal colonic bacteria should the enterohepatic circulation of conjugated bile salts be interrupted by ileal resection) causes release of C^{14}-labelled glycine which is converted into C^{14}-labelled CO_2 and then exhaled. The amount of C^{14}-labelled CO_2 in the breath is a direct reflection of the amount of bacterial deconjugation of bile salts.

Chronic Intestinal Ischaemia

Chronic incomplete narrowing of the superior mesenteric artery may result in intestinal ischaemia; this may also occur with chronic venous congestions as in congestive heart failure or constrictive pericarditis. The main symptoms are "abdominal angina"—abdominal pain developing soon after a meal and relieved before the next meal, weight loss and sometimes malabsorption.

Narrowing of the mesenteric vessels may result in ischaemia of the colon. The important clinical features are sudden abdominal pain, rectal bleeding and signs of left-sided peritonitis. The attacks may be transient, or may lead to gangrene; in a third group the ischaemia results in stricture formation, the strictures being most frequent in the region of the splenic flexure and often surprisingly extensive. The main distinction is from Crohn's disease, in which additional similar lesions are usually present, and carcinoma, which usually causes a shorter stricture. The characteristic feature of intestinal ischaemia on the barium enema is "thumb printing" of the outline. This is due to local oedema in folds of mucosa. It can occasionally be seen at sigmoidoscopy and usually disappears when collateral circulation is established in 4–6 weeks.

The disease may occur in early adult life when it usually presents as haemorrhagic colitis and is frequently right-sided. Stricture formation is unusual when the disease occurs in this age group.

Protein-losing Gastro-enteropathy

Low serum albumin may result from diminished synthesis as in cirrhosis, excessive breakdown as in post-operative states, Cushing's syndrome, or excessive loss from the body as in the nephrotic syndrome, severe burns and exfoliative dermatitis; decreased intake of protein may also be responsible. However, occasionally hypoalbuminaemia occurs in the presence of normal absorption and *increased* synthesis. Some conditions are associated with exudation of protein into the gut—this has been demonstrated by recovering plasma protein from the intestinal contents by direct intubation.

From a practical clinical point of view in order to detect the presence of excessive protein loss into the gut albumin is labelled with [131]I. Following an injection of radio-active labelled albumin the level in the serum declines rapidly as albumin is distributed to the total protein pool—this takes 5 days; after this, the serum level falls slowly as the radio-active labelled albumin is metabolised and is replaced by recently synthesised albumin. This later rate of decline is a measure of the rate of albumin synthesis and albumin loss. The serum level falls rapidly if there is excessive loss into the gut. Fortunately for clinical purposes this test is sufficiently accurate. However, for research purposes attempts have been made to assess the exact amount of protein lost. One of the problems is that when radio-active labelled albumin is lost into the gut the albumin is digested and the radio-active iodine is reabsorbed. In an attempt to circumvent this problem a technique using a resin which would bind radio-active iodine was introduced. The resin was fed by mouth at the same time as an intravenous dose of ^{131}I-labelled albumin was given.

A further improvement was suggested using a synthetic substance which is metabolised in much the same way as albumin except that once in the gut the radio-active iodine is not split from it, this substance is ^{131}I labelled polyvinyl pyrrolidone (PVP). The main conditions causing protein exudation into the gut are:

Giant rugal hypertrophy of the stomach (Ménétrier's disease)
Ulcerative lesions of the gut
Neoplasms of the gut
Idiopathic steatorrhoea
Crohn's disease
Stagnant-loop syndrome
Radiation
Intestinal lymphangiectasia
Cardiac failure or constrictive pericarditis
Idiopathic hypoproteinaemia.

THE SIGNIFICANCE OF FIBRE IN THE DIET

Some diseases common in developed countries are rare in under-developed countries. It was suggested by Cleave, Trowell and Burkitt that the reduced amount of undigestible fibre in the diets of developed countries might be a factor in causing many of the diseases more prevalent there. The main hypothesis started by postulating that reduced stool volume led to straining at defaecation which led to such conditions as hiatus hernia, diverticulitis, varicose veins and piles; the increased time in transit, because of the small volume of faeces, might predispose to carcinoma of the colon by leaving possible carcinogens in the faeces in contact with the mucosa for a longer time. Since the first suggestion in the late 1960's that dietary fibre is important, its physicochemical properties and metabolic effects have also been studied. The plant celluloses are largely undigested (crude fibre); there are in addition other non-digestible dietary constituents such as polysaccharides, and pectins these are hemicelluloses and contribute to the total dietary fibre. Dietary fibre and crude fibre have a number of properties which may be relevant:

Ability to absorb water
Ability to adsorb bile salts
Ability to absorb solutes, e.g. carbohydrate, intestinal absorption
   of which may be reduced or delayed because solutions of sugars
   are held by fibres and are not so readily available for rapid or
   complete absorption by the small bowel.

The possible beneficial effects of fibre are:

Reduction in appetite by fatigue of mastication muscles, delayed
   gastric emptying and production of satiation
Reduction of calorie requirements by slowing carbohydrate
   absorption and so reducing insulin surges which, in their turn,
   promote hunger
Effect on bile acids and blood lipids by binding bile salts
Reduced saturation of bile with cholesterol, thus reducing the
   likelihood of gall-stone formation
Altered colonic bacterial content, which may be responsible for
   detoxicating potential carcinogens.

CROHN'S DISEASE (REGIONAL ILEITIS)

There is evidence to support a genetic predisposition to Crohn's disease—the disease being commoner in HLA A 11 people; there is also evidence of an immune basis in that there is anergy to DNCB and increase in complement levels suggesting a continuing immune process.

The disease usually begins in early adult life and in the majority, onset is gradual—symptoms have often been present for several years before the patient attends his doctor. Diarrhoea is the commonest early symptom, pain comes later and is often worse before defaecation. The pain is usually colicky and is often localised to the right iliac fossa. Other features which may be present are fever, anaemia, weight loss, iritis, erythema nodosum, clubbing and arthritis. Complications include fistulae, obstruction, malabsorption and ischiorectal abscess. The presence of a chronic anal fissure with fever or abdominal pain should suggest the probability of Crohn's disease. The perianal skin is often a bluish-red colour and swollen, and sometimes ulcerated skin tags are present.

Widespread involvement of the terminal ileum will result in a megaloblastic anaemia as this is the part of the ileum from which vitamin B_{12} is absorbed. It should be noted that diarrhoea does not invariably occur but sometimes diarrhoea is profuse and is accompanied by blood and mucus; under these circumstances the colon is usually but not invariably involved.

Crohn's disease most commonly affects the ileocaecal region or terminal ileum, however, any part of the gut from the duodenum to the anus may be affected. About 10 per cent of cases of Crohn's disease affect the large bowel alone while in 20 per cent of the remainder the large bowel is involved to a variable extent. The incidence of pathological anal skin tags is much higher when the colon is involved.

The x-ray appearances consist of narrowing of the lumen—"the string sign"; the lesions are usually separated by normal bowel—"skip lesions". If the mucous membrane is swollen and oedematous there may be a "cobble-stone" appearance. Small fissures may be seen as spikes of barium projecting at right angles from the lumen, sometimes a fistula may fill with barium. In the colon the x-ray appearances may resemble those of ulcerative colitis except that there is often a segment of normal bowel between two affected areas; strictures are very uncommon in ulcerative colitis; the ascending colon is more frequently involved in Crohn's disease. Narrowing of the terminal ileum with changes in the colon is highly suggestive of Crohn's disease rather than ulcerative colitis. Involvement of the ascending colon alone is suggestive of Crohn's disease; evidence of shortening of the colon is more suggestive of ulcerative colitis.

Comparisons between Crohn's disease and ulcerative colitis.—Both conditions tend to run in families, some members suffering from one and some from the other. Occasional patients have typical Crohn's disease of the terminal ileum with typical changes of ulcerative colitis in the colon. There are documented instances of the same patient developing both diseases.

In their classical forms there are distinctive pathological differences. Crohn's disease consists of non-caseating granulomata with giant cells, involving the submucosa of the terminal ileum. There is oedema and fibrosis involving the whole of the bowel wall with enlargement of the regional lymph glands. The fibrosis predisposes to stricture formation; the swollen oedematous loops of bowel adhere to each other and predispose to fistula formation.

In ulcerative colitis the mucosa is primarily affected, firstly in the sigmoid colon or upper rectum. The mucosa becomes hyperaemic and infiltrated with inflammatory cells, ulceration occurs which later spreads into the submucosa; the ulcers often heal by granulation tissue which becomes epithelialised, forming pseudopolyps.

Management of Crohn's Disease

Certain aspects of treatment are uncontroversial, viz:

Affected patients who are symptom-free need no treatment

Steroids are indicated for severe systemic manifestations (fever, eye, skin or joint involvement)

Steroids are indicated when small-bowel involvement is extensive

Steroids are indicated in patients who have a recurrence of the disease after having more than one small-bowel resection

Surgery is indicated for surgical complications such as fistulae, perforation, ischiorectal abscess or bowel stenosis

Laparotomy may be indicated in rare instances of doubt about the diagnosis. Ileocaecal tuberculosis still occurs although the Mantoux test will then be positive. The Mantoux test is frequently negative in Crohn's disease.

Treatment of the Acute Attack

Corticosteroids by mouth usually result in symptomatic and objective improvement. Steroids never cure the ileal lesion and they do not prevent recurrence when given continuously. It has been estimated that symptomatic relapse at five years occurs in about one-third and at ten years in about half the patients. The proportion requiring further resection is about one-sixth at five years and a quarter at ten years. The probability of recurrence following a second recurrence is probably higher. Sulphasalazine is used in the acute attack, and may prevent relapse in ileal disease; however, it appears to be of more value in preventing relapse of colonic Crohn's disease. Azathioprine seems to be more useful in preventing recurrence of Crohn's disease. Metronidazole may also be effective in some cases of colonic Crohn's.

For Crohn's disease of the colon resection is usually performed; ileorectal anastomosis is possible in a much higher percentage of patients with Crohn's disease of the colon than with ulcerative colitis. Recurrence of the disease in the terminal ileum following colectomy for colonic involvement is probably less common than recurrence when a localised segment of Crohn's disease has been removed from the ileum. Crohn's disease of the colon may heal when a temporary bypass ileostomy is performed.

ULCERATIVE COLITIS

The disease usually starts in the upper rectum and sigmoid colon and then spreads proximally. The rectum is usually, but not invariably, involved. It is uncommon for the appearances at sigmoidoscopy to be normal provided a good view is obtained.

The first symptom is usually bright red blood passed per rectum following defaecation, later the stools become more liquid and more frequent and are accompanied by blood and mucus. Abdominal pain is also a common early symptom, as in Crohn's disease. When the disease is limited to the rectum (granular or distal proctitis) constipation is usual. Occasionally the disease presents in an acute fulminating form or, rarely, with one of its complications. In a patient who has evidence of ulceration and bright red blood passed per rectum for the first time, it is essential to exclude other causes of rectal bleeding. The main alternative infections and conditions which should be considered are:

Entamoeba histolytica
Dysentery (Shigella)
Staphylococci
Viruses
Salmonella
Pathogenic E. coli
Tuberculosis
Crohn's disease

Granular proctitis (a form of
    ulcerative colitis)
Carcinoma
Haemorrhoids
Ischaemic colitis
Spastic colon
Purgative abuse
Post-dysenteric diarrhoea.

Sigmoidoscopy

Sigmoidoscopy should *always* be performed on patients admitted with diarrhoea or with loss of bright red blood per rectum. Four characteristics should be considered:

1. The overall impression of normality or abnormality
2. The presence or absence of a vascular pattern
3. The presence or absence of contact bleeding
4. The presence or absence of oedema.

Important appearances in the rectum which may suggest ulcerative colitis are:

Abnormally red or abnormally pale mucosa	Oedema
Absent vessel pattern	Ulceration
Contact bleeding	Rigidity
Granularity	Free blood, liquid faeces.

Local Complications

Haemorrhage	Fistula
Perforation	Stricture
Acute dilatation of the colon	Pseudopolyposis
Paracolic abscess	Carcinoma.
Ischiorectal abscess	

Radiological Signs

The reliable radiological signs of ulcerative colitis seen on the barium enema are:

Narrowing of the bowel	Loss of haustrations
Shortening of the bowel	Fine serration
Decreased distensibility	Polyps
Decreased tone	Longitudinal folds after evacuation
Ulceration	Double outline.

Remote Complications

Skin disorders.—Erythema nodosum, erythema multiforme and purpura are the commonest. Pyoderma gangrenosum is a skin lesion only seen in ulcerative colitis, and despite its name it is not due to pyogenic organisms. The lesion consists of bulla formation which usually involves the legs and results in ulceration and necrosis of the skin. The lesions are usually sterile and closely resemble pressure sores, except that they often occur in areas other than pressure areas. Many of the drugs used in treatment of ulcerative colitis may result in skin rashes. Aphthous ulcers in the mouth are also common.

Liver damage.—The liver is frequently involved in severe ulcerative colitis. The types of liver disease are:

Fatty infiltration

Pericholangitis with the inflammation around the bile canaliculi within the liver. This is probably due to portal pyaemia, which is a frequent finding in ulcerative colitis. Portal hypertension may ensue

Chronic active hepatitis

Cirrhosis

Sclerosing cholangitis.

The liver damage does not depend on the severity of the colitis and may progress even though the colitis is in remission or has been cured by a colectomy.

Eye complications.—Conjunctivitis, iritis and episcleritis occur. When eye complications are present there are usually other systemic manifestations of the disease. The eye complications usually improve when the condition is treated surgically but not so frequently with conservative treatment.

Arthritis.—This is usually a recurrent monoarticular arthritis affecting a large joint of the lower limbs, the rheumatoid factor is absent, nodules do not occur and the arthritis is cured when the colon is cured. Ankylosing spondylitis and sacro-iliitis also occur more commonly than in the general population. The spondylitis may precede the colitic symptoms and may continue to progress when the colon is cured. Unlike classical ankylosing spondylitis the spondylitis of ulcerative colitis is equally common in both sexes.

Nutritional deficiencies and anaemia.

Renal calculi.—Several series have shown an increased incidence of renal calculi in patients with ulcerative colitis. The incidence probably increases if the patient has an ileostomy. The postulated causes are many, dehydration, low urinary sodium and increased oxalate absorption. Hyperoxaluria occurs in malabsorption and ileal resection because calcium binds to free fatty acids acids and is unavailable to form insoluble calcium oxalate. Instead, soluble oxalate salts are formed and are absorbed, leading to hyperoxaluria.

Course of Ulcerative Colitis

The natural history of ulcerative colitis follows two distinct pathways. Some patients are free of symptoms between the acute attacks—chronic intermittent type; while others are never free of symptoms once the disease has presented—chronic continuous type. The mortality of ulcerative colitis is greatest in patients under the age of 20 or over 60, and it increases with the number of attacks. The mortality is much higher if the whole of the colon is involved.

Management of Ulcerative Colitis

Bed rest

Correction of dehydration and electrolyte depletion

Correction of anaemia

High calorie and protein intake. If there is dehyration, parenteral feeding can be used to supply enough calories and proteins. The colon should be rested by reducing the volume of indigestible roughage. If necessary, methyl cellulose can be given two or three times a day.

Corticosteroids. Prednisone 40–60 mg daily by mouth, by local application to the colon through a rectal drip, or by retention enemata. There is no evidence that steroids increase the incidence of perforation or affect subsequent surgical mortality, although they undoubtedly mask the signs of perforation.

Sulphasalazine (Salazopyrin). 0·5 g tablets in a dose of 1–3 g 3–6 times a day. This drug is chemically allied to the salicylates and sulphonamides and has been shown to be beneficial in shortening an acute attack of colitis.

Antibiotics are usually given—they should be administered *parenterally* so as not to sterilise the colon, which predisposes to super-infection with staphylococci.

Daily abdominal x-rays to detect dilatation of the colon. This can be suspected clinically if there is a sudden decrease in the number of stools, loss of gut sounds with a markedly distended and tympanitic abdomen, and abdominal pain.

Features Suggesting an Acute Exacerbation

More than six bowel actions per day
Macroscopic blood in the stool
Fever and tachycardia
Anaemia
Raised sedimentation rate
Lowered serum albumin
Colon greater than 6 cm in diameter on plain x-ray of the abdomen.

Surgical Treatment of the Acute Attack

The mortality of an emergency colectomy is much higher than that of an elective one; however, the mortality in an acute attack of colitis treated medically is closely related to its severity and duration. Some argue that it is better to persist with medical treatment in the hope that the patient will improve enough for elective operation; others argue that it may be better to operate early in an acute attack after a short period of intensive medical treatment. The mortality of severe attacks treated medically is over 10 per cent; when severe cases are treated with early colectomy, the mortality is just over 1 per cent. Early operation means within 2–3 days in the elderly and within 4–5 days in younger patients. Despite differences with regard to its timing most would agree that the indications for surgery in the acute attack are:

Involvement of the whole colon
Severe haemorrhage
Perforation
Acute dilatation of the colon

Sudden deterioration under medical treatment

Failure to improve after *three* days in patients over 60 years of age

Failure to improve after *six* days in young patients.

Long-term Management

Not all acute attacks of ulcerative colitis are severe enough to present the dilemma of surgical or medical treatment; many are of moderate severity and can nearly always be controlled by the medical regime.

Recurrence of acute attacks can seldom be prevented by therapeutic doses of corticosteroids; the risks of steroids in therapeutic doses usually outweigh the possible advantages. Small doses of steroids are totally ineffective in preventing recurrences. It is *not* now recommended that steroids be used when the patient is in remission, although the occasional patient is seen who appears to relapse when steroids are withdrawn. It is reasonable to make a general working rule to withdraw steroids when a patient goes into remission but to bear in mind that there are occasional exceptions. *Sulphasalazine is much more effective than steroids in preventing relapses.*

Diet.—There is some evidence that a proportion of patients with ulcerative colitis are sensitive to the proteins of cows' milk. In these patients the colitis improves when milk is withheld, but relapse occurs if the milk is reintroduced.

Patients with attacks of ulcerative colitis may have a deficiency of lactase in the affected colon so that they suffer from intolerance to the disaccharide lactose which is present in milk. There is evidence that withdrawal of lactose from the diet of some patients with ulcerative colitis leads to an improvement. The deficiency of lactase becomes less marked when the disease goes into remission.

Factors Favouring Surgery

1. Increasing frequency of acute attacks (whether severe or moderate).

2. Chronic continuous type of ulcerative colitis with continuing symptoms.

3. Involvement of the whole colon.

4. Severe remote complications particularly iritis and liver damage.

5. Prevention of carcinoma. The main factors associated with the development of carcinoma are a history of over 10 years involvement of the whole of the colon and an onset in childhood. The appearance of a stricture on the x-ray should be assumed to be carcinomatous until proved otherwise. Pseudopolyps indicate severe disease but are not pre-malignant.

Parenteral Nutrition

There is evidence that moderate protein and calorie deficiency is harmful because of:

Reduced immune defence
Reduced resistance to infection
Reduced wound healing
Reduced healing of inflammatory conditions
Less resistance to portasystemic encephalopathy in liver disease
Electrolyte disturbances, particularly hyponatraemia
Disturbed acid-base balance.

Following severe trauma, inflammation or operation there is an increase in metabolism affecting the whole body which results in excessive breakdown of protein and also diminished excretion of sodium and water.

There are a number of hazards of parenteral nutrition in addition to the possibility of introducing infection; these are:

Jaundice.—The precise cause is not always clear but jaundice probably occurs more frequently when fat emulsions are used
Hyperosmolar dehydration
Lactic acidosis.—This arises when calorie requirements in excess of those which can be metabolised are given
Acute folate deficiency. This may arise quickly and may be due to the fact that methionine is contained in many parenteral nutritional preparations. Methionine is normally involved in the metabolism of one-carbon fragments which are also involved in the final stages of folate metabolism—thus an excess of methionine may require additional folate if folate deficiency is to be avoided.
Fatty liver from excess glucose infusion
Essential fatty acid deficiency.

Planning an Intravenous Diet

Basic guidelines:

60% of the total calories (about 3000) should be given as carbohydrate (1 g glucose produces 4 calories)
Fat emulsion should not exceed 2 g/kg body weight
200 carbohydrate calories are required for every gram of nitrogen
Protein intake may need to be higher if there is excessive protein breakdown (2 g of urine urea requires 1 g of nitrogen)

PROPRIETARY INFUSION FLUIDS FOR PARENTERAL FEEDING

Preparation	Manufacturer	Nitrogen g/litre	Fat g/litre	Energy kcal/litre	Electrolytes mmol/litre				
					K^+	Mg^{2+}	Na^+	Acet$^-$	Cl^-
Aminoplex 12	Geistlich	12·4			30	2·5	35	5	67·2
Glucoplex 1000	Geistlich			1000	30	2·5	50		67
Intralipid 10%	KabiVitrum		100	1100					
Intralipid 20%	KabiVitrum		200	2000					
Plasma-Lyte M (dextrose)	Travenol			190	16	1·5	40	12	40
Synthamin 14	Travenol	14·3		2574	60	5	73	130	70
Synthamin 17	Travenol	16·9		3042	60	5	73	150	70
Vamin glucose	KabiVitrum	9·4		650	20	1·5	50		55

Glucose is probably a better source of carbohydrate calories than either fructose or sorbitol

More than 150 g carbohydrate per day requires insulin to be given in addition.

A suitable 24-hour maintenance regime would be:

1·0 l glucose 50% (Travenol) (2000 calories; 500 g glucose)
1·0 l Intralipid 10% (KabiVitrum) (1100 calories; 100 g fat)
1·0 l Vamin N (KabiVitrum) (250 calories; 9·4 g nitrogen)

An alternative regime, using less fluid, would be:

1·0 l Synthamin 9 (Travenol) (9·3 g nitrogen; 1667 calories)
or 1·0 l Synthamin 14 (14·3 g nitrogen; 2574 calories) adding either Intralipid 10% or glucose 20–50%

These solutions do not provide all the electrolytes, vitamins or micronutrients necessary. Many of the commercial amino acid solutions also contain a carbohydrate source other than glucose (e.g. alcohol, sorbitol or laevulose). These regimes may have to be modified to suit the particular metabolic requirements of individual patients, and the fluid and electrolyte losses.

Spastic Colon

This term is used to signify abnormal colonic function as a result of emotion, anxiety or mental stress. The symptoms are abdominal pain with constipation which may alternate with diarrhoea. There are a large number of synonyms for the condition many of which are misnomers; these include irritable colon, nervous diarrhoea and colonic spasm. The term mucous colitis is also a synonym and refers to the large amounts of mucus which very occasionally accompany the stools.

Pressure recordings from different positions in the lumen of the colon show that there may be localised increased intraluminal pressure during emotional stress – the hyperactivity can be reduced by anticholinergic drugs. The barium enema appearances reflect the hyperactivity of the colon – the lumen is diminished, haustral markings are prominent and numerous; these changes can usually be reversed with anticholinergics.

The pain is usually worse before defaecation after which it generally disappears. The pain may be felt anywhere over the course of the colon; when it occurs in relation to the splenic flexure it is sometimes known as the splenic flexure syndrome. Sometimes palpation of the caecum produces pain in the transverse and descending colon. Patients with this condition often complain of excessive abdominal gurgling—in some patients the small bowel is also hypermotile. Constipation is commoner than diarrhoea although often the two alternate; the stools are usually small no matter what their consistency. Clinical features identical to those of spastic colon occur after attacks of dysentery, after vagotomy and in ulcerative colitis. The mandatory sigmoidoscopy also frequently reproduces the patient's symptoms.

Treatment is with anticholinergic drugs and psychotherapy if the symptoms are severe and protracted.

ENDOCRINE CAUSES OF DIARRHOEA

Diarrhoea may be caused by disorders of the major endocrine glands:

Addison's disease
Thyrotoxicosis
Hypoparathyroidism (and hypocalcaemia)
Diabetes
Phaeochromocytoma.

Diarrhoea may also be produced by other humoral agents:

Zollinger-Ellison syndrome (gastrinoma). Non-beta-cell tumour of pancreatic islets
Carcinoid syndrome
Medullary carcinoma of thyroid
Vasoactive intestinal peptide excess (Werner-Morrison or pancreatic cholera syndrome.) This leads to profuse, watery diarrhoea.

Zollinger[22]-Ellison[23] Syndrome

In 1955 Zollinger and Ellison described a syndrome consisting of a triad of peptic ulceration at an unusual site, or recurrent anastomotic ulcers, gastric hypersecretion and a non-insulin-secreting islet cell tumour of the pancreas. In about half the cases there is a profuse watery diarrhoea and sometimes steatorrhoea, which is probably due to intestinal hurry as a result of inability of the pancreas to neutralise the excessive quantities of acid gastric juices. The diarrhoea may be present for several years before other manifestations of the syndrome are apparent.

About 10 per cent of patients with the syndrome have adenomata in other endocrine glands, the commonest being the parathyroids and adrenals—the "pluriglandular" syndrome. There is a high familial incidence of the pluriglandular syndrome and the Zollinger-Ellison syndrome.

The diagnosis is suggested by the presence of multiple peptic ulcers particularly if they are in unusual sites such as the postbulbar region of the duodenum or in the jejunum. In the stomach there is usually giant hypertrophy of the mucous membrane. Excessive gastric acidity should be demonstrated in a 12-hour nocturnal collection of the gastric juice—more than 100 mEq per 12 hours (10 mmol/hour) is highly suggestive. The pentagastrin test is lesser value. The most important diagnostic finding is a high level of serum gastrin. With regard to treatment there are several important factors to be considered: two-thirds of the tumours are in the body or tail of the pancreas; 10 per cent are in aberrant pancreatic tissue; about 30 per cent are multiple; approximately half the tumours are malignant and of these about a third have metastasised by the time diagnosis is made. However, the metastases are always very slow growing so that it is usually worthwhile to remove the primary tumour if this can be found. Total gastrectomy carries a better prognosis than operations on the pancreas. There is evidence that some pancreatic tumours regress and serum gastrin levels return to normal after operations on the stomach.

Carcinoid Syndrome

The carcinoid syndrome consists of a variable combination of flushing, diarrhoea, asthma and valvular heart lesions. The syndrome is usually caused by humoral substances produced by the metastases of tumours arising from the ileum. The cells of the tumours stain with silver salts hence the alternative name—argentaffinomata. The primary tumour and its metastases contain large quantities of 5-hydroxy-tryptamine (5HT) and this is excreted in the urine as 5-hydroxyindole acetic acid (5HIAA). 5HT is synthesised from tryptophan which is an essential amino acid and is a precursor of nicotinamide (vitamin B_6). There may be a deficiency of the vitamin leading to pellagra if excessive 5HT is produced. Many but not all the clinical features of the carcinoid syndrome are produced by release of the 5HT into the circulation. Other substances are produced by carcinoid tumours.

> 5-hydroxytryptophan—this is a precursor of 5HT and is produced by carcinoids arising from the embryological foregut
> Histamine—this is occasionally produced by carcinoids arising from the stomach
> Bradykinin—some carcinoid tumours produce a proteolytic enzyme, kallikrein, which splits a circulating α_2-globulin (kininogen) to produce bradykinin.

The type of flush varies from patient to patient depending on which humoral substance predominates. 5HT alone rarely produces a flush—when it does the flush is cyanotic; bradykinin tends to produce an erythematous flush. The flushes may be provoked by cheese, alcohol or emotion.

The diarrhoea is almost certainly due to 5HT and can usually be controlled with a 5HT antagonist such as methysergide. The cardiac effects of the carcinoid syndrome are an increase in cardiac output due to vasodilatation and endocardial fibrosis which leads to tricuspid and pulmonary stenosis in many instances of liver metastases. In the rare instances of a pulmonary carcinoid the valve lesions may be in the left side of the heart. Asthma may occur during attacks of flushing.

The clinical diagnosis of the carcinoid syndrome is confirmed by demonstrating the primary tumour and metastases by radiology and by demonstrating a high urinary excretion of 5HIAA. Flushing may be provoked by small intravenous injections of noradrenaline.

Treatment The carcinoid syndrome usually only develops after metastases have occurred; however, these are usually very slow growing. Methysergide is a 5HT antagonist and may control the asthma and diarrhoea (side-effects include vascular spasm and retro-peritoneal fibrosis).

The stimulating effects on the tumours of catecholamines may be prevented with α-methyldopa (Aldomet) and the peripheral effects of the humoral substances produced by the tumour may sometimes be inhibited by an α adrenergic blocking drug such as phenoxybenzamine.

REFERENCES

MEDICAL CLINICS OF NORTH AMERICA (1978) Vol **61**, No. 1.
TOPICS IN GASTROENTEROLOGY, Numbers 1–8. Ed. Truelove, S. C. Oxford: Blackwell Scientific Publications.

EPONYMS

1. BURRILL BERNARD CROHN (b. 1884)

Regional enteritis was first recognised by Crohn, Ginzburg and Oppenheimer in 1932. Crohn himself subsequently published extensively on his eponymous disease. He had qualified at Columbia University and was an intern in the Mount Sinai Hospital with Emanuel Libman. He was head of the gastro-enterology division of the hospital from 1925 to 1969.

2. HENRY STANLEY PLUMMER (1874–1937)

Plummer was Professor of Medicine at the Mayo Foundation Graduate School, University of Minnesota, and was largely responsible for the innovations incorporated into the construction of the Mayo Clinic. He published mainly on diseases of the thyroid.

3. PORTER PAISLEY VINSON (1890–1959)

Physician, Rochester, Minnesota.

4. SIR JONATHAN HUTCHINSON (1828–1913)

Hutchinson qualified at the medical school in York and then studied under Sir James Paget at St Bartholomew's Hospital. He became surgeon to the London Hospital and is said to have seen over a million cases of syphilis. He was one of the outstanding clinicians of the nineteenth century.

5. ALBERT MASON STEVENS (1884–1945)

New York paediatrician, who qualified at Columbia University at the same time as Crohn.

6. F. C. JOHNSON (1894–1934)

American physician.

7. HULÚSI BEHÇET (1889–1948)

Turkish dermatologist.

8. JOHANNES LAURENTIUS AUGUSTINUS PEUTZ (1886–1957)

Dutch physician.

9. HAROLD JOSEPH JEGHERS (b. 1904)

Professor of Genetics, Harvard.

10. GEORGES THIBIERGE (1856–1926)

Thibierge studied under Rendu and Besnier (of the prurigo) and specialised in dermatology. He published extensively and contributed the section in dermatology and syphilis to Charcot and Bouchard's *Traite de Medecine*. He published his observations with Weissenbach in 1911.

11. CHARLES ÉMILE TROISIER (1844–1919)

Troisier qualified in Paris, and became Professor of Medicine in 1880.

12. BERNARD MORITZ CARL LUDWIG RIEDEL (1846–1916)

Jena surgeon.

13. GIOVANNI BATTISTA MORGAGNI (1682–1771)
Morgagni became Professor of Anatomy in Padua having studied with Valsalva at Bologne. Morgagni was the first regularly to perform post-mortems and to relate pathology to clinical features. He wrote his famous work *De Sedibus* describing 600 post-mortems in the form of letters to friend. He was elected to the Royal Society, but he failed to recognise the significance of the recently introduced microscope.

14. VINCENZ ALEXANDER BOCHDALEK (1801–1883)
Professor of Anatomy, Prague.

15. FRANTISEK CHVOSTEK (1835–1884)
Chvostek was Professor of Medicine in the Imperial Austrian Army. He published papers covering the whole of medicine.

16. ARMAND TROUSSEAU (1801–1867)
Trousseau qualified in Paris. He was greatly influenced by Pierre Bretonneau (1778–1862) (who had clearly differentiated typhoid fever from diphtheria, and who was among the earliest to accept the germ theory of disease), and also by Corvisart (Napoleon's physician). Trousseau wrote a textbook on therapeutics which tried to establish rational therapy. He performed the first tracheotomy in Paris, and was the first to apply Addison's name to adrenal insufficiency.

17. EUGENE PÓLYA (1876–1944)
Pólya was born in Budapest, where he became Professor of Surgery. In the revolution in Hungary after the First World War he stayed at his post, but was later accused of radicalism and removed for two years. During the Russian siege of Budapest in the Second World War he had to go into hiding, but in December 1944 his identity was discovered by Hungarian Nazis and he died in a concentration camp; his body was never recovered.

18. ABRAHAM VATER (1684–1751)
Vater was born in Wittenberg but qualified in Amsterdam. He eventually returned to Wittenberg to become Professor successively of Anatomy and Botany and then Pathology and Therapeutics.

19. CHRISTIAN ALBERT THEODOR BILLROTH (1829–1894)
Billroth was a great friend of Brahms, who dedicated two string quartets to him. He was a surgeon in Zurich before becoming Professor of Surgery in Vienna; he was responsible for introducing antiseptic surgical methods on the Continent.
    In 1881 he resected a pyloric carcinoma and demonstrated thereby the possibility of gastric surgery. (It had previously been thought that the sutures would be digested by gastric juices.)

20. KIYOSHI SHIGA (1870–1957)
Shiga qualified in Tokyo and worked with Kitasato who, with von Behring, discovered tetanus toxin. Shiga also worked with Ehrlich and described the dysentery bacillus in 1898. He eventually became Professor of Bacteriology in Seoul (Korea).

21. GEORG HOYT WHIPPLE (1878–1976)

Whipple studied in Yale and Johns Hopkins. He received the Nobel Prize in 1934 with G. R. Minot (1885–1950) and W. P. Murphy (b. 1892) for their discovery of dietary factors which affect anaemias (particularly vitamin B_{12} and pernicious anaemia). Whipple eventually became Professor of Pathology at the University of Rochester.

22. ROBERT MILTON ZOLLINGER (b. 1903)

Professor of Surgery at Columbus, Ohio.

23. EDWIN HOMER ELLISON (b. 1918)

Surgeon at Columbus, Ohio.

4

LIVER AND PANCREAS

FUNCTIONS OF THE LIVER

Excretion of bilirubin
Excretion of bile salts and cholesterol
Synthesis of glycogen
Synthesis of albumin and urea
Storage of vitamins A, D and B_{12}
Detoxification of drugs such as opiates, barbiturates, salicylates, quinine and heavy metals.
Detoxification of hormones such as aldosterone, oestrogens and antidiuretic hormone

Excretion of bilirubin.—Bilirubin is a waste product resulting from destruction of worn-out red cells or their precursors. The iron and protein (globin) of the haemoglobin are metabolised and re-used, the remainder of the haemoglobin is a waste product and becomes bilirubin. The destruction of red cells takes place throughout the reticulo-endothelial system, including the bone marrow. Bilirubin is carried to the liver attached to serum albumin—in this form it is insoluble in water. In the liver, bilirubin is removed from the albumin and conjugated with glucuronic acid. Once it is removed from the albumin and conjugated it becomes soluble in water. This difference in solubility before and after passage through the liver is the basis of the van den Bergh[1] reaction. Water-soluble conjugated bilirubin changes the colour of the diazotised sulphanilic acid; water-insoluble bilirubin (unconjugated) will not change the colour until it has been removed from the serum albumin by the addition of alcohol—unconjugated bilirubin is, therefore, referred to as indirect-acting bilirubin. Conjugated bilirubin is referred to as direct-acting.

In the gall bladder the bile is concentrated by the removal of water, thence conjugated bilirubin passes down the small intestine unchanged. In the colon it is reduced by coliform and other organisms to stercobilinogen which when oxidised gives the brown colour to the faeces. Some stercobilinogen is absorbed, some of it is excreted in the urine as urobilinogen and some is re-excreted by the liver (entero-hepatic circulation).

In obstructive jaundice, direct-acting (conjugated) bilirubin is forced back through the liver cells into the blood as a result of increased pressure in the biliary system. In haemolytic jaundice indirect-acting (unconjugated) bilirubin accumulates in the blood because red cells are being broken down faster than the liver can excrete the bilirubin. In addition, increased amounts of stercobilinogen are present, more is absorbed from the colon but the ability to re-excrete urobilinogen is limited; therefore, more has to be excreted in the urine, accounting for the increased urinary urobilinogen which appears in haemolytic anaemias.

In hepatocellular jaundice two things are happening; one is that damaged liver cells cannot conjugate bilirubin in the normal amounts so that there is a rise in indirect (unconjugated) bilirubin in the blood and the other is that the damaged liver cells swell and block the bile canaliculi, causing intrahepatic biliary obstruction, which will cause a rise in direct-acting (conjugated) bilirubin, provided the liver cells are still capable of conjugating some bilirubin. In hepatocellular damage due to infective hepatitis the obstructive element generally comes first and is followed by failure of the liver cells to conjugate bilirubin.

Excretion of bile salts and cholesterol.—Bile salts are the end-product of cholesterol metabolism; however, they are essential for the emulsification and hence absorption of fats (and the fat-soluble vitamins A, D and K), and they also activate pancreatic and intestinal lipase. In obstructive jaundice the excretion of bile salts is prevented, they accumulate in the serum and are responsible for the skin irritation of obstructive jaundice. Cholesterol exists in the serum as free cholesterol or as cholesterol esters—this esterification takes place in the liver. In hepatocellular damage the liver loses its ability to esterify cholesterol; hence the proportion of esterified to free cholesterol in the serum falls. In chronic biliary obstruction there is usually a marked rise in serum cholesterol.

Bile contains several bile acids, each conjugated with glycine or taurine. The two primary bile salts are cholates and deoxycholates and are produced by the liver; the secondary bile salts are the deoxycholates produced in the intestine by bacterial action, but absorbed and excreted by the liver into the bile.

Maximum bile-salt absorption occurs from the distal ileum. Bile salts aid in the absorption of fats by forming micelles. The physical chemistry of this is very complicated, but basically a micelle consists of a steroid ring, soluble in fatty acid, and a hydroxyl group, soluble in water; thus the whole micelle is a way of rendering fatty acids soluble in water and suitable for absorption through the enterocyte. Inside the cell, fatty acids reform triglycerides, which are transported in the blood as chylomicrons. Medium-length triglycerides can be absorbed without fatty acids being formed first, and without micelle formation.

Bile salts are almost completely reabsorbed in the distal ileum and take part in an enterohepatic circulation. Diseases which affect the distal ileum will prevent reabsorption of bile salts which are, therefore, not re-excreted—this may cause failure of emulsification of fats and exaggerate the effects of malabsorption.

Synthesis of glycogen and carbohydrate.—Glycogen is stored in the liver cells and can be synthesised from and metabolised to glucose. In hepatocellular damage this ability is impaired and may result in hyperglycaemia if glycogen is not formed quickly enough, or hypoglycaemia if glycogen is not broken down to glucose quickly enough.

Synthesis of albumin and urea.—Urea is the waste product of amino-acid metabolism within the liver. Severe liver damage is associated with impaired production of urea, a low blood urea and increased amino acids in the blood leading to aminoaciduria.

Albumin is manufactured by the liver, whereas most of the globulins are produced by the reticulo-endothelial system. Other proteins are manufactured in the liver; the most important of these are prothrombin and other protein factors concerned with blood coagulation. In obstructive jaundice the serum lipids are raised, many of them are attached to β globulins so that in obstructive jaundice there may appear to be an increase in β globulins.

Bilirubin is transported attached to the plasma albumin; many drugs are also transported in the same way. Substances which are bound to the plasma proteins are not pharmacologically active, and it is the concentration of the free drug in the plasma which determines its activity. Some substances are more readily displaced from protein-binding sites than others. In newborn babies there are relatively small amounts of plasma albumin and all the binding sites are occupied by bilirubin. If sulphonamides are given to premature babies, bilirubin is displaced from the albumin and is then free in the serum to enter the brain and cause kernicterus. For this reason neonates should never be given sulphonamides or salicylates.

There are many examples of one drug displacing another from the albumin-binding sites, giving rise to toxic concentration of the displaced drug in the serum.

The following list shows drugs which are attached to plasma albumin; phenylbutazone will displace most of the others. The most important examples clinically are potentiation of anticoagulants in patients given phenylbutazone and potentiation of tolbutamide causing hypoglycaemia by most of the others in this list:

Phenylbutazone	Sulphonamides
Warfarin	Penicillin
Salicylates	Tolbutamide.

Several hormones are transported attached to plasma proteins, e.g. thyroxin, corticosteroids and insulin. Many of the antirheumatic drugs may have their effect by displacing corticosteroids from the binding plasma protein. Tolbutamide may act in a similar way with regard to insulin. It has been noted that patients with rheumatoid arthritis may improve if they develop obstructive jaundice, probably as a result of displacement of corticosteroids from their binding sites by bilirubin.

Storage of vitamins.—Patients with cirrhosis sometimes develop night blindness due to deficiency of vitamin A. A macrocytic anaemia occurs in cirrhosis but is probably not related to inability to store vitamin B_{12}; by far the commonest causes of anaemia in cirrhosis are iron deficiency or haemolysis.

Detoxification of drugs.—Liver damage results in a reduced ability to excrete those drugs normally handled by the liver. This will produce a serious overdosage if these drugs are inadvertently used.

Detoxification of hormones.—The diseased liver may be responsible for a large number of clinical manifestations related to other systems, and these include the endocrine system. Carcinoma of the liver, in common with carcinomas in other sites, may produce excess quantities of peptides which closely resemble normally occurring peptides such as parathyroid hormone, erythropoietin and ACTH. The commonest endocrine manifestations are due to failure to metabolise hormones normally, and alterations in the plasma proteins which alter the binding of normally circulating hormones.

The main endocrine manifestations of liver failure are:

Increased renin and aldosterone.—Sodium excretion is low in cirrhosis and the main stimulus for the sodium retention is raised renin concentration which gives rise through the angiotensin system to secondary aldosteronism. It is believed that in cirrhosis there are alterations in renal blood flow which reduces perfusion of the juxtaglomerular apparatus.

Hypogonadism.—There are several reasons for hypogonadism and feminisation. Sex-hormone binding globulin binds more testosterone; testosterone production in the testes is decreased. There is also evidence of hypothalamic impairment in that FSH and LH are low, particularly in view of the low testosterone levels which would normally lead to an increase in FSH and LH. In cirrhosis there is increased conversion of testosterone to oestrogens.

Hypoglycaemia.—This occurs as a result of reduced gluconeogenesis in the damaged liver. In the rare primary liver carcinoma, hypoglycaemia may occur because of deficiency of glucose-6-phosphatase and phosphorylase.

Hyperglycaemia.—Glucose intolerance occurs and is usually due to hyperglucagonaemia, due to failure to detoxify glucagon which may also be produced in excess.

Osteomalacia.—This occurs in cirrhosis and is now thought to be due to a simple deficiency of vitamin D. Failure of hydroxylation of cholecalciferol in the liver does not usually occur until later in the progression of liver disease.

Hypothyroidism.—This may be missed in liver disease because of the galaxy of other clinical features and because the conventional thyroid biochemistry may not be abnormal. There may be an alteration in the conversion of T4 to T3, which is the metabolically active thyroid hormone in the tissues; in cirrhosis more is formed of the so-called "reverse T3". In liver disease there is also an increase in plasma protein binding of T4 and T3, giving rise to higher-than-normal levels, although the unbound, free circulating hormone is reduced. In patients with liver disease the TSH level and TRH test may be necessary to elucidate the exact thyroid status.

Liver Function Tests

The patient's description of alteration of colour of his urine and stools is still one of the most useful pointers in the diagnosis of liver disorders. The urine should always be examined for bilirubin before embarking on formal biochemical tests of liver function. The main tests are:

Serum bilirubin	Plasma prothrombin and fibrinogen
Urinary urobilinogen	Amino acids in blood and urine
Excretion tests	Blood ammonium
Serum proteins	Serum lipids
Serum enzymes	Galactose tolerance.

Serum bilirubin.—Indirect-acting (unconjugated) bilirubin increases in haemolytic jaundice. Direct-acting (conjugated) bilirubin accumulates in obstructive jaundice.

Urinary urobilinogen.—This will be increased in haemolytic jaundice and absent in complete obstruction of the bile ducts. The reappearance of urobilinogen in the urine in infectious hepatitis is a good prognostic sign, because it means that the swelling of the liver cells is subsiding allowing some bile through the bile canaliculi. Urobilinogen is found in the urine mainly in the afternoon or evening, hence early morning specimens of urine are not so suitable for estimation of urinary urobilinogen.

Excretion tests.—Bromsulphthalein (BSP) is a dye which is more or less completely excreted by the liver in 45 minutes. Retention of more than 5 per cent of the original dose at this time indicates some impairment of liver function. The test will always be abnormal in the presence of obstructive jaundice. A number of other conditions may give false high readings at the end of 45 minutes, e.g. congestive heart failure, anaemia (by causing hepatic anoxia), fever, recent meal, shock and chronic debilitating diseases.

Serum proteins.—The serum albumin is usually reduced in liver damage. The γ globulin is sometimes raised in cirrhosis. The flocculation tests of liver functions depend on alterations in the proportions of the various plasma proteins.

Serum enzymes.—Hepatocellular damage causes leakage of intracellular substances into the blood, and these include iron and various enzymes. The main enzymes are the transaminases and the dehydrogenases (glutamic oxaloacetic, glutamic pyruvic transaminases, SGOT and SGPT and lactic and iso-citrate dehydrogenases, LDH and ICD). SGPT and ICD are the most sensitive as indicators of liver impairment.

Alkaline phosphatase is excreted by the liver cells and by the mucosal cells of the biliary tree. The serum level is generally higher in biliary obstruction than in hepatocellular damage. Levels above 150 iu/l indicate biliary obstruction.

Carcinoma of the biliary epithelium results in extremely high levels of alkaline phosphatase in the serum. Alkaline phosphatase is also found in bone and in the gastro-intestinal tract. It is possible to differentiate the different alkaline phosphatases biochemically. An enzyme similar to alkaline phosphatase, 5-nucleotidase, is specific for liver disease.

Plasma prothrombin and fibrinogen.—Plasma prothrombin may be reduced because the hepatocellular damage is so severe that it cannot be synthesised, or because vitamin K from which it is formed is not absorbed because of lack of bile salts. Lack of fibrinogen may also be responsible for excessive bleeding.

Amino acids in blood and urine.—There is increased aminoaciduria in severe cirrhosis, particularly of cystine. The raised level of amino acids in the blood may be partly responsible for hepatic coma.

Blood ammonium.—There is some correlation between the blood ammonium level and hepatic coma; however, the exact cause of hepatic coma remains obscure.

Serum lipids.—The serum cholesterol is increased in obstructive jaundice. The proportion of esterified cholesterol may fall in liver impairment.

Galactose tolerance.—The rate at which galactose is metabolised to glycogen is measured by the rate of decrease in serum levels of galactose following a loading dose.

Isotopic Scanning of the Liver and Biliary System

There are now available several isotopes and carriers which are of value in the diagnosis of liver disease. The carriers include:

Colloid
Methionine
BSP
Ethyl or butyl imino diacetic acid (HIDA), which behave like bile salts
Rose bengal.

The isotopes include:

^{131}Iodine: γ and β emitter (half-life 8 days)
^{123}Iodine: γ emitter (half-life 13 hours)
Technetium: γ emitter (half-life 6 hours)
^{67}Gallium (half-life 3 days)
^{75}Selenium (half-life several months).

Colloid labelled with technetium, rose bengal labelled with iodine, and methionine labelled with selenium are mainly excreted by the Kupffer cells of the reticulo-endothelial system of the liver. Most space-occupying lesions in the liver, such as regeneration nodules, dilated bile ducts, metastases or hepatomas, will therefore show up as relatively "cold" areas on the scan. The limits of resolution are about 1–2 cm.

For detecting deep-seated lesions the gamma camera may be less satisfactory than rectilinear scanning because with the latter it is possible to focus the detector at a depth, whereas with the gamma camera resolution is best at the surface. Gallium concentrates preferentially in malignant tissues, so that hepatomas and metastases tend to be "hot", whereas regeneration nodules and dilated bile ducts tend to be "cold". HIDA and BSP are excreted into the bile canaliculi. Hence technetium-labelled HIDA (using a gamma camera) or ^{123}I-labelled BSP are of value in distinguishing cholestatic from post-hepatic jaundice. HIDA has the disadvantage of being also excreted through the kidneys and hence, if the jaundice is severe and of long standing, HIDA will not be excreted by the liver as well as BSP, which is not excreted at all by the kidneys. Labelled HIDA and BSP scans can be used to demonstrate isotopes in the biliary tree, gall bladder and the intestinal tract after they have been excreted by the liver.

In the distinction between cholestasis and post-hepatic obstructions, HIDA, BSP and rose bengal scans may show the following features:

	Persistence of activity in the liver	Appearance of activity in the biliary tree or gastro-intestinal tract	Speed of uptake and activity by liver
Cholestasis	Yes	No or delayed	Delayed
Post-hepatic obstruction	Less than in cholestasis	Depends on severity & position of obstruction but more tends to appear in gut than with cholestasis	Normal if bilirubin level not excessive

HIDA scans, because the isotope is technetium, have the great advantage that the gamma camera can be used to detect radioactivity. In tumour localisation or detection the following differential features may be helpful:

	Colloid	HIDA	BSP	Gallium	Selenio-methionine
Regeneration nodules	cold	cool	hot	cold	cold
Hepatomas	cold	cool	cold	hot	warm
Dilated bile ducts	cold	hot	hot	cold	cold
Metastases	cold	cool	cold	hot	cold
Type of scan	γ camera or rectilinear, depending on isotope label	γ camera	rectilinear (^{131}I label) γ camera (^{123}I label)	γ camera or rectilinear	
Radiation dose (compare barium meal dose of 1·5 rads)	0·7	1·8	12·3 (^{131}I) 1·3 (^{123}I)	2·7	6·7

JAUNDICE

Increase in Unconjugated Bilirubin

1. Increased production as in haemolytic anaemias.
2. Impaired handling of bilirubin by the liver.

(a) Impairment of entry of bilirubin into hepatic cells (Gilbert's[2] disease). This is characterised by mild fluctuating jaundice present from childhood. The condition may be exacerbated by acute infections, the increased bilirubin is always the unconjugated type; it is the commonest of the congenital hyperbilirubinaemias. Nevertheless, it should only be diagnosed by exclusion of all other causes of a raised bilirubin, particularly haemolysis. Liver biopsy is always normal.

(b) Failure of conjugation of bilirubin inside the hepatic cell (Crigler-Najjar syndrome). This condition is always fatal in infancy.

(c) Impairment of excretion of conjugated bilirubin by the hepatic cells (Dubin-Johnson and Rotor syndromes). These are benign, rare conditions associated with an increase of conjugated bilirubin in the serum. Liver biopsy shows brown pigmentation of the liver cells.

Gilbert's disease can be positively confirmed by a rise in unconjugated bilirubin occurring with reduced calorie intake (Owens and Sherlock, 1973).

Increase in Conjugated Bilirubin

This is always due to obstruction of the biliary tree, which may be intrahepatic in the case of "drug cholestasis" or extrahepatic in the case of obstruction to the bile duct.

Increase in Conjugated and Unconjugated Bilirubin

This means liver-cell damage as well as biliary-tree obstruction and is exemplified by virus hepatitis.

Jaundice Caused by Drugs

Drugs may produce jaundice in the following ways:

1. Liver-cell necrosis, which is usually fatal. Examples are chloroform, carbon tetrachloride, heavy metals, hypothermia and hyperthermia. Tetracycline, when outdated and in large doses, may produce a rapid, severe fatty infiltration which is fatal and resembles acute liver necrosis. Paracetamol in large doses overloads the normal excretory pathways, and its metabolites are retained and are hepatotoxic.

2. Hepatitis-like syndrome. This usually improves if the drugs are withdrawn. There may be evidence of generalised hypersensitivity (urticaria, asthma and eosinophilia). Examples are phenindione, sulphonamides, MAO inhibitors, phenlybutazone, barbiturates, penicillin and phenytoin.

3. Hypersensitivity cholestasis, i.e. intrahepatic biliary obstruction, occurs in hypersensitive patients only and is not dose dependent. Examples are phenothiazines, chlorpropamide, tolbutamide and anti-TB drugs (isoniazid, PAS, rifampicin and ethambutol).

4. Non-hypersensitivity cholestasis, i.e. biliary obstruction, will occur in anyone who takes the drugs for long enough. Examples are methyltestosterone and norethandrolone.

5. Haemolytic jaundice. In G-6-PD-deficient subjects, haemolytic crises develop with some drugs. Examples are primaquine, aspirin, sulphonamides, methyldopa and phenacetin.

6. Hepatitis transmitted by blood transfusion or unsterile syringes.

7. Chronic hepatitis and cirrhosis. Methyldopa, methotrexate and introfurantoin have all been implicated.

8. Gall stones. There is now clear evidence that clofibrate is associated with an increased incidence of gall stones.

The reaction of antituberculous drugs is complex. Isoniazid and rifampicin often produce a transient rise early in treatment but this usually subsides. With isoniazid the reaction is greater in patients who are *fast* acetylators presumably because of rapid accumulation of hepatotoxic metabolites. Rifampicin may also interfere with bilirubin metabolism, causing a rise in unconjugated bilirubin.

Hepatitis

The clinical range of acute or chronic hepatitis varies from sub-clinical asymptomatic to rapid progression and death. Acute hepatitis generally refers to infection with either hepatitis A or B virus, although some cases of chronic active hepatitis can present and progress with an acute hepatitis-like illness. There are also cases of acute viral hepatitis in which neither the A nor B virus is found. (Non-A, Non-B hepatitis).

Acute Viral Hepatitis

It is usually not possible on clinical grounds to distinguish between the A and B virus. The characteristic features of clinical acute hepatitis is jaundice; this is usually preceded by a period of general malaise and non-specific systemic symptoms such as occur with many viral illnesses. The characteristic urine and stool changes of obstructive jaundice usually result from the intrahepatic bile-duct obstruction which occurs with the inflamed hepatic cells. The liver and spleen are usually enlarged. (If splenomegaly is considerable, glandular fever is a more likely cause of the illness than viral hepatitis.) Infection with hepatitis A virus results in recovery usually within a month, although it can be delayed for as long as a year. The relapse rate and progression to chronic acute hepatitis or fulminating hepatitis depends on whether infection is due to hepatitis A or B. The diagnosis is confirmed by finding a raised bilirubin (often both conjugated and unconjugated, because of (a) biliary obstruction, and (b) failure of the inflamed liver to excrete unconjugated bilirubin). The transaminases are usually raised but the level does not always correspond with the severity of liver damage; the level of bilirubin is a better guide to this.

It is important to establish the exact cause of the hepatitis and therefore a careful history of alcohol intake is essential, for alcohol can produce an acute hepatitis-like picture; the Australia antigen (HB$_s$Ag) and the EB virus antigen in the serum should be sought, and any antecedent drug intake established. Hepatitis A virus can be found in the stool using electron microscopy. A number of antibody tests are available. The differences between the two types of hepatitis are:

	Hepatitis A	Hepatitis B
Incubation time	30 days	120 days
Age predilection	young	none
Severity of illness	usually mild	often severe
Progression to chronic hepatitis of cirrhosis	hardly ever	5–10% of clinical cases
Transmission	enteric	parenteral/sexual

Nomenclature in Hepatitis (Bianchi *et al.* 1977)

The liver biopsy appearances are of increasing value in predicting the progression from acute to chronic hepatitis and in predicting the progress of chronic hepatitis. The biopsy appearances in the chronic disease may be crucial in deciding what treatment is best. Some knowledge of the histological appearances is necessary for clinicians.

Types of Necrosis

Piecemeal necrosis refers to necrosis of liver cells between inflamed connective tissue and normal liver cells; *confluent* or *bridging necrosis* refers to necrosis crossing between two vascular structures, e.g. central vein to portal tract at the edge of each acinus; *spotty necrosis* refers to small areas of necrosis of liver cells.

Patterns of Necrosis

In acute hepatitis the pattern of necrosis (e.g. portal-portal, central-central, or central-portal) may be important in predicting progression to chronic hepatitis (Table VII, Bianchi *et al.* 1977).

TABLE VII

LIVER-CELL NECROSIS IN ACUTE HEPATITIS IN RELATION TO ACINAR CONCEPT OF HEPATIC STRUCTURE

Necrosis pattern	Acinar location	Necrosis type	Outcome in non-fatal acute cases
Central-central bridging	Periphery of complex acinus	Confluent	Healing, usually without fibrosis
Central-portal bridging	Periphery of simple acinus	Confluent	Usually heals, with or without fibrosis, unless associated with piecemeal necrosis
Multilobular necrosis	Multiple acini	Confluent	Healing with fibrosis, unless associated with piecemeal necrosis
Portal-to-portal connections	Mainly around terminal portal tracts	Piecemeal	Often associated with chronic liver disease.

Serological Findings in Virus Hepatitis

Hepatitis A virus.—The virus was first isolated from faeces in 1973. Excretion of the virus occurs only during the incubation period, and ceases when jaundice develops. Several serological tests are useful in determining previous infection (and therefore the value of immune serum in contacts of proven cases). Following an acute infection IgM antibodies remain for about 60 days, whereas IgG antibodies remain indefinitely. Failure of IgM levels to fall or IgG antibodies to develop suggests persisting viral infection.

Hepatitis B virus.—The Australia antigen was discovered in 1965 and it is now known to be the surface antigen of hepatitis B virus (hence HB_sAg or hepatitis B surface antigen). This antigen appears during the pre-icteric period and is replaced by the core antigen, followed by antibodies to the core antigen (anti-HB_c) which much later are followed or accompanied by antibodies to the surface antigen (anti-HB_s). The carrier state is characterised by persistence of the HB_s antigen and failure to produce anti-HB_s. The HB_c antigen may also persist in the carrier state.

Management of Acute Hepatitis

Bed rest.—Patients usually feel better if rested but several controlled studies have shown that physical activity does not always have an adverse effects on recovery. However, recent evidence suggests that bed-rest is often advantageous.

Steroids.—There is now incontrovertible evidence that steroids have no benefit, even in severe cases.

Liver biopsy.—This may be indicated if there is doubt about the initial diagnosis or if the hepatitis is slow to resolve. Some cases of chronic active hepatitis present with a remittent acute hepatitis-like illness.

Infectivity.—Isolation is not necessary *provided* adequate safeguards are taken for disposal of excreta, and when blood is being taken. Immune serum is available for both hepatitis A and B prophylaxis. Hepatitis A prophylaxis is recommended for non-immune travellers to the tropics.

Chronic Hepatitis

Chronic active hepatitis is defined pathologically (Bianchi *et al.* 1977) as "a chronic inflammatory and fibrosing liver lesion of varied aetiology and variable histological features. The features common to all untreated examples are: piecemeal necrosis together with new fibre formation and lymphocytic infiltration of portal tracts and lobules. Other infiltrating cells may also be found, and features of acute hepatitis, such as spotty necrosis (hepatocytolysis) may be superimposed. Passive septa formed by collapse after bridging or multilobular liver-cell necrosis may be present. Cirrhosis is not a defining criterion but can develop. Signs of liver-cell regeneration are usually seen in CAH and the borderline between CAH and cirrhosis in the more severe cases is not sharp. The severity of CAH varies with the degree of piecemeal and confluent necrosis and the density of the inflammatory infiltrate."

Chronic persistent hepatitis is defined pathologically as "chronic inflammatory infiltration, mostly portal, with preserved lobular architecture and little or no fibrosis. Piecemeal necrosis is absent or slight. Features of acute hepatitis may be superimposed." Chronic hepatitis is characterised clinically by continuation of evidence of liver inflammation for six months. The two varieties of chronic hepatitis—persistent and active—may be *indistinguishable by clinical and biochemical criteria*. The distinction has to be made on histological appearances; in essence, periportal inflammatory cell infiltration without necrosis characterises chronic persistent hepatitis, which has a good prognosis untreated, whereas the presence of periportal necrosis indicates chronic active hepatitis which may, untreated, have a poor prognosis. Chronic hepatitis is also characterised clinically by recurrent jaundice, malaise and often fever. The laboratory features of chronic hepatitis are raised bilirubin, transaminases and immunoglobulins. Some distinctive features of chronic persistent and chronic active hepatitis are shown below.

	Chronic persistent hepatitis	*Chronic active hepatitis*
Onset	Often like acute viral hepatitis	Gradual
Recurrent acute episodes	Rare	Common
Involvement of other systems (e.g. serous membrane joints)	Rare	Common
Bilirubin	Up to twice normal	Above twice normal
Transaminases	Up to 4 times normal but variable	10 times normal but variable
HB$_s$ antigen	Rare	20-30%
Raised immunoglobulins	Slight	Polyclonal; often twice normal
Smooth-muscle antibodies	Rare	70%
Positive rheumatoid factor and LE factors	Rare	20%
Anti-mitochondrial antibodies	Rare	20%

The agreed nomenclature for chronic hepatitis is shown in Table VIII.

TABLE VIII
FORMS OF CHRONIC HEPATITIS

Morphological categories	Terms recommended by international group, 1976	Clinical terms in current use	Salient morphological features	Likelihood of direct progression to cirrhosis
Chronic persistent hepatitis	Chronic persistent hepatitis	Chronic persistent hepatitis	Portal inflammation	0
Chronic active hepatitis	Chronic active hepatitis	Chronic active hepatitis, Chronic active liver disease with subacute hepatic necrosis (when bridging present)	Portal and periportal inflammation, periportal necrosis. Severe periportal lesion or chronic hepatitis with bridging necrosis	+ to ++ ++ to +++
Chronic lobular hepatitis	Acute hepatitis lasting more than six months	Prolonged, persistent unresolved hepatitis, etc.	Predominantly intralobular inflammation and necrosis	0

Management of Chronic Hepatitis

It is important to be sure of the diagnosis; the main conditions which give rise to confusion are Wilson's disease, alpha 1 antitrypsin deficiency, and unusual forms of primary biliary cirrhosis. In Wilson's disease there may be a family history, Kayser-Fleischer rings may be present, serum caeruloplasmin levels are low, urinary copper excretion is increased and copper deposition is seen in liver biopsy specimens. Kayser-Fleischer rings are always present if there are associated neuropsychiatric manifestations, but may be absent even with quite marked hepatic impairment.

Chronic persistent hepatitis requires no treatment, although patients with persistent elevation of the transaminases should be followed up. Chronic active hepatitis should probably always be treated to prolong survival and prevent progression to cirrhosis. When chronic active hepatitis is severe, treatment with prednisolone is indicated. The response is less good in those patients who are $HB_s Ag$ positive. The value of treatment in mild cases is still uncertain. Treatment can be with prednisolone alone or a combination of prednisolone and azathioprine. Treatment is usually necessary for six months or more and should be monitored by symptoms, transaminases and evidence of liver-biopsy resolution.

The Halothane Problem

Hepatic necrosis occurs occasionally in the post-operative period. Chloroform was known to do this particularly after repeated administration. Halothane was suspected of doing the same but less frequently—nevertheless its continued use was more than justified by the fact that it is in other ways a safe anaesthetic agent. Once the drug was suspected the question arose whether the drug was causally related to the hepatic necrosis or only an associated factor in it. In order to try and resolve the problem the National Halothane Study was established in the U.S.; in a retrospective survey it could not be established that halothane is causally related to post-operative hepatitis. However, the case against halothane as a very rare cause of hepatitis still remains—particularly after repeated administration. There are proven instances of halothane (and other anaesthetic agents) producing acute hepatocellular damage. Despite analysis of nearly a million cases the National Halothane Study still stress the need for collecting more information on the subject. However, the fact that the case against halothane is so difficult to bring to court implies that the dangers of its use are remote and its safety in other respects justify its continued use. There is no evidence to suggest that the dangers of post-operative hepatic necrosis are greater when operations are performed on the biliary system.

OTHER INFECTIONS

The liver may be involved in septicaemia and almost all viraemias; the most important are yellow fever, glandular fever, Q fever, influenza and Coxsackie infections. The liver is usually involved in Weil's disease, which is due to *Leptospira icterohaemorrhagiae* acquired from contact with infected rat's urine. A similar illness may be caused by *Lept. canicola* acquired from dogs. The important clinical features of leptospirosis are abdominal pain, muscle pains, meningitis, conjunctivitis, haemorrhagic tendency, nephritis and carditis. The clinical diagnosis can be confirmed by demonstrating and culturing the spirochaetes from the blood, a rising antibody titre and intraperitoneal guinea-pig inoculation. The leptospiroses are treated with penicillin or tetracycline.

Worldwide, the two commonest infective diseases affecting the liver are malaria and schistosomiasis. Schistosomiasis gives rise to "pipe stem" cirrhosis in which the lesions are predominantly in the portal tracts. It is the commonest cause of presinusoidal portal hypertension.

The liver is the site of election for many parasitic infections; particularly amoebiasis (*Entamoeba histolytica*) and hydatid disease (*Echinococcus granulosus*) acquired from the excreta of dogs who have eaten infected sheep. Amoebiasis is said never to result in cirrhosis although there may be impairment of liver function tests. Liver function tests are often abnormal in infections remote from the liver. Liver histology in these cases shows "non-specific reactive hepatitis". Where liver function tests are abnormal due to infection within the liver the serum B_{12} is often raised.

CIRRHOSIS

The liver in common with many other organs can only react in a limited number of ways to disease processes. Liver cells may become damaged and necrotic and replaced by fat and fibrous tissue; the portal tracts and central zones may become infiltrated with fibrous tissue and inflammatory cells. The architecture of the liver is dislocated by fibrous tissue and the hepatic cells cease to function because they are directly damaged by the disease, compressed by fibrous tissue and deprived of their blood supply. The liver cells are capable of considerable regeneration, but unfortunately this tends to occur in localised areas and although liver cells may regenerate, the architecture of the liver is not restored. These regeneration nodules may in turn become necrotic if their blood supply is not adequate. The fibrosis and distorted architecture constricts the portal venules, causing a rise in pressure in the portal veins. In the absence of normal liver cells blood is able to flow direct from the portal vein through the sinusoids into the central veins, without coming into contact with viable liver cells, causing a shunt between the portal and systemic veins. These changes explain the main manifestations of liver disease:

Portal hypertension due to obstruction of portal venules within the liver

Hepatocellular failure due to loss of functioning liver cells

Portasystemic encephalopathy due to shunting of blood from the portal vein into the hepatic vein and thus the systemic circulation

Ascites due to a combination of portal hypertension and hepatocellular failure.

PORTAL HYPERTENSION

The portal vein is formed by union of the splenic and superior mesenteric veins. The inferior mesenteric vein drains into the splenic vein. There are several situations where there is a capillary connection between the portal and systemic venous systems. At these sites capillaries and venules become dilated if the pressure in the portal system rises. The most important sites are the lower end of the oesophagus and the anus. The superficial veins on the anterior abdominal wall also dilate; in the normal person the direction of flow in these veins is always away from the umbilicus. The direction of flow is *not* altered in portal hypertension but the veins are dilated and easy to see. If there is obstruction of the inferior vena cava the direction of flow in the veins below the umbilicus is towards the umbilicus and in the veins above the umbilicus the direction of flow remains normal, i.e. upwards. In the rare instances of thrombosis of the portal vein blood reaches the liver through remnants of the umbilical vein (the falciform ligament) and the direction of flow in all the dilated veins is towards the umbilicus. Increased flow of blood in these veins may result in a venous hum.

The spleen enlarges as a result of increased portal vein pressure and congestion. An enlarged spleen from any cause may result in hypersplenism which is characterised by a pancytopenia in the peripheral blood with a normoblastic bone marrow; occasionally only one of the cellular elements of the blood is reduced (Banti's[3] syndrome).

Portal hypertension should rarely be diagnosed unless the spleen is palpable or seen to be enlarged on x-ray. In the extremely rare instance of thrombosis of the splenic vein the spleen may not enlarge. It may also be small and fibrotic as a result of repeated splenic infarcts.

The intrasplenic pressure accurately reflects portal vein pressure;

percutaneous splenic puncture is a convenient way of measuring the portal venous pressure, which should not normally exceed 10 mm Hg. It is also a convenient way of performing portal venography to demonstrate the anatomy of the portal venous system or the site of a blockage.

Obstruction of the hepatic vein is known as Chiari's syndrome, the appearances of the liver are those of severe congestion. The same appearance occurs in veno-occlusive disease, a condition caused by ingesting brews containing Senecio (ragwort) or bush teas commonly drunk in Jamaica. Occlusion of the hepatic veins may be caused by invasion by tumour, thrombophlebitis migrans and thrombosis secondary to polycythaemia or inferior vena cava thrombosis. Two clinical features are important: one is the presence of gross ascites and the other is the absence of hepatojugular reflux due to obstruction of the hepatic vein.

Portal hypertension results from obstruction of the portal venous system inside or outside the liver; extrahepatic portal obstruction is rare in this country. Within the liver the block may be before the portal blood reaches the sinusoids or after the sinusoids (pre- or post-sinusoidal portal hypertension). Portal cirrhosis results when obstruction is post-sinusoidal. The commonest example of pre-sinusoidal portal hypertension is the fibrosis which results from schistosomiasis. It is possible to distinguish between pre- and post-sinusoidal block by measuring the hepatic vein wedge pressure. A catheter wedged tightly in the hepatic vein will measure the pressure in the sinusoids, hence in post-sinusoidal block the wedge pressure will be high and in pre-sinusoidal block the wedge pressure will be low.

Management of Bleeding Oesophageal Varices

Although bleeding from oesophageal varices is usually severe, death is often due to hepatocellular failure and electrolyte disturbances which the loss of blood will almost inevitably produce in a patient with portal hypertension and barely adequate liver function. In this country extrahepatic portal hypertension is a rare cause of oesophageal varices. Patients with cirrhosis causing portal hypertension and oesophageal varices may bleed from a chronic peptic ulcer, to which they are more prone than normal people, or occasionally they may bleed from alcoholic gastritis.

The first essential is to restore blood volume and to institute treatment of hepatocellular failure at the same time. Vitamin K should be given in case there is prothrombin deficiency. The patient may need sedation; the most suitable drugs are chloral, phenobarbitone or chlorpromazine. Paraldehyde, opiates and short-acting barbiturates should not be used.

Control of Haemorrhage

Vasopressin (Pitressin).—Posterior pituitary extract lowers portal venous pressure by constricting splanchnic arterioles, it is useful in reducing portal blood flow and promoting haemostasis. Pitressin is given intravenously, 20 units in 5 per cent dextrose are given over 20 minutes, and it is effective for about an hour. Widespread arteriolar constriction occurs resulting in pallor, a rise in blood pressure and narrowing of the coronary arteries; it should, therefore, be used with caution in patients with coronary artery disease. Another effect is to cause colic and stimulation of the colon which results in diarrhoea. As well as reducing blood flow in the portal vein it also reduces hepatic artery flow which may lead to further anoxia of the liver and hepatocellular damage. Prolonged use of Pitressin results in tachyphylaxis—repeated doses have to be increased in order to have the same effect. The therapeutic dose is the same as the dose which produces side-effects, hence the drug is probably not fully effective until pallor of the skin and colic have been produced.

Sengstaken oesophageal tube (oesophageal tamponade).—The bleeding veins are compressed by an oesophageal balloon kept in place by a balloon in the stomach. Asphyxia and aspiration pneumonias as well as ulceration of the stomach and oesophageal mucosa are common complications.

Gastric hypothermia.—This is available in some centres and may control bleeding.

Emergency surgery.—The main operations used are:

Ligations of varices
Emergency portacaval shunt
Oesophageal and gastric transections.

In transection operations oesophagus or stomach are cut across and resutured. The dilated veins are thereby divided, reducing the pressure at the site at which they are bleeding. Unfortunately, new varices develop very quickly.

Injection of varices with sclerosing substances. This procedure is particularly useful for bleeding varices due to extrahepatic portal hypertension.

Elective portacaval shunt.—Anastomosis of the portal vein to the inferior vena cava will reduce the pressure in the portal veins and oesophageal varices may disappear. The most favoured operation is anatomosing the end of the portal vein to the side of the inferior vena cava. Before the operation a splenoportogram is performed to demonstrate the presence of a patent portal vein. Careful selection of patients for this elective operation is essential. Important features to be considered with regard to operation are:

Serum albumin over 30 g/l
Serum bilirubin below 17 μmol/l
Age under 50
Absent neurological signs during haemorrhage.

Portacaval anastomosis undoubtedly reduces the incidence of further bleeding from varices. However, there is a high incidence of portasystemic encephalopathy—probably about 20 per cent even with rigid selection for operation; the 5-year survival is about 50 per cent. Nevertheless, there is still some doubt whether a portacaval shunt materially improves the mortality rate as compared with conservative management of well-compensated cirrhosis with portal hypertension. The mortality following the first haemorrhage from oesophageal varices is much higher than following subsequent bleeds—in other words a patient who survives his first bleed has already had his most dangerous haemorrhage. Prophylactic shunt operations do not influence survival and they carry the risk of portasystemic encephalopathy although they do reduce the frequency of bleeding.

Hepatocellular Failure

The main causes of hepatocellular failure are:

Acute viral hepatitis
Paracetamol overdose
Other drugs, such as:
    Methyldopa
    Rifampicin
    Halothane
Chronic liver damage
Infarction of the liver.

The precipitating features are often:

Sedation
Excess protein intake
Gastro-intestinal haemorrhage
Infection of ascitic fluid
Diuretics, leading to hypovolaemia
Renal failure.

As soon as acute liver failure is evident it is important to screen for hepatitis B and Wilson's disease, both of which are potentially reversible.

The main features of hepatocellular failure relate to the main functions of the liver:

Jaundice due to failure to conjugate and excrete bilirubin. Severe jaundice is unusual in chronic liver failure except as terminal event. Many causes of cirrhosis are complicated by a haemolytic anaemia which will exaggerate the retention of bilirubin.

Impaired synthesis of proteins, glycogen and glucose leading to weight loss, loss of muscle bulk, hypoglycaemia and a low plasma albumin. Other plasma proteins such as prothrombin and other coagulation factors are also affected, leading to a haemorrhagic tendency. This may be exaggerated if associated portal hypertension causes splenomegaly and hypersplenism with a reduction in platelets.

Hyperkinetic circulation due to:

Increased blood volume

Associated anaemia, which may be caused by haemorrhages, impaired conversion of folic acid into effective folinic acid and impaired metabolism of vitamin B_{12}. The serum levels of folic acid and B_{12} may be normal. Haemolysis may also contribute to the anaemia

Arteriovenous shunting within the lungs

Excessive vasodilator material (VDM) causing peripheral vasodilatation, possibly due to failure of detoxification by the damaged liver

Associated alcoholism may cause beri beri with peripheral vasodilatation and high cardiac output. The hyperkinetic circulation may result in tachycardia, warm peripheries and an ejection-type systolic murmur at the aortic area.

Fever.—A low-grade fever is very common in chronic liver damage, but the exact cause is not known; it has been postulated that the liver fails to detoxify a pyrogenic steroid, or that damaged liver cells release a pyrogen. Gram-negative septicaemias are more common in severe liver disease, due to shunting of blood direct from the portal system to the systemic circulation.

Ascites is due to a combination of hepatocellular failure and portal hypertension. The principal mechanism of formation of ascites is:

Increase in portal vein pressure

Decrease in osmotic potential of plasma, due to decreased serum albumin

Increased production of lymph by the liver

Sodium retention due to hyperaldosteronism from failure of the liver to detoxify aldosterone

Increased water retention due to failure to detoxify antidiuretic hormone

Reduced renal blood flow

Intrarenal shunting.

Ascites is often accompanied by a pleural effusion. Ascitic fluid contains 1–2 g/100 ml protein, in contrast to ascites due to malignant disease and tuberculosis, which usually contains at least 3 g per cent of protein. In a patient with cirrhosis, the presence of a raised protein content and bloodstaining of the ascitic fluid may be due to a hepatoma. There is a rapid interchange between ascitic fluid and the extracellular fluid. Ascites should not be tapped unless the patient is distressed; removal of large amounts of ascitic fluid will deplete the patient's already reduced protein pool; it will also remove a large amount of sodium. Albumin infusions and steroids may be necessary to induce a diuresis and tide the patient over a temporary episode of liver impairment. They are of little value for long-term use.

In the treatment of ascites, the aldosterone antagonist spironolactone may be useful, but its beneficial effect may not be seen for several days; if the ascites is very resistant, amiloride or bumetanide should be used. Sometimes ascites is difficult to improve because of:

Portal-vein thrombosis
Hepatoma
Chronic peritoneal infection.

Portasystemic encephalophathy.—Severe liver-cell damage enables portal blood arriving at the liver to pass through the liver sinusoids directly into the hepatic vein. With the development of portal hypertension there are additional communications between the portal and systemic venous systems. Portal blood contains toxic substances which are normally metabolised in the liver; with extensive porta-systemic shunting these substances pass direct into the systemic circulation.

The clinical features range from minimal mental deterioration to deep coma. The picture is often a mixture of neuropsychiatric manifestations; however, in the early stages the mental changes may predominate, they include personality change, disturbance of sleep rhythm, intellectual deterioration and slurred speech.

The most common neurological abnormality is the "hepatic flap", which is a coarse tremor of the outstretched arms—it is not specific for liver disease. Other neurological abnormalities seen in portasystemic encephalophathy are:

Cerebellar and basal ganglia disturbances
Paraplegia
Motor neuropathy
Epilepsy
Cortical degeneration
Muscle spasms.

Some of these improve with treatment of the primary condition, but others are due to permanent damage and will not improve. The two which usually do not improve are the paraplegia and the focal cortical degeneration.

The CSF may show an increase in protein and the EEG may show slowing of the normal waves. In the normal the dominant wave in the EEG is the α wave with a frequency of 8–13 per second. In portasystemic encephalopathy the speed is about 3–5 per second (delta waves). These changes are also seen in other conditions causing coma, but their appearances in a conscious patient is virtually diagnostic. The EEG is useful in assessing the influence of treatment. One of the best ways of recording progression of cerebral changes is to record the patient's ability to make certain shapes out of match sticks or to draw symmetrical objects, e.g. making a star out of match sticks or drawing a clock face in the notes. Encephalopathy generally leads to constructional apraxia.

The toxic substance producing encephalopathy is not known but there is some correlation with increased blood ammonium levels, although occasionally both blood and CSF ammonium levels are normal in the presence of deep coma.

Peripheral neuropathy occurs in primary liver disease with surprising frequency. In some instances it is impossible to be certain that the neuropathy is not caused by the frequently associated alcoholism, uraemia or diabetes.

Hepatocellular failure may be precipitated by:

> Gastro-intestinal haemorrhage
> High-protein diet
> Infections
> Anaesthesia and operations
> Hypnotic drugs
> Diuretic therapy and hypokalaemia
> Paracentesis abdominis.

Treatment of Hepatocellular Failure and Portasystemic Encephalopathy

Bed rest.

High-calorie and low-protein diet with vitamin supplements.

Correction of electrolyte disturbances.—Hypokalaemia may occur as a result of reduced dietary intake, diuretics and purgation; hypokalaemia may precipitate liver failure by causing an increase in blood ammonium.

Patients with ascites and oedema may have a low serum sodium, due to excessive retention of water. Despite the low serum sodium, they should not be given sodium, but should be treated with sodium and water restriction and an osmotic diuretic. This is followed by oral diuretics; in general it is better to combine a diuretic which acts on the proximal renal tubule, such as the thiazides or frusemide, with one which acts on the distal tubule and conserves potassium, such as spironolactone. However, patients with hyponatraemia *without* ascites and oedema may be sodium depleted and require hypertonic saline. Paracentesis abdominis may precipitate hyponatraemia. A rise in blood urea may occur and is often associated with hypotension or gastro-intestinal haemorrhage. However, the pressure of ascites on renal veins may be responsible for the rise in blood urea in which case some improvement may be obtained by removing some of the ascitic fluid.

Following prolonged use, the effectiveness of the standard diuretics may decline; in some cases it is possible to obtain a diuresis with prednisone or salt-free albumin infusion, although prolonged albumin injections are of no value.

Avoidance of precipitating factor.—Drugs excreted by the liver, such as morphia and the short-acting barbiturates, are never used.

Colonic washout and neomycin enemata.

Antibiotics to sterilise the colon and destroy ammonia-producing organisms. The antibiotic most commonly used is neomycin in a dose of 4 g daily. It should be noted that enough neomycin may be absorbed to cause damage to the eighth nerve.

Colonisation of the colon with non-ammonia-producing organisms resistant to neomycin.—Enpac consists of a dried preparation of *Lactobacillus acidophilus* and has been used for this purpose.

Milk and cheese diet.—The proteins in milk and cheese do not cause as much elevation of blood ammonia as other proteins because they undergo less degradation by ammonia-producing colonic organisms. Milk and cheese are also rich in non-ammonia-producing organisms which tend to displace the ammonia-producing organisms from the colon.

Lactulose.—This is a synthetic disaccharide which is split into lactose and lactic acid. The lactose acts as an osmotic purgative and induces diarrhoea and the lactic acid decreases the pH, inhibiting ammonia-producing organisms.

Consider levodopa or bromocriptine, which is a dopamine agonist. It is proposed that part of the cause of hepatic coma is the production of a false neurotransmitter, octopamine, which diverts precursors away from noradrenalin synthesis. Dopaminergic drugs increase the availability of noradrenalin precursors and, hopefully, reduce the production of false neurotransmitters.

CLASSIFICATION OF CIRRHOSIS

Cirrhosis is best classified as Portal, Biliary, or Cardiac.

Portal Cirrhosis

Portal cirrhosis is so called because the pathological changes are mainly in the portal tracts. In the majority of cases no antecedent cause for the cirrhosis can be found; however, known causes of portal cirrhosis include:

Alcohol
Virus hepatitis (post-necrotic cirrhosis)
Malnutrition
Haemochromatosis
Wilson's disease.

The liver has a limited number of ways in which it can react to injury. There are no specific histological features which distinguish alcoholic from post-necrotic portal cirrhosis. Both types have a diffuse, disorganising fibrosis, liver-cell necrosis and regeneration nodules. There are minor pathological differences between some cases of portal cirrhosis which are suggestive, but not diagnostic, of alcoholic cirrhosis:

The liver is more uniformly affected
Nodules are finer
Fatty change is more pronounced
Cytoplasmic eosinophilic inclusion bodies (Mallory[4] bodies) are commoner. There is a tendency for alcoholic and post-necrotic cirrhosis to present initially in different ways. Alcoholic cirrhosis tends to present with features of hepatocellular failure and hepatomegaly, whereas post-necrotic cirrhosis tends to present with portal hypertension with splenomegaly and oesophageal varices.

The incidence of alcoholism among cirrhotics is about 50 per cent, and the incidence of cirrhosis among alcoholics is about 10 per cent. No particular liquor is more hepatotoxic than any other.

Nutritional liver disease, such as occurs in kwashiorkor, has many similarities with the liver disease occurring in alcoholics. Both are characterised by fatty infiltration and portal cirrhosis, although fatty infiltration is much commoner than cirrhosis in malnutrition. Many alcoholics exist on a diet that is vitamin deficient and low in proteins; this is probably the cause of the fatty liver in most alcoholics. However, the fatty change in the livers of alcoholics has never been shown to proceed to cirrhosis, and furthermore cirrhosis can develop in an alcoholic who has never had a fatty liver.

Alcoholic cirrhosis is reputed to be more commonly associated with a number of extrahepatic manifestations than other forms of cirrhosis. These are: parotid gland enlargement, gynaecomastia, Dupuytren's[5] contracture and leuconychia. Other manifestations of alcoholism are likely to be present in alcoholic cirrhosis—these include peripheral neuropathy with tender calves, gastritis, pancreatitis, myopathy and cardiomyopathy.

In the case of a fatty liver or very mild cirrhosis the liver may revert to normal if the patient totally abstains from alcohol. Abstention from alcohol should be supplemented with B vitamins and a high-protein diet, provided there is no evidence of hepatocellular failure.

Acute alcoholic hepatitis.—The liver may be affected acutely by a high intake of alcohol. There is a sudden onset of hepatocellular failure accompanied by a tender enlarged liver, fever, leucocytosis and cholestasis. Pre-existing cirrhosis need not be present, the condition may occur in a previously normal liver.

Zieve's[6] syndrome.—In 1958 Zieve defined a syndrome which consists of jaundice, haemolytic anaemia and hyperlipaemia or hyper-cholesterolaemia. The syndrome develops following a bout of alcoholic drinking and is commoner in males; it always recedes with abstinence from alcohol; the histology of the liver may be normal or may show fatty infiltration or mild portal cirrhosis. There may be a pyrexia but the transaminases are usually normal. From a practical point of view the syndrome is important because the presence of jaundice with hypercholesterolaemia is highly suggestive of biliary obstruction and secondly because the haemolytic anaemia may not be recognised and an unrewarding search be made for bleeding from the gut.

Other complications of portal cirrhosis include:

Peptic ulcer	Primary hepatoma
Intercurrent infections	Gram-negative septicaemias
Thrombosis of the portal vein	Haemochromatosis.

Haemochromatosis

Iron is carried in the blood bound to a beta 1 globulin (transferrin). Transferrin can transport about $350\,\mu g/dl$ of iron. Normally the serum iron is about $125\,\mu g/dl$. The transferrin is only transporting one-third of the amount of iron that it is potentially capable of carrying, i.e. it is normally 33 per cent saturated. In iron-deficiency anaemia the serum iron is low, the percentage saturation of transferrin is low, but the iron-binding capacity (amount of transferrin) is normal. In haemochromatosis there is increased iron absorption and the serum iron is high, the percentage saturation is increased but the iron-binding capacity is normal.

Some conditions are associated with an iron-deficiency anaemia even though enough iron is being ingested—the main ones are uraemia, carcinomatosis and rheumatoid arthritis. The reason for this is that there is in these conditions either a reduction in the iron-binding capacity or there is a reduced ability to remove iron from the transferrin.

In haemochromatosis, excessive iron is absorbed from the gastro-intestinal tract and is deposited intracellularly as ferritin in certain sites, particularly liver, pancreas, heart and skin. Its deposition is accompanied by fibrosis and an increase in lipofuscin which is partly responsible for the "bronzed" appearance of the skin which gave this condition its original name of "bronzed diabetes". The incidence of mild iron and lipofuscin deposition in the siblings of patients with haemochromatosis is high. Patients with alcoholic cirrhosis also absorb more iron and have a higher serum iron than normal. Excessive iron storage is, therefore, associated with both an inherited defect in the intestinal mucosa and an acquired disease. The controversy about the relative importance of genetic or environmental causes in the development of haemochromatosis has not yet been resolved.

Haemosiderosis is the condition which results from excessive iron ingestion in the presence of a normal small-bowel mucosa, such as occurs in Bantus who cook in iron vessels, or chronic haemolytic anaemias and multiple blood transfusions (usually more than 100). The distribution of ferritin is usually similar to that of haemochromatosis; it may, however, be confined to the reticulo-endothelial system, which, in the liver, is represented by the Kupffer[7] cells.

Clinical features.—The disease is rare but not unknown in women; it does not occur before the menopause unless menstruation has stopped for some other reason. There is a higher incidence of the disease among siblings of affected patients. Occasionally the serum iron is normal and liver biopsy is often necessary to confirm the diagnosis and to check progress. Haemosiderin is frequently found in the liver in cirrhosis and is increased following portacaval shunt operations. The sites most frequently affected are the liver, pancreas, skin and endocrine glands, particularly pituitary, adrenals and testes. Abdominal pain occurs and may be due to stretching of the capsule of the liver. Patients frequently die in shock due to widespread arteriolar dilatation caused by release from the liver of ferritin, which has strong vasodilator properties. Haemochromatosis is one cause of cardio-myopathy, the myocardium becomes fibrotic; involvement of the conducting tissue leads to conduction defects and arrhythmias.

Diagnosis.—Important diagnostic tests are:

Serum iron
Saturation of transferrin
Biopsy appearances of liver, skin and bone marrow
Demonstration of increased iron absorption
Increased urinary excretion of iron with iron-chelating agents
Screening of relatives.

Treatment.—Still the most effective method of removing iron is by repeated phlebotomy. On average the body contains about 50 g of iron in haemochromatosis. One pint of blood contains 250 mg iron. For severe cases, a pint of blood is removed at weekly intervals, until the haemoglobin and serum iron begin to fall. Treatment may have to continue for two years.

Iron-chelating agents (*Gk.* chele—a claw) such as desferrioxamine can only remove about 15 mg of iron per day. Nevertheless, desferrioxamine is a useful adjunct to phlebotomy; its main use, however, is in the treatment of iron overdosage in children who accidentally swallow iron tablets.

Wilson's[8] Disease

Hepatolenticular degeneration is characterised by deposition of copper in liver, basal ganglia and cornea, increased copper secretion in the urine, aminoaciduria, glycosuria and phosphaturia. In the plasma there is a deficiency of the copper-carrying protein caeruloplasmin, an alpha globulin; in its absence copper is loosely bound to albumin and easily deposited in the tissues. Deposition of copper in the cornea is in the form of copper-containing pigment in Descemet's[9] membrane in the posterior surface of the cornea. The deposition is in the form of a ring, separated from the limbus (the corneoscleral junction) by a small zone of clear iris. This clear zone distinguishes Kayser[10]-Fleischer[11] rings from arcus senilis. Portal hypertension is commoner than in haemochromatosis.

Diagnosis.—Important diagnostic findings are:

Low serum copper
Low caeruloplasmin
High urinary copper after penicillamine
Copper content of liver or muscle biopsy
Aminoaciduria
Screening of relatives.

Treatment is with penicillamine (dimethylcysteine) and must continue for at least two years. Toxic effects are similar to those of penicillin. Wilson's disease should be considered as a cause in any patient who develops cirrhosis under the age of 30.

CHRONIC INTRAHEPATIC CHOLESTASIS

Despite considerable advances which have been made in the understanding of the pathophysiology of liver disease and bile production, one clinical question remains fundamental: In the presence of evidence of cholestasis, is the obstruction intrahepatic or extrahepatic?

Once the excretory products of the hepatocytes reach the bile canaliculi the further flow of bile results from its high osmotic pressure due to the bile salts it contains, its high sodium content and the active secretion of fluid by the biliary epithelium under the control of secretin from the duodenal mucosa.

The clinical features of biliary obstruction are often similar irrespective of the level of obstruction; hence a knowledge of the usefulness and limitations of the investigations is essential in order to make a precise diagnosis. One of the practical problems is that other forms of primary liver damage may present as, or be complicated by, cholestasis. Extrahepatic obstruction is always due to gall-stones, stricture, compression from neoplasms or cholangiocarcinomas.

The causes of intrahepatic cholestasis are:

Cirrhosis
Drugs
Viral hepatitis
Pregnancy
Primary biliary cirrhosis
Ascending cholangitis
Inflammatory bowel disease.

Clinical features in all cases of biliary obstruction which has lasted more than a few weeks will include jaundice, itching, dark urine and pale stools. The liver is usually palpable, the patient jaundiced, with scratch marks and xanthomata if the obstruction is long-standing.

The Distinction Between Intrahepatic and Extrahepatic Obstruction

A history of previous attacks, suggestive of cholecystitis, will favour the diagnosis of gall stones. However, enlargement of the liver, if rapid or gross, will cause right hypochondrial pain which may be mistaken for dyspepsia or pleuritic pain. A palpable gall bladder suggests extrahepatic obstruction due to pancreatic or Vaterian carcinoma (Courvoisier's[12] law). Most cases have a raised direct-acting bilirubin, bile in the urine, raised alkaline phosphatase and raised transaminases. Investigations should include a barium meal and hypotonic duodenography to demonstrate the possibility of an abnormal duodenal loop due to a pancreatic carcinoma. If the bilirubin level is not too high it is still worth considering a high-dose intravenous cholangiogram to demonstrate the extrahepatic biliary tree; if positive, the cholangiogram may expedite surgery. Radioisotope scanning may show filling defects, but care should be taken in interpreting multiple filling defects as these may be due to dilated bile ducts. Isotope scanning using different isotopes may give some useful information; for example, hepatomas tend to concentrate selenium-labelled methionine or gallium-labelled citrate, whereas biliary carcinomas result in filling defects. Other scans such as ^{131}I-labelled rose bengal or HIDA scans concentrate in dilated bile ducts, and therefore suggest extrahepatic obstruction. The most useful tests are:

> An ultrasound scan
> Isotopic scanning
> Transhepatic cholangiography using a Shiba needle (skinny needle)
> ERCP
> CAT scan.

Other helpful investigations include:

> Antimitochondrial antibodies (M antibodies). These are present in all patients with primary biliary cirrhosis, although there is an overlap in that they may also be present in other forms of cirrhosis and in some normals;
> Carcinoembryonic antigen (CEA) often present in cholangiocarcinoma;
> Alphafetoprotein is frequently present in patients with hepatocellular carcinoma (hepatoma);
> Liver biopsy. The dangers of liver biopsy in jaundice are probably less than was previously feared.

Management of Chronic Cholestasis

1. Avoidance of surgery and corticosteroids.
2. Preventions of vitamin deficiencies, particularly vitamin K and vitamin D.
3. Cholestyramine. This is given as an orange-flavoured drink—4 g daily with meals so that it can mix with and be excreted with the postprandial bile. Cholestyramine may aggravate vitamin D deficiency, and will only be of value in preventing itching if biliary obstruction is not complete. Itching is due to excessive levels of bile salts in the blood and tissues, because the liver is unable to excrete bile salts normally in the presence of cholestasis. Normally, the gall bladder empties after a meal and delivers up to 3 g of bile salts into the intestine; all of this is rapidly absorbed and cleared by the liver, so that bile-salt concentrations in the peripheral circulation seldom rise after a meal (although of course levels in the portal circulation do rise). In the presence of cholestasis the liver has to excrete bile salts

slowly all the time; hence, it follows that it is better to avoid bile reaching the intestines for as long a period as possible. Patients should therefore be advised to allow as much time as possible between an evening meal and breakfast.

4. Consideration of an H_2-receptor antagonist, because of the high incidence of associated duodenal ulceration.

5. Consideration of penicillamine. There is an increased deposition of copper in all forms of cholestasis, but particularly in primary biliary cirrhosis. It has been assumed by analogy with Wilson's disease that the accumulation of copper may be harmful and that its removal would be beneficial; however, in contrast to Wilson's disease the copper is not present in hepatocyte mitochondria and there is no correlation between the quantity of copper in biopsy specimens and the extent of liver fibrosis. Penicillamine is therefore not indicated in primary biliary cirrhosis.

ACUTE PANCREATITIS

In most cases the aetiology of an attack of acute pancreatitis is not known, but there is an association between attacks of acute pancreatitis and a number of known factors. These are:

Cholelithiasis	Hyperparathyroidism
Alcoholism	Steroid therapy
Pancreatic-duct obstruction	Hypothermia
Trauma	Septicaemia
Vascular insufficiency	Virus infections, such as mumps.

Clinical Features

In the classical case there is a sudden onset of severe epigastric pain which is constant in intensity but may be relieved by the patient leaning forward or by kneeling forward on the bed. The pain does not always radiate to the back, is not usually relieved by opiates, and is accompanied by vomiting. The physical signs depend on the stage of the disease. In the early stages there may be a resemblance to acute cholecystitis, with upper abdominal pain and guarding; at this stage there is no ileus, and bowel sounds may be normal. Some hours later the patient becomes shocked, there is peritonitis with widespread rigidity and absent bowel sounds. In the early stages the diagnostic clue may be mild tenderness in the flanks, which usually becomes obvious in the later stages.

The level of serum amylase is helpful but it is essential to realise that raised serum amaylase is not diagnostic. Levels over 1000 Somogyi[13] units are highly suggestive but do occur in other causes of peritonitis, possibly as a result of associated pancreatic damage.

Conditions in which a raised serum amylase may occur are perforated ulcer, paralytic ileus, acute cholecystitis, cirrhosis, mumps, parotitis and renal failure. The rise in serum amylase may be transient but the urinary amylase is raised for longer; in addition, the serum lipase shows a more sustained rise than the amylase in acute pancreatitis.

Other clinical features which may be present are hyperglycaemia, tetany—due to a reduction in the serum calcium possibly as a result of combination with liberated fats in the peritoneum—electrocardiographic changes, and an x-ray appearance of an isolated distended loop of small intestine. The other condition in which an isolated distended loop may be seen is localised ischaemia due to occlusion of a branch of the mesenteric artery.

Treatment

If possible laparotomy should be avoided if the diagnosis is reasonably certain as the mortality of acute pancreatitis is increased following an operation. Pain is treated with analgesics which will not constrict the sphincter of Oddi[14] or cause contraction of the gall bladder. Vagal stimulation of the pancreas can be prevented by blocking the vagi with atropine or propantheline. Continuous gastric suction will prevent gastric contents causing hormonal stimulation of the pancreas by means of secretin and pancreozymin.

Pain may also be relieved by epidural or paravertebral block. Broad-spectrum antibiotics are usually given; corticosteroids are justified if all else seems to be failing.

Aprotinin (Trasylol) is a proteolytic enzyme inhibitor, and there has been one double-blind controlled trial which has confirmed that Trasylol reduces mortality and may reduce the severity of the illness. Nevertheless the mortality in the controlled group was 25 per cent, which seems unusually high, although the mortality in the treated group was 7·5 per cent, which would suggest that when used according to the scheme advocated by these authors Trasylol may be beneficial.

Peritoneal lavage to remove extruded proteolytic enzymes may also be helpful.

Glucagon produced by the islet α-cells is known to reduce both the volume and enzyme content of exocrine pancreatic secretion. Furthermore glucagon levels are raised in acute pancreatitis. It is suggested that following any acute injury to the pancreas there is a rise in glucagon levels which protects the pancreas against auto-injury—only when endogenous glucagon levels fall does pancreatic damage progress. This would account for the delay frequently noted between pancreatic injury and the onset of pancreatic symptoms and signs. It is suggested that on this basis glucagon infusion is logical and worthwhile in the management of acute pancreatitis.

CHRONIC PANCREATITIS

The commonest features are constant, dull, upper abdominal or back pain and weight loss; rarely, jaundice, diabetes or pancreatic cysts occur.

Pancreatic exocrine insufficiency can be confirmed by measuring the volume, bicarbonate and enzyme content of pancreatic juice obtained by duodenal intubation. Secretin causes the pancreas to produce an increased volume of juice with a high bicarbonate content; pancreozymin increases the enzyme content. In the presence of diffuse damage to the pancreas as a result of chronic pancreatitis, secretin and pancreozymin produce a juice of normal volume but of reduced bicarbonate and enzyme content, whereas in the presence of duct obstruction the volume falls off but the concentration of bicarbonate and enzymes remains roughly normal. The serum levels of amylase and lipase are measured before and after injection of secretin and pancreozymin—a rise in serum enzymes indicates obstruction of the pancreatic duct. If the pancreas is completely replaced by fibrous tissue there will be no response to secretin and pancreozymin as measured either by the serum enzymes or by duodenal intubation.

Pancreatic insufficiency should be suspected in malabsorption with a normal intestinal biopsy. It is always worth looking for microscopically visible meat fibres in the stool. These are present in chronic pancreatic insufficiency because of the absence of proteolytic enzymes. They are not found in malabsorption of intestinal origin.

In severe chronic pancreatitis there may also be pancreatic calcification visible radiologically, and mild diabetes. Chronic pancreatitis also results in B_{12} deficiency; the postulated mechanism is excessive binding of B_{12} to proteins which are normally destroyed by pancreatic proteolytic enzymes. Treatment is with pancreatic extract; if this is not successful it may be because it is destroyed in the stomach by acid gastric juice, in which case cimetidine may be helpful.

A new test being evaluated is the benzoyl-tyrosyl-PABA test; PABA appears in the urine if it is split off the complex by pancreatic proteolytic enzymes.

REFERENCES

BIANCHI, L. et al. (1977) Acute and chronic hepatitis revisited. (Review by an International Group.) Lancet, 2, 914.

INTERNATIONAL GROUP (1976) Diseases of the Liver and Biliary Tract. Washington: D.H.E.W. Publication No. (N.I.H.) 76–725.

OWENS, D. and SHERLOCK, S. (1973) Brit. med. J., 3, 559.

ZIEVE, L. (1958) Ann. intern. Med., 48, 471.

EPONYMS

1. Albert Abraham Hujmans Van Den Bergh (1869–1943)
Utrecht physician.

2. Nicolas Augustin Gilbert (1858–1927)
Gilbert became Professor of Medicine at the Hotel Dieu, Paris in 1910. He described his syndrome in 1907.

3. Guido Banti (1852–1925)
Banti was Chief of the Institute of Pathology in Florence, and described his anaemia in 1883.

4. Frank Burr Mallory (1862–1971)
Mallory, Professor of Pathology in Harvard, popularised haematoxylin and aniline blue stain for collagen; he also devised methods of tracing the embryonic origin of tumours. He was the first pathologist to perfect techniques of photomicrography.

5. Baron Guillaume Dupuytren (1777–1835)
Dupuytren was lucky to qualify; in the middle of his education the French Revolution started and he had to return home. All the medical schools in France were abolished until Napoleon re-established three of the older schools. Dupuytren successfully exploited the tortuous political climate of Revolutionary, Napoleonic and Restoration Paris. He was created a Baron by Louis XVIII. The wounded from Waterloo provided him with extensive experience. The 1830 Revolution also added to his unrivalled experience in dealing with the surgery of violence. He is said to have purloined his assistant's own treatise on the treatment of trauma; the assistant was Prosper Menière.

6. Leslie Zieve
Minneapolis physician.

7. Karl Wilhelm Von Kupffer (1829–1902)
Kupffer qualified in Munich and became Professor of Anatomy successively in Kiel, Königsberg and Munich. He made a study of the blood and bone marrow using the newly introduced stains derived from aniline dyes. He studied the electric organs of electric eels, and while in Königsberg he studied the skull of Immanuel Kant who had been Professor of Philosophy there.

8. Samuel Alexander Kinnier Wilson (1877–1937)
Born in New Jersey, Wilson qualified in Edinburgh and then worked with Marie and Babinski. He then went to Queen's Square as a physician. In 1912 he published his M.D. thesis on lenticular degeneration associated with cirrhosis. He was an influential figure who wrote and taught well.

9. Jean Descemet (1732–1810)
Descemet was both physician and botanist; he was one of the first teachers at Napoleon's newly created lycées.

10. Bernhard Kayser (b. 1869)
Kayser qualified in Tübingen and Berlin. He eventually worked in Stuttgart.

11. Bruno Fleischer (1874–1965)
Fleischer qualified in Tübingen in 1904 and specialised in ophthalmology. Kayser discovered the rings in 1901 but it was Fleischer who linked them with Wilson's disease. Much of his work was done on the inheritance of red/green colour blindness and other eye diseases.

12. Ludwig Courvoisier (1843–1918)
Basle surgeon.

13. Michael Somogyi (1883–1971)
Biochemist, Jewish Hospital, St Louis, Missouri.

14. Ruggero Oddi (1845–1906)
Physiologist, Perugia, Italy.

5

AUTOIMMUNE AND JOINT DISEASES

The clinical significance of disorders related to immune mechanisms has increased with greater understanding and technical achievements. The factors which affect the current importance of immunology are the greater understanding or discovery of:

Cellular and humoral immune mechanisms
Human leucocyte antigens (HLA system)
Differential lymphocyte function (T and B lymphocytes)
The structure and function of immunoglobulins
The mediators of inflammatory changes such as prostaglandins and complement
The immune processes of transplantation and neoplasia.

The starting point in the study of immunity was the well-known observation that people who survived one of the infectious diseases seldom developed the same disease a second time. Pasteur[1] was concerned with attenuating virulent organisms, particularly anthrax and rabies, and vaccinating prophylactically, trying to induce the same immunity that naturally occurring infectious diseases induce. It was later shown for some diseases, for example cholera, that when cell-free filtrate of serum from patients who had recovered was injected into other individuals, it could prevent development of the disease, indicating that it was a circulating substance and not the organism itself which was responsible for immunity. In the case of typhoid fever Widal[2] in 1896 found that the protection was due to a circulating antibody which could be detected *in vitro*. At the same time actual cases of diphtheria were sometimes cured by injecting the serum from a horse previously immunised with diphtheria, and the concept of antitoxins as well as circulating antibodies developed. However, the suggestion that circulating antibodies and antitoxins were mainly responsible for immune protection was challenged by Metchnikoff[3] who almost accidentally discovered cellular phagocytosis in an organism devoid of blood vessels (and so therefore devoid of humoral antibody). So was born the controversy over the relative importance of humoral against cellular mechanisms in immune protection.

It had always been understood that immunity was protective until

Richet in 1902 discovered the harmful effects of anaphylaxis and in 1906 Von Pirquet suggested the term allergy to cover both immunity and hypersensitivity. Thus, immunology should strictly be allergology, but allergy usually now refers to the state of hypersensitivity.

Further fuel was provided for the humoral-versus-cellular basis for immunity by the observation of Arthus in 1903 that second and subsequent injections of antigen into the skin produced a local skin reaction involving lymphocytes, and the observation of Schick that repeated injections of horse serum containing diphtheria antibodies resulted in systemic illness called serum sickness. Both of these observations supported the cellular mechanism of immunity.

The two postulated principal immune mechanisms became largely reconcilable with the discovery of histamine by Sir Henry Dale in 1909. The anaphylactic reaction could be explained by histamine release from an antibody-antigen complex, even if the antibody was attached to cells and so not detectable in the serum before the antigen which produced the anaphylactic shock was given.

In the 1920s and 1930s there were glimmerings of the concept of immune mechanisms causing disease, as opposed to immunity being protective or harmful as with anaphylaxis or serum sickness. It was noted that the lesions of rheumatic fever (Aschoff[4] nodes) closely resembled those of the Arthus reaction. In 1934 a Japanese pathologist (Musugi) succeeded in inducing glomerulonephritis in response to injection of antiserum raised against kidney, and so was born the concept of autoimmunity, or immune mechanisms directed against the body's own tissues. It was known that tissues and blood from one individual could not be successfully transplanted into another individual and that rejection occurred as a result of local immune mechanisms, but attempts to induce generalised and harmful immune reactions as a result of injection of tissues from the same species were unsuccessful and it was not until 1945 that Coombs and others demonstrated that in acquired haemolytic anaemia there were antibodies against the patient's own red cells. Soon other disorders were produced as a result of injecting testicular and brain tissue. The concept of autoimmune diseases was now established. The enigma of why the body does not generally develop immunity to its own tissues remained. In 1949 it was predicted by Burnet that the ability to recognise "self" was due to the fact that the antibody-producing cells were exposed to the "self" antigen during fetal life and the cells learnt not to produce this anti-self antibody. This was soon confirmed experimentally in mice by Medawar, and it was shown that acquired tolerance was due to failure to manufacture antibody rather than a mechanism to destroy self-mutilating antibody. The clonal selection theory of Burnet postulated the inheritance of innumerable cell genotypes each of which can respond by producing a line of phenotypes capable of producing only a specific antibody in response to a specific antigen; acquired tolerance would be due to suppression of those primitive cells with genotypes capable of producing antibody-producing phenotypes against any of the body's protein already encountered in fetal life. The theory has stood the test of time and is additionally supported by the occurrence of disturbances of cell proliferation such as myeloma in which plasma cells over-produce a morphologically normal globulin. The concept that immune mechanisms have developed to protect mainly against external antigens must be expanded considerably to include the concept that the most important aspect of immunity may be to protect against antigens occurring within the body as a result of spontaneous malignant change in some of the body's own cells—a process which is probably continuous. The need for this constant immune surveillance has led to the development of an immune system which has well-developed afferent and efferent components.

Certain technical as well as conceptual developments have also contributed greatly to the understanding of the importance of immune mechanisms. In 1937 Tiselius showed by electrophoresis that the plasma proteins could be separated into different components and that the gamma component contained antibodies. In 1953 Graber and Williams demonstrated that further separation of the gamma globulins could be made if electrophoresis was combined with precipitation of the globulins with already prepared antigens—a process known as immunoelectrophoresis. In 1959 Porter reported that gamma globulin could be split by a process of papain digestion into three separate components, two of which contained the antibody-binding sites and the third of which gave the molecule other properties such as the ability to pass through cell membranes or combine with complement.

As a result of investigation into transplant rejection it is known that rejection involves local cellular reactions as well as generalised serum-sickness type of reactions, and it is known that most cells contain inherited and specific antigens responsible for rejection; these are the histocompatibility antigens.

HLA System

The genetic control of immunity is of fundamental importance. In man chromosome 6 carries the genes controlling antigens associated with histocompatibility. There are four groups of histocompatibility leucocyte antigens (HLA A, B, C and D). These antigens were discovered as a result of histocompatibility studies in transplant work. The antigens occur on most tissue cells but can be detected most easily on lymphocytes. The role of the HLA system in man is:

Control of cell membrane antigens
Control of genes concerned with immunoglobulin function
Regulation of lymphocyte development
Regulation of complement
Association with disease susceptibility.

A number of diseases are known to be associated with certain HLA antigens, but the evidence is conflicting that the disease is due to the presence of a particular antigen. For example, the HLA B27 antigen, which is found in up to 96 per cent of patients with ankylosing spondylitis, has no related immunological activity. Some of the suggested mechanisms of disease association with the HLA system are:

Micro-organisms can incorporate HLA antigens onto their surfaces so that the body recognises the virus as self, does not mount an antibody response, and is therefore susceptible to infection.

Individual tissue may lack some HLA antigens and therefore may not be recognised as self. Platelets, and endocrine tissue may lack HLA B8.

Similarity of HLA and viral antigens may also allow viruses to enter cells through an HLA window.

The presence of particular HLA antigens may simply be associated with another gene which is the fundamental cause for the increased disease susceptibility.

Table IX shows the main histocompatibility-antigen-associated diseases, but it should be noted that there is often not enough information to answer the most important question "What is the risk of an individual who carries a specific associated HLA antigen (e.g. B27) developing the associated disease (e.g. ankylosing spondylitis)?"

HLA B27

This HLA antigen is of great importance in the seronegative arthritides. The antigen is present in 5–10 per cent of the population. Its incidence varies in different races from zero in Maoris to 50 per cent in some Indian tribes. About 20 per cent of those with HLA B27 will develop sacro-iliitis; it is present in over 90 per cent of patients with ankylosing spondylitis. The frequency is probably similar for Reiter's disease. The frequency of complications following Reiter's disease is also related to the presence of HLA B27; it may become a chronic disease in about 10 per cent of those who develop it; nearly all of these will be HLA B27 positive.

TABLE IX

HLA-ASSOCIATED DISEASES

HLA-B27-related diseases	Frequency (per cent)
Normals	8
Ankylosing spondylitis	90
Reiter's syndrome	80
Psoriatic arthritis	50
Juvenile rheumatoid disease in boys	80
Colitis with spondylitis	80
Yersinia arthritis	90
Anterior uveitis	60

Other HLA-associated diseases

B8	Coeliac disease
	Dermatitis herpetiformis
	Myasthenia gravis
	Graves' disease
	Chronic active hepatitis
B7	Multiple sclerosis

Immune-Complex Disease

This term refers to those clinical states which result from deposition of antigen-antibody complexes and complement as a result of continued production of immune complexes long after the initiating stimulus. The clinical features vary, but include fever, arthralgia, lymphadenopathy, vasculitis, uveitis and nephritis. Diseases which are thought to be caused by immune complexes are Henoch-Schönlein purpura, polyarteritis nodosa and Reiter's disease. More non-specific manifestations may follow most infectious diseases. One possible mechanism for immune-complex diseases is partial failure of T-lymphocytes to eliminate the offending antigen. This allows continuous antigenic stimulation of B-lymphocytes and an excess of humoral antibody, which then form insoluble immune complexes with the circulating antigen. Rheumatoid factor is an antibody directed against a circulating specific IgM in most patients with rheumatoid arthritis.

Autoimmunity

A number of diseases are caused by the production of antibodies against patients' own tissues. There are several possible mechanisms:

By mutation, clones of lymphocytes develop which are directed against self as a result of failure of the normal mechanism acquired in fetal life by which lymphocytes capable of producing antibody against self are suppressed.

By failure of the normal mechanism by which anti-self antibodies are normally destroyed.

By the introduction of an antigen very similar to some tissue within the body so that the resulting antibodies are also directed against this similar body tissue.

Types of Immune Reaction

There are four main reactions by which immune responses are mediated.

Type I or anaphylactic reactions.—The body's first defence against a foreign protein is usually the skin or one of the mucous membranes. The mucous membranes are coated with a secretory immunoglobulin known as IgA. The next defence is the presence of reaginic antibody (IgE) in the lymphocytes of the submucous layers; IgE is attached to mast cells and the combination of antigen with cell-bound IgE leads to local cell damage and release of histamine and prostaglandins.

The commonest antigens responsible for Type I reaction are pollens, moulds, house-mite dust, animal fur, some foods, and drugs such as penicillin and iodides. The reactions may be generalised if the allergen is injected, or local, resulting in asthma, urticaria or food allergies, depending on the site of absorption.

Desensitisation is often possible if only one or two allergens produce a reaction. Desensitisation results in the production of circulating IgG antibody which combines with the offending allergen before it gets a chance to react with IgE antibody attached to mast cells.

Type II reaction or direct damage by circulating antibodies.— These are cytotoxic immune reactions involving circulating antigen which reacts with cell surface antibodies, leading to destruction of the cell. This process involves complement as well and is mainly intravascular. In most of these reactions complement is used up and it is this type of reaction that immobilises or destroys invading micro-organisms; again, B lymphocytes are mainly involved. This type of reaction is also involved with drug hypersensitivities, particularly those causing haemolytic anaemia. The drug may act as a hapten and becomes attached to the cell membrane of the red cells, rendering them antigenic; antibodies to the red cell or drug antigen then arise, resulting in destruction of the red cell.

Type III or immune complex reactions.—Immune complexes are large antibody/antigen combinations, their solubility, and hence their distribution, may vary according to whether the antibody or antigen is in excess. This may also affect the cellular immune response. Depending on their solubility they may deposit in:

Vessel walls, causing an arteritis.—The deposition may also be affected by mediators which affect vascular permeability.

Diseases probably associated with vessel-wall deposition are: polyarteritis, necrotising vasculitis, Wegener's granulomatosis, Behçet's disease, and glomerulonephritis.

Extravascular tissue (and joint cavities).—This occurs in several conditions associated with a transient arthritis, and also in rheumatoid arthritis in which the situation is known to be very complicated, with IgG, rheumatoid factor behaving both as an antigen and an antibody.

Immune complexes produce disruption of tissues by several mechanisms:

Activation of complement, some components of which are cell destructors

Activation of cells which release harmful enzymes

Production of hyperviscosity of the blood

Direct interference with function simply by deposition, e.g. impairment of glomerular filtration by immune-complex deposition.

The possible therapeutic implication of the above mechanisms are the removal of immune complexes by plasmapheresis, the direct effect on immune complexes of penicillamine, and the possibilities of removing or interfering with complement and cell mediators of inflammation. Antibody production following the admission of antigen takes several days to build up, and Type III or serum-sickness reactions can only occur if the antigen remains for this length of time in the plasma; usually, therefore, the antigen has to be a protein. Penicillin and other drugs produce a Type III reaction by forming complexes with circulating plasma proteins and acting as haptens.

Type IV, or delayed hypersensitivity reactions, or cell-mediated immune reactions.—This type of reaction is mediated by the T-lymphocytes, and is characterised by lymphocyte infiltration; this type of reaction is responsible for graft rejection. The antigens of the graft stimulate the production of T-lymphocytes which contain antibody to graft antigen, and the host lymphocytes infiltrate, causing graft rejection.

Role of the Lymphocytes

The lymphocytes are involved in all immune responses, whether humoral or cellular. The humoral antibodies are derived from B-lymphocytes which mature into plasma cells, and the cell-mediated immune responses are mediated by lymphocytes derived from the thymus, known as T-lymphocytes. The T-lymphocytes have antibodies firmly attached to the cell surface and the whole lymphocyte therefore becomes involved in any antibody-antigen reaction, whereas the plasma cells derived from B-lymphocytes produce antibody which acts unattached to cells, and at a distance, having been carried to the site of the antigen in the blood stream. T- and B-lymphocytes are located in different parts of lymph nodes: the T-lymphocytes are in the deepest layer of the cortex of lymph glands. B-lymphocytes differ from T-lymphocytes in that they have receptors for the Fc fragment of antibodies and for the C3 component of complement. The exact mechanism of antibody production, of recognition of previously encountered and self antigens, and of the afferent or detection system are still obscure. It is known that the T- and B-lymphocyte systems are mutually interdependent and that T-lymphocytes are necessary for the B-lymphocytes to be able to manufacture antibodies; furthermore, following an antigenic stimulus the initial antibody response is often an IgM antibody, followed some days later by an IgG antibody. The B-lymphocytes become programmed to react with antigens, but the proliferation of B-lymphocytes is profoundly affected by T-lymphocytes which may enhance B-lymphocyte production ("helper" cells) or may suppress B-lymphocyte production ("suppressor" cells). In addition, T-cells act as "cytotoxic" cells in cell-mediated immune reactions and produce lymphokines, which inhibit movement of macrophages and so localise the macrophage response to the site of immune injury. The "cytotoxic" T-cells recognise and destroy host cells which have antibody attached to them. "Suppressor" cells limit the hosts response to programmed B-cells, especially if this response may itself be harmful.

The Complement System

Most B-lymphocytes are coated with monomeric IgM attached to the cells by their Fc fragment, leaving the antibody-reactive part of the IgM molecule free to react. The B-lymphocytes also have receptor sites for the Fc portion of IgG and for components of the complement series. The complement series consists of about 15 separate circulating plasma proteins; when activated each of the components of the complement series is the trigger which induces different parts of the inflammatory response, for example:

Histamine release	Leucocyte immobilisation
Neutralisation of viruses	Promotion of phagocytosis
Cell-membrane destruction	Promotion of fibrinolysis
Release of kinins	Promotion of coagulation.
Vascular permeability	

The complement system is activated by two separate mechanisms:
1. The classical pathway, activated by antibody/antigen complexes, which binds $C1_q$ to the free Fc fragment of the immunoglobulins which make up the immune complex; the Fc fragment is not

involved when antigen reacts with antibody. Cl_q normally prevents the activation of C1 but when "neutralised" by being bound to the Fc fragments complement activation occurs. The classical pathway activates C1 C2 C4 and C3 which binds the immune complex to cell membranes and promotes vascular permeability.

2. The "alternative" pathway is activated by endotoxins and IgA. The two pathways both activate C3 and the remainder of the complement cascade. The later components of the complement series all contribute to cell-membrane dissolution.

Complement components can be measured individually but in practice it is usual to measure only C3 C4 and Cl_q. The integrity of the whole complement cascade is measured by the "CH_{50}", which is a measure of the haemolytic activity of the complement series.

Septicaemic shock and glomerulonephritis are characterised by activation of the alternative pathway which causes reduced C3, reduced overall function of the complement series (therefore reduced CH_{50}) but normal C4. There are certain inherited conditions in which individual components of the pathway are deficient.

C3 complement component deficiency:	recurrent bacterial infections
C1 inhibitor activity:	angioneurotic oedema
C2:	SLE syndromes and other connective-tissue diseases
C6 and C8:	Neisseria infections

Diseases Produced by Immune Processes

Type I:
  Asthma
  Acute allergic phenomena.
Type II (require activation of complement):
  Autoimmune haemolytic anaemia in which the circulating antibody damages the red cell membrane in the reticulo-endothelial system; the weakened red cell is haemolysed when it returns to the circulation
  Thrombocytopenic purpura
  Goodpasture's syndrome
  Penicillin-induced haemolytic anaemia.
Type III (immune-complex mediated):
  Serum sickness
  Vasculitis
  SLE, rheumatoid arthritis, thyroiditis
  Hypersensitivity pneumonitis, e.g. farmer's lung

Post-streptococcal glomerulonephritis
Other post-infectious nephritis (e.g. SBE, glandular fever, malaria)
Hepatitis-B-associated nephritis, and connective-tissue diseases
Henoch-Schönlein purpura
Polyarteritis
Tumour antigen nephritis.

Type IV:
Allograft transplant rejection
Tumour-cell destruction
Resistance to intracellular pathogens, e.g. toxoplasmosis
Resistance to chronic mucocutaneous candidiasis.

The Laboratory Diagnosis and Assessment of Immunological Disorders

1. Circulating auto-antibodies and antigens.—Radioimmunoassay involves using pure antigen which is isotopically labelled, and incubating with the test serum. Any immune complex then formed will contain radioactivity, and this is detected by filtering or precipitating out the immune complex. In connective-tissue diseases there are circulating antibodies to normal cell components such as DNA and other nuclear components.

2. Complement levels.—Circulating immune complexes usually depress total complement levels. The CH_{50} measures the overall complement system (the CH_{50} refers to the fact that the test result is related to normal serum complement haemolysing 50 per cent of red cells *in vitro*). Individual complement components such as C3 and C4 can also be measured.

3. Circulating immune complexes

1. *Indirect measurement* by finding low complement levels or raised levels of complement breakdown products, e.g. C3c and C3d.
2. *Labelled* Cl_q *binding.* Labelled Cl_q globulin is incubated with test specimen and the amount of radioactivity incorporated in any immune complexes can be measured.
3. *Rajii cell immunoassay.* Rajii cells are lymphoid cells which have complement receptors and receptors for the Fc fragment of IgG. Labelled anti-IgG will react with the free ends of IgG attached to the Rajii cell by the Fc component.

4. Cryoglobulins.—Immune complexes tend to precipitate at temperatures below blood temperature. Monoclonal cryoglobulins of IgA, IgG or IgM occur in lymphomas. The cryoglobulins of connective-tissue diseases are polyclonal, often mixtures of IgM and IgG immune complexes.

5. Tests of cell-mediated immunity

1. *E rosette test*. Normally about 75 per cent of circulating lymphocytes are T-lymphocytes. The E rosette test uses sheep erythrocytes to bind on to leucocytes to form the E rosette.

2. *Lymphocyte transformation*. Lymphocytes incubated with tritiated thymidine are grown in culture with and without phyto-
haemagglutinin. Transformation to lymphoblasts is indicated by
the incorporation of tritiated thymidine into newly synthesised
DNA.

3. *DNCB sensitisation*. Dinitrochlorobenzene acts as a hapten and
in a normal individual with normal functioning T-lymphocytes
skin sensitisation occurs after 10 days.

4. *Inhibition of leucocyte migration*. Lymphocytes which are
immunologically active will, when challenged with a ubiquitous
antigen, release lymphokinins which inhibit further leucocyte
migration.

Immunoglobulins

There are three main groups of immunoglobulins designated
immunoglobulins G, M and A or IgG, IgM and IgA. The normal
amounts of these in the serum are:

IgG : 700–1500 mg per cent
IgM : 60–170 mg per cent
IgA : 150–250 mg per cent

The structure of immunoglobulins can be represented diagrammatically as four chains of polypeptides, parallel to each other, with the
shorter, light chains enclosing a pair of larger, heavy chains. All four
chains are joined at intervals by sulphydryl bonds (Fig. 27). All the

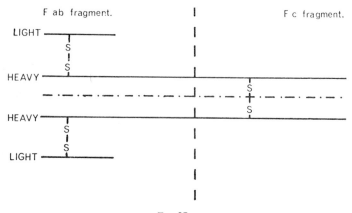

FIG. 27.

immunoglobulins have the same basic structure, except that IgM (macroglobulins) consist of aggregates of five of the basic units. There are only two types of light (L) chains, known as κ(kappa) and λ(lambda) chains; these are never mixed in the same *molecule*. Normally, two-thirds of immunoglobulins contain κ L chains and one-third contain λ L chains. IgG contains 4 different types of H chain which are antigenically distinct.

The 4 antigenically different H chains on IgG are designated a, b, c and d. IgA contains only one antigenic type of H chain, designated an α (alpha) H chain, as does IgM, which is designated a μ (mu) H chain. It should be noted that there are probably hundreds of different antibodies contained in the few antigenically distinct H chains, thus there are six basic types of H chain, containing 300–400 amino acids; the different antibodies are produced by jiggling around with the last, say, dozen amino acids in the chain; the vast bulk of the chain remains unchanged and is responsible for producing the recognisable six basic types of H chain.

Individual molecules of immunoglobulins can be split by papain digestion, as shown in Fig. 27. This produces two fragments which still have antigenic properties and are therefore called the antibody fragment (Fab), and one fragment which crystallises (Fc). Note that it is the Fc fragment which is responsible for antigenic differences between the immunoglobulins. The Fab fragment is the part that binds antigen. IgG contains about 80 per cent of the antibodies, including antibacterial and antiviral antibodies; IgG alone has other properties which it owes to its Fc component, viz:

Ability to cross the placenta
Ability to initiate complement fixation (IgM is more able to mobilise complement)
Fixation to skin receptor sites for sensitisation in the passive cutaneous anaphylactic reaction.

IgG is a smaller molecule than IgM and can pass into the body fluids. The initial immune response usually involves IgM, which, being a larger molecule than IgG, remains in the circulation.

IgM is a macroglobulin because it consists of 5 standard immuno-globulin molecules attached at their Fc ends. IgM is especially good at mobilising complement. Because of its large size it is confined to the vascular system. It is the first antibody to increase when there is a foreign antigen present.

IgA is found in high concentrations in secretions such as saliva, tears and bronchial mucus. IgA found in secretions contains an additional unit, the T-chain, which presumably allows it to pass into these secretions. IgA found in secretion is not antigenically identical to serum IgA. Secretion IgA has some antibacterial and antiviral activity.

1gM contains 5–10 per cent of antibody. IgM constitutes about one-third of macroglobulin normally present, the remaining two-thirds are an α_2 and a γ globulin—this α_2 macroglobulin is *not* an immunoglobulin.

It is important to note that there are immunoglobulins other than IgG, IgA and IgM; already IgD and IgE have been discovered.

In normals, a small amount of IgG globulin (not IgA or IgM) is found in the urine mainly as Fab fragments.

The immunoglobulins are synthesised in the plasma cells and probably the lymphocytes; each cell can only produce one type of H or L chain.

Acute-Phase Proteins

Following acute infection there are immediate changes in the plasma proteins, which lead to the production of acute-phase proteins, in contrast to the changes in immunoglobulins which occur more slowly. The acute-phase proteins are all produced in the liver; they are:

Prompt:	Fibrinogen
	Haptoglobin
	C-reactive protein
Intermediate:	Antitrypsin
	Orosomucoid
Slower:	Complement (C3)
	Caeruloplasmin

Fibrinogen.—The erythrocyte sedimentation rate (ESR) relates to increased levels of fibrinogen and reduced levels of albumin; it is also affected by some of the other acute-phase proteins as well as by IgG levels.

Haptoglobin.—This protein carries any loose haemoglobin in the plasma to the reticulo-endothelial system. It has a very short half-life. The haptoglobin level is reduced if haemolysis is present. This is a sensitive test of any haemolytic process. The level remains low for 2–3 days after an acute haemolytic episode.

C-reactive protein.—This is so named because it used to be tested by precipitating with the C polysaccharide of the pneumococcus. Its function is disputed.

Alpha₁ antitrypsin.—This acute-phase protein rises more slowly than fibrinogen, haptoglobin or C-reactive protein. There may be a congenital deficiency especially in women which may lead to emphysema because of the uninhibited action of proteases on the alveoli.

Orosomucoid.—This is a reliable guide of acute and chronic inflammation but does not reach a peak for about 5 days. It may be the transport protein for progesterone.

Complement.—This is mainly C_3, the rise is slow and not quantitatively very great.

Disorders of Immunoglobulins

Increase in the immunoglobulins (paraproteinaemia) may affect all components (i.e. diffuse increase) or it may affect only one component (i.e. local increase). Any local increase in immunoglobulins is known as an M component. This terminology has given rise to confusion; an M component is *not* the same as macroglobulinaemia or an increase in IgM; an M component merely means a local increase in one of the immunoglobulins whether it be IgA, IgG, IgM, etc. An M component is believed to indicate that only one clone of cells is producing an excess of protein; it is therefore referred to as monoclonal gammopathy. Increase in several proteins (diffuse increase) suggests that several clones are involved, i.e. polyclonal gammopathy. It should be noted that the protein produced need not be abnormal qualitatively, it may only be increased in quantity.

Causes of Diffuse Increase in Globulins

Infection and neoplasia.—Usually an increase in IgG.

Hepatic disease.—The increase may be in IgG, IgA or IgM; in cirrhosis there is a loss of a clear distinction between beta and gamma globulin (so-called "beta-gamma bridging").

Causes of Paraproteinaemia

Myeloma in which in 50 per cent of cases the M band is IgG, in 25 per cent of cases it is IgA, and in 1 per cent of cases IgM.

Not all patients with myeloma with an M band have Bence Jones protein in the urine and occasionally in myeloma there may be no M band, the presence of Bence Jones protein in the urine being the only evidence of a protein abnormality. The Bence Jones protein appears when the urine is warmed and disappears when it is brought to boiling point, although this may be difficult to see if there is associated albuminuria. Bence Jones protein consists of light chains, either κ or λ, but never both in the same patient; these can be detected by paper electrophoresis and immuno-electrophoresis. The particular L chain in the urine is the same as those occurring in the protein of the M band. For some reason the conditions causing proliferation of the plasma cells (plasma-cell dyscrasias) produce both κ and λ L chain proteins in excess, but when there is Bence Jones protein either in the blood or urine excessive amounts of only one type of L chain are produced. This may be important diagnostically: abnormalities of the plasma cells with a good prognosis produce the two types of L chains in the proportion normally found in the body, but those plasma cell dyscrasias with a poor prognosis produce only one type of L chain.

Management of myeloma.—Factors adversely affecting prognosis are a Hb below 8·0 g/dl, calcium over 11·5 mg per cent, IgG over 7·0 g per cent or IgA over 5·0 g.

Cyclophosphamide and melphalan are equally effective. Combination therapy can be given with an intermittent regime of alternating melphalan and prednisolone. There seems to be no advantage in a maintenance regime once the patient has responded. In patients who do not respond or who relapse there may be benefit from Adriamycin (doxorubicin), BICNU (bichloronitrourea) or Oncovin (vincristine).

The plasma cells in this condition more closely resemble large lymphocytes, the serum contains an M band in the IgM component. Bence Jones protein occurs in 10–15 per cent of patients. Features of the condition are hepatosplenomegaly, lymphadenopathy, anaemia, coagulation disorders, cryoglobulins and increased blood viscosity.

Cryoglobulins are a feature of myeloma and Waldenström's macroglobulinaemia; they give rise to Raynaud's phenomenon, vascular occlusion and peripheral gangrene. The increased blood viscosity causes heart failure, dyspnoea and localised bulging of the retinal veins which may be associated with retinal haemorrhages and exudates. Transient limb paresis, neuropathies and myelopathies may occur. Unlike myeloma in Waldenström's macroglobulinaemia the following are rare:

> Renal impairment
> Hypercalcaemia
> Osteolytic bone lesions
> Amyloidosis.

The treatment of Waldenström's macroglobulinaemia is plasmapheresis for the viscosity-induced manifestations, and corticosteroids for the bleeding disorders, followed by chlorambucil.

Benign M bands (essential paraproteinaemia).—These occur in patients with no evidence of malignant disease; the incidence is 1 per cent over 50 years of age and 5 per cent over 70. The M band may be permanent or transient and associated with a wide variety of diseases other than those causing a diffuse increase in globulins. The main problem of M bands is to decide whether they are truly benign or are a manifestation of myeloma, macroglobulinaemia, plasma-cell leukaemia or Hodgkin's disease. Contrary to previous reports there is no evidence that paraproteins are more common in other malignancies than in the general population.

The factors suggesting that M bands are associated with malignant disease in a particular patient are:

Presence of Bence Jones protein in the urine
Diminution in the other immunoglobulins
A high level of paraprotein greater than Ig/dl for IgA and IgM and greater than 2 g/dl for IgG
A rapid rise in the level of paraprotein
Presence of anaemia, leucopenia or thrombocytopenia
Presence of bone-marrow infiltration or osteolytic lesions.

Heavy-chain disease (Fc fragment disease).—A few cases have been described of patients with a lymphoma-like illness with an M band and urinary protein consisting of the Fc fragment of IgG

IMMUNOLOGICAL DEFICIENCY SYNDROMES

Congenital.—Agammaglobulinaemia, sex-linked and seen only in male children
Wiskott-Aldrich syndrome; eczema, infections, bleeding
Ataxia telangiectasia
Congenital rubella-induced agammaglobulinaemia
Late-onset hypogammaglobulinaemia (higher than normal incidence of hypogammaglobulinaemia in relatives).
Acquired.—Primary hypogammaglobulinaemia; occasionally patients have a thymoma, rarely there may be a high family incidence, usually IgG, IgA and IgM reduced, occasionally only one immunoglobulin reduced and others increased (a situation known as dysgammaglobulinaemia).

Secondary immunoglobulin deficiencies

Physiological—IgG is low in premature babies; the normal adult levels are usually reached by age 3. Occasionally there is delay in producing IgG and other immunoglobulins.
Excess catabolism—mainly IgG:
Nephrotic syndrome
Malnutrition
Protein-losing enteropathy
Dystrophia myotonica.
Marrow disorders—mainly IgG:
Hypoplasia
Metastases
Myelosclerosis.

Immunoglobulin deficiencies probably due to toxic factors—IgM usually affected first followed by IgA then IgG:
Uraemia
Corticosteroids
Cytotoxic drugs
Gluten-sensitive enteropathy
Severe infection
Diabetes
Thyrotoxicosis.
Reticulo-endothelial neoplasia—again IgM first followed by IgA or IgG:
Reticulosarcoma
Mycosis fungoides
Hodgkin's disease
Lymphosarcoma
Giant follicular lymphoma
Lymphatic leukaemia
Myeloma
Macroglobulinaemia.

The lymphoid disorders leading to disturbed cellular immunity are:

Acute leukaemia
Chronic lymphatic leukaemia
Lymphosarcoma
Hodgkin's disease
Irradiation
Antimetabolite and corticosteroid administration
Thymoma
Thymic aplasia.

The main causes of reduced or abnormal polymorphs are:

Myeloid leukaemia
Lymphatic leukaemia
Hypersplenism
Uraemia
Toxic drugs
Bone marrow depression or replacements.

RADIOLOGY OF BONES AND JOINTS

BONES

Increase in Bone Density (Sclerosis)

Paget's[5] disease.—This may be localised or widespread. The bone involved may become deformed, but the involved area does not project above the surface of the bone—unlike secondary deposits which may grow outside the confines of the bones. The trabecular pattern of the bone is replaced by dense structureless bone. Bone deformity causes bowing of the tibia and a triradiate pelvis. In the skull, Paget's disease may cause an area of rarefaction which is well circumscribed (osteoporosis circumscripta) or platybasia in which the soft skull is indented by the vertebral column. Normally the odontoid process of the axis should not project more than 5 mm above the straight line drawn backwards from the hard palate (Chamberlain's line).

Secondary deposits.—The only common primary carcinoma which produces sclerotic secondaries is prostatic. Rarely sclerotic secondaries occur from a breast carcinoma or in the reticuloses. Sclerotic secondaries occur mainly in vertebrae, pelvis and ribs, the long bones are rarely involved.

Chronic Osteomyelitis

Myelofibrosis (often but not invariably due to secondary carcinoma).

Avascular area of bone, e.g. infarction, or damage to blood supply (via the periosteum) as in a fractured scaphoid.

Marble bone disease (osteopetrosis or Albers-Schönberg[6] disease).

Fluorosis due to ingestion of fluoride, usually in drinking water. The vertebrae are usually sclerotic and there is calcification of vertebral ligaments (in contradistinction, the vertebrae in ankylosing spondylitis are rarefied).

In the skull, sclerosis may be due to a meningioma or hyperostosis frontalis (interna or externa) in which the frontal bone is thickened as well as sclerotic.

Skeletal scintiscanning may be useful in detecting bone secondaries. There is an increased uptake of the isotope by osteolytic and osteosclerotic secondaries except for multiple myeloma. There is also an increased uptake in osteo-arthritis and Paget's disease.

Decreased Bone Density

Osteomalacia and Osteoporosis

In *osteomalacia* there is loss of mineral from the bone but the protein matrix remains relatively intact. If the mineral loss is sustained the protein matrix may become secondarily diminished and the radiological features of osteoporosis are superimposed. Osteomalacia is exemplified by the bone disorder which occurs due to lack of vitamin D. One of the features of this bone disease is an excess of osteoid tissue. Conditions other than lack of vitamin D can cause an increase in osteoid tissue, e.g. renal failure, renal tubular defects, hyperparathyroidism, hyperthyroidism and Paget's disease. Causes of osteomalacia are nutritional deficiency, partial gastrectomy, malabsorption and obstructive jaundice.

In *osteoporosis* there is a decrease in the protein matrix of the bone, but the matrix which remains calcifies normally. Causes of osteoporosis are old age, Cushing's syndrome (and corticosteroid treatment), immobilisation and thyrotoxicosis. In intestinal malabsorption in which calcium and protein are malabsorbed, osteomalacia and osteoporosis may coexist.

Radiological signs which unequivocally indicate *osteomalacia* are: the Milkman[7] fracture, or Looser[8] zone which is a tongue of radiotranslucency extending about a centimetre into the bone from the surface; they are most frequently seen in the upper end of the femur and humerus or lower end of the tibia. Bending of the bones usually indicates osteomalacia.

Radiological signs which indicate *hyperparathyroidism* are:

> *Subperiosteal erosions*, usually best seen in the middle phalanges of the fingers and in the femoral necks. The cortex of the phalanges may become fragmented and lace-like.
> *Multiple bone cysts* which may project from the surface of the bones (von Recklinghausen's[9] disease).
> *Loss of the lamina dura* round the teeth.
> *Mottling of the skull*—"pepper-pot skull".

In hyperparathyroidism the radiological appearances of osteomalacia usually appear later.

The changes of *osteoporosis* are most marked in the vertebrae. There is increased translucency of the bones with loss of trabeculae. However, the trabeculae that do remain usually appear sclerotic, particularly in lines of stress—thus in the vertebrae the vertical trabeculae appear sclerotic whereas the horizontal trabeculae may be difficult to see. The width of the cortex of the bones is reduced, it is also more irregular than normal, but in contrast with the increased translucency (rarefaction) of the cancellous bone the cortex may appear sclerotic. Osteoporosis usually involves some bones while sparing others, thus wedge-shaped collapse of a few vertebrae is highly suggestive. *Osteomalacia* is a disease which affects the whole skeleton evenly so that any deformity tends to affect all the vertebrae equally. It also tends to cause the "cod fish" spine in which the intervertebral discs indent the surface of the vertebrae more or less equally. Collapse of a single vertebra or localised Schmorl's[10] nodes favours *osteoporosis*. As a working rule osteoporosis affects the axial skeleton (spine and limb girdles) more than the long bones, therefore, osteoporosis should only be diagnosed from an x-ray of the lumbar spine (preferably a lateral view).

There are two causes of bone disease secondary to renal disease (renal osteodystrophy). The first is due to renal failure in which the kidneys fail to excrete phosphate. This is accompanied by an acidosis; there is diminished absorption of calcium from the gut and increased resistance to vitamin D. The lowered serum calcium may stimulate the parathyroids, causing hyperparathyroidism; thus the bone abnormalities will be those of rickets in children or osteomalacia in adults with the addition of hyperparathyroidism. In addition to the effects of osteomalacia on the spine there are often areas of sclerosis in relation to the intervertebral discs ("rugger-jersey spine").

The other type of renal osteodystrophy occurs in tubular defects in which there is a tubular inability to reabsorb phosphate, amino acids and glucose (Fanconi syndrome). The tubular loss of phosphate results in hypophosphataemia and failure to calcify bone, resulting in osteomalacia and rickets which is resistant to vitamin D. Both these types of renal osteodystrophy may require large doses of vitamin D.

Causes of Localised Translucency of Bone

In relation to arthritis.

Simple bone cysts.—These are usually in the upper end of humerus and are surrounded by a rim of sclerotic bone. The cyst may be divided by bony septa and is usually filled with fluid. If the "cyst" is filled with fibrous tissue it is called fibrous dysplasia. When this condition is seen in many bones it is called polyostotic fibrous dysplasia.

Secondary deposits particularly from thyroid, bronchus, breast and kidney. They are usually irregular in outline. Myeloma causes widespread areas of translucency which are often well defined.

Reticuloses usually look like secondaries but leukaemia may cause numerous pin-point translucent areas.

Sarcoidosis seen particularly in the phalanges.

Histiocytosis X (lipoidoses).

Tumours of the bone.

Causes of Periosteal Calcification (Periostitis)

Subperiosteal haemorrhage which may be due to trauma or spontaneous bleeding such as in leukaemia or haemophilia.

Following a fracture.

Bone infections: pyogenic, tuberculous or syphilitic.

Pulmonary osteo-arthropathy.

Bone neoplasms and secondary deposits.

Schmorl's nodes in the vertebrae due to bulging of the intervertebral discs into the vertebral bodies.

RADIOLOGY OF ARTHRITIS

The radiological sign common to all forms of arthritis is narrowing of the joint space. Changes occurring in association with a narrowed joint space are:

Osteophyte formation at the edges of the joint
Areas of bone resorption which may be erosions of the joint surface or be entirely within the substance of the bones
Decalcification of bones
Periosteal calcification
Periarticular thickening of adjacent soft tissues.

Rheumatoid arthritis.—The distribution of joints involved is a valuable pointer. The interphalangeal joints (except the distal), second and third metacarpophalangeal joints and wrist are involved most frequently. The joint space is narrowed and there are erosions of the joint surfaces and "spindling" of the fingers, due to associated inflammation causing thickening of periarticular structures. A rheumatoid nodule may be seen in the soft tissues. Usually there is decalcification of the bones whose joints are affected. Later in the disease the joint becomes distorted and the joint cavity entirely disappears because of fibrous or bony alkylosis. A very severe form of joint deformity occurs particularly after Still's disease and is known as arthritis mutilans.

Psoriatic arthritis.—This is similar to rheumatoid arthritis except that all the interphalangeal joints (including the distal) are involved, but involvement of metacarpophalangeal joints is rare. Rheumatoid nodules, arteritis and neuropathy do not occur. Involvement of the nails with psoriasis is almost always present in psoriatic arthritis.

Arthritis with ulcerative colitis.—The arthritis is similar to rheumatoid except that knees, ankles and sacro-iliac joints are more frequently involved. The rheumatoid factor is absent and the arthritis improves as the primary condition improves.

Reiter's syndrome.—The arthritis is similar to rheumatoid except that periosteal calcification is commoner and that calcification of the plantar fascia, particularly at its attachment to the os calcis, is very common (calcaneal spur).

SLE.—Similar to rheumatoid except that, like psoriatic arthritis, all the interphalangeal joints are often affected.

Ankylosing spondylitis (rheumatoid spondylitis).—Widening of the sacro-iliac joint space occurs because of joint erosion. Later there is narrowing of the joint space, calcification of intervertebral discs and longitudinal ligaments of the spine, and kyphosis ("bamboo spine").

Osteo-arthritis.—Narrowing of the joint spaces, particularly of hips, knees, and lumbar spine, occurs together with osteophytic formation at the joint margins and calcification of synovial membranes and ligaments. Cyst-like areas are often seen near the joint surface but do not become sclerotic in relation to the joint; later, bony ankylosis occurs.

Charcot's[11] arthropathy.—This is a severe form of osteo-arthritis with synovial calcification, often calcified intra-articular loose bodies and severe joint deformity. Diminished sensitivity to deep pain is responsible. The condition occurs with tabes dorsalis and peripheral neuropathy in the lower limbs, with syringomyelia and peripheral neuropathy in the upper limbs. An identical x-ray appearance may occur in joints which have been frequently injected with intra-articular steroids.

Gout.—Narrowing of the joint spaces occurs with well-defined "punched-out" circular erosions of the bones in relation to the joint. The periarticular soft tissues are usually swollen, by inflammation or tophi. Only one joint at a time is affected in acute gout. However, following many attacks of gout, chronic gouty arthritis occurs in which several joints are involved—there are usually tophi in relation to the deformed joints.

Alkaptonuria.—This causes calcification of the intervertebral discs and dark pigmentation of cartilage (seen in the ear) and tendons (seen on the back of the hand).

Infective arthritis.—Early there is slight opacity of the joint space and swelling of soft tissues compared with the opposite side due to intra-articular fluid. The development of an effusion causes widening of the joint space. After about two weeks the surrounding bone becomes decalcified and periosteal calcification begins, bony ankylosis is common. The x-ray appearances are similar in tuberculous arthritis.

Diagnostic Classification of Arthritis

A useful classification of arthropathies from a diagnostic view-point is according to the number of joints involved, viz:

Single joint	Acute	Haemarthrosis
		Crystal arthropathy
		Pyogenic arthritis
	Subacute	Rheumatoid disease
		Ankylosing spondylitis
		Reiter's disease
		Tuberculosis
Three to four joints	Ankylosing spondylitis	
	Reiter's disease	
	Arthritis secondary to Crohn's disease or ulcerative colitis	

Multiple joints	Transient	Rheumatoid disease
		Systemic lupus erythematosus
		Rheumatic fever
	Subacute	Rheumatoid disease
		Ankylosing spondylitis

RHEUMATOID DISEASE

Diagnosis

The American Rheumatism Association has devised a useful method of making a "definite" diagnosis. Joint symptoms must be present for at least six weeks and at least five of the following findings must occur:

1. Morning joint stiffness
2. Pain on movement of a joint
3. Soft tissue thickening over a joint
4. Soft tissue thickening over a second joint
5. Spontaneous symmetrical joint swelling
6. Subcutaneous nodules
7. Characteristic x-ray findings
8. Presence of rheumatoid factor
9. Characteristic histological changes in the synovial membrane
10. Characteristic histological changes in the nodule.

Extra-articular Manifestations

In addition to the joint involvement there are a number of important manifestations of the disease outside the joints.

Anaemia.—Most frequently this is normochromic normocytic and is similar to the anaemia of infection. Haemolysis or iron deficiency may also occur (due to gastro-intestinal bleeding from drugs) and a macrocytic anaemia which is due to folate deficiency.

Subcutaneous nodules.—These occur most frequently around the elbow; they may appear suddenly or gradually, and can ulcerate badly. They can occur in any part of the body including the ears (and may resemble tophi), the nervous system (where they may compress nerves), in the heart (where they may cause bundle-branch block) and in the lungs.

Lung involvement.—In addition to rheumatoid nodules which may occur and cavitate, rheumatoid disease may also cause pleural effusions (which contain the rheumatoid factor and may be chylous), fibrosing alveolitis, and arthritis (which can lead to pulmonary infarcts). In coal-miner's pneumoconiosis rheumatoid nodules occur readily even if the associated rheumatoid disease is mild (Caplan's syndrome).

Vasculitis.—This can be severe and lead to areas of skin necrosis, myocardial infarction and mesenteric infarction. It is common in the digital arteries but may only be recognised by arteriography. When severe the rheumatoid factor is usually IgG, not IgM as in most seropositive cases of rheumatoid disease. Vasculitis may develop when steroids are stopped too abruptly.

Hyperviscosity and cryoglobulinaemia.—Hyperviscosity occurs more frequently if the rheumatoid factor is IgG and is due to polymerisation (combining together) of individual IgG molecules. It may result in excessive bleeding, retinopathy and neurological involvement, due to occlusion of small vessels leading to small infarcts. The bleeding may be due to competitive inhibition of some clotting factors.

Lymphadenopathy.—Histologically, lymph-gland involvement in rheumatoid disease is very frequent although the glands are not often clinically enlarged.

Amyloidosis.

Peripheral neuropathy and/or entrapment neuropathies.—From a clinical point of view it is important *not* to assume that all peripheral nerve lesions in a patient with rheumatoid arthritis are due to a rheumatoid neuropathy. Readily remediable compression neuropathies due to deformed and swollen joints and extra-articular soft tissues occur frequently.

Carpal tunnel syndrome.

Eye complications.—Kerato-conjunctivitis sicca (Sjögren's[12] disease), corneal ulceration, uveitis, cytoid bodies in the retina and scleromalacia perforans.

Pathogenesis

The disease affects the synovium of joints, in which immune complexes are found which activate complement and other mediators of inflammation. The synovium is infiltrated with lymphocytes, and eventually granulation tissue is formed which results in the production of proteolytic enzymes, leading to destruction of the articular cartilages and adjacent bone. The continued presence of immune complexes in progressive disease and the continued production of immunoglobulins implies the constant availability of the causative antigen. *This antigen has not been identified.* The abnormal IgG occurring in rheumatoid disease is a marker for the disease but is not the antigen which initiates and sustains it, neither is the rheumatoid factor which is an IgM immunoglobulin directed against the abnormal IgG "marker" of the disease.

It has been proposed that the whole complex of "marker" IgG plus its IgM antibody may be involved in the complement-releasing component of the disease. (If complement is activated it leads to inflammation.) Normally when small amounts are activated they are "mopped up" by the Fc portion of IgG; if this is already occupied by IgM, damaging activated complement roams free, causing complement-mediated damage and *reduced* blood levels of all the normally inactive circulating complement components.

The search for the presumed infective agent causing rheumatoid disease had been based on the finding of diphtheroids, mycoplasmas and viruses in rheumatoid joints, but it is not yet established whether these are merely commensals, as they have also been found in non-rheumatoid patients. The links between joint disease and infection are strong, e.g.

Rheumatic fever and its known association with streptococcal infections

Reactive arthritis

Reiter's disease and mycoplasma infection

Hepatitis-B-associated rheumatic disease

Yersinia-enterocolitica-induced arthritis, which resembles ankylosing spondylitis and is common in Scandinavia

Arthritis associated with Whipple's disease, for which there is now strong evidence of a microbial cause

Rubella-induced arthritis in adults

Leucovirus-induced lupus syndrome in New Zealand mice.

Rheumatoid Factors

The rheumatoid factors are endogenous normal immunoglobulins against other endogenous but abnormal immunoglobulins. The abnormal immunoglobulin is always IgG but it is not thought that this IgG is the main immunological cause of rheumatoid arthritis. The most frequent immunoglobulin against the abnormal IgG is an IgM antibody, but occasionally it is an IgG or an IgA antibody. The two methods used for detecting the IgM antibody (the rheumatoid factor) against abnormal IgG are:

1. SCAT (sensitised sheep cell agglutination test or Rose Waaler test), in which the IgG antibody is coated onto sheep red cells which will then agglutinate with the patient's serum if it contains the rheumatoid factor (IgM).
2. DAT (differential agglutination test or latex fixation test), in which the abnormal IgG is produced in rabbits and coated onto latex particles.

A proportion of cases have an IgG or IgA immunological response to the abnormal IgG. These immunoglobulins are not detected in the conventional tests for IgM rheumatoid factors.

Assessment of Rheumatoid Disease

There are many different methods of trying to assess progression of disease rather than an effect on symptoms. The most reliable are:

Radiological changes
ESR, C reactive protein and titres of rheumatoid factor.

Other tests such as pain scoring, articular index and grip tests measure only symptoms or function. It is thought that gold and penicillamine have more effect than steroids in slowing progression.

Drug Treatment of Rheumatoid Disease

There is now a consensus about the drug treatment of rheumatoid disease:

1. Once the diagnosis is made the patient is encouraged to take aspirin to relieve pain. Many rheumatologists still use aspirin as a first line drug but all agree that for it to be effective a minimum of 4·0 g per day are required and often as much as 7·0 g are necessary. Some argue that compliance when taking aspirin is so low (over a third of patients will have side-effects) that it is better to start with one of the other non-steroidal anti-inflammatory drugs, and reserve aspirin until later.

2. There are a wide variety of non-steroidal anti-inflammatory drugs (Table X). These should be used in the order given; there is

TABLE X

NON-STEROIDAL ANTI-INFLAMMATORY DRUGS

Non-proprietary name	Proprietary name	Tablet/ Capsule size	Common daily dose
Aspirin	Aspirin	300 mg	4·0 g
Indomethacin	Indocid	25, 50 mg	75 mg
Phenylbutazone-like			
Feprazone	Methrazone	200 mg	200–600 mg
Azapropazone	Rheumox	300 mg	1200 mg
Propionic acid derivatives			
Flurbiprofen	Froben	50, 100 mg	200–300
Fenoprofen	Fenopron	300 mg/600	2400 mg
Naproxen	Naprosyn	250 mg/500	750 mg
Sulindac	Clinoril	100 mg/200	400 mg
Diflunisal	Dolobid	250 mg/500	500–750 mg
Ketoprofen	Alrheumat	50 mg	200 mg
	Orudis	50, 100 mg	200 mg
Ibuprofen	Brufen	200, 400 mg	1600 mg
Diclofenac	Voltarol	25, 50 mg	100–150 mg

often great individual variation in response and it is important to try each drug until a response is obtained; usually one knows within a week or 10 days whether one has found the correct drug for that patient.

3. If the patient has pain and stiffness at night indomethacin should be used.

4. Phenylbutazone is not now used because of its side-effects; there are, however, two drugs which have a similar action but probably fewer side-effects: these are feprazone and azapropazone. If these drugs do not work then indomethacin or aspirin should be the main drug.

5. The next line of treatment is penicillamine, chloroquine or gold.

6. Steroids are indicated if the disease continues to progress or if there are severe systemic features such as haemolytic anaemia or lung involvement.

7. Azathioprine may be used to try to reduce a high steroid dosage, or if vasculitis is present.

Possible Mechanisms of Action of Anti-Rheumatic Drugs

Stimulation of endogenous cortisol production.—The disadvantage of this hypothesis is that a number of substances without anti-rheumatic activity also increase cortisol production.

Lysosome inhibition.—Intracellular lysosomes, which contain many hydralases and proteolytic enzymes, are known to be disrupted in the inflammatory process and their enzymes damage protein-polysaccharide complexes of articular cartilage. Against this hypothesis is the fact that not all the effective anti-rheumatic drugs affect the lysosomes.

Enhancement of endogenous anti-inflammatory agents.—It is known that acute inflammation is accompanied by the production of endogenous anti-inflammatory substances. Anti-rheumatic drugs may act by displacing this substance from binding proteins, so increasing the free and effective endogenous anti-inflammatory substances.

Inhibition of mediators of inflammation.—These include histamine and prostaglandins. Some drugs inhibit prostaglandin synthesis as well as blocking prostaglandin receptors once it is formed.

The mechanism of the non steroidal anti-inflammatory drugs was thought to be inhibition of a widely distributed chemical mediator such as histamine or bradykinin. It was demonstrated in 1969 that inflammation was associated with activation of enzymes responsible for synthesis of prostaglandins. These are naturally occurring fatty acid derivatives, widely distributed in almost every cell in the body. Excessive prostaglandin production occurs in many forms of inflammation, including allergy, burns and rheumatoid arthritis. Prostaglandins are present in all inflammatory exudates and are known to be responsible for pain and fever in addition to inflammatory responses. They increase vascular permeability and enhance the action of other inflammatory mediators. In 1971 it was shown by Vane that aspirin and other non-steroidal anti-inflammatory drugs inhibit the enzymes responsible for the synthesis of prostaglandins.

Felty's[13] **syndrome** is rheumatoid arthritis with splenomegaly and leucopenia.

Sjögren's syndrome is rheumatoid arthritis with kerato-conjunctivitis sicca due to deficient secretion of the lachrymal glands. The salivary glands are also involved.

Still's disease is an acute form of rheumatoid arthritis occurring usually between the ages of 2 and 4. Systemic and constitutional effects are much more in evidence than in rheumatoid arthritis. Lymphadenopathy and a leucocytosis are common. Corticosteroids are used much earlier than in adult rheumatoid arthritis.

Palindromic rheumatism.—This term is used to describe recurrent acute attacks of arthritis and inflammation of the periarticular structures. There is no permanent joint deformity, even after many attacks. The ESR may be raised but the rheumatoid factor is always absent. A small proportion of patients who have had numerous attacks of palindromic rheumatism will develop true rheumatoid arthritis.

THE SEROLOGY OF CONNECTIVE TISSUE DISORDERS

Rheumatoid Arthritis

The rheumatoid factor is a circulating immunoglobulin, IgM; it is associated with circulating immune complexes and can be detected by the sheep-cell agglutination test (SCAT or the Rose Waaler test) and the differential agglutination test (DAT) or latex fixation test. Less commonly there is an IgG rheumatoid factor not detectable by these tests.

Antinuclear Factors (ANF) in Connective Tissue Diseases

Antinuclear factors are detected by immunofluorescence. The standard ANF test measures a variety of nuclear components some of which can now be separately identified and their clinical relevance clarified. The pattern of immunofluorescence is of some value in deciding which of several antinuclear factors is present. Nuclear and cytoplasmic components may act as antigens and be either pathogenic or markers of disease. The most significant antinuclear factor is anti-native double-stranded DNA. Normally native DNA is non-antigenic; there is no clear reason why it and other normal cell components become antigenic in SLE and other connective diseases.

Antinuclear Antibodies in SLE

Anti-native double-stranded DNA.—This is highly specific for SLE and is sometimes a good index of disease activity. Anti-heat denatured DNA or single-stranded DNA is not exclusive for SLE but may give positive ANF test. The DNA binding test is a measure of the amount of anti-native double-stranded DNA, i.e. it helps in eliminating false positives. Some patients have both positive ANF and positive LE cell tests, but negative DNA binding. In the assessment of progress of SLE, DNA binding and a fall in complement level are important, although increased DNA binding may precede clinical exacerbation of SLE by many months, and treatment should be decided on the basis of clinical symptoms and signs.

Anti-DNA histone.—This is an IgG antibody which is responsible for the LE cell phenomenon.

Sm antigen.—Specific for SLE but cannot be used for assessing activity.

Antinuclear antibodies in other connective-tissue disorders

Anti-extractable nuclear antigens (ENA): raised in mixed connective tissue disease (MCT)

Anti-ribonucleoprotein (anti-RNP): present in MCT but associated with a good prognosis

Anti-histone: raised in drug-induced SLE

Anti-PM$_1$: a nuclear antigen specific for polymyositis

Hepatitis B antigen occurs in about a third of patients with polyarteritis.

Seronegative arthritis

Ankylosing spondylitis	Ulcerative colitis and Crohn's disease
Reiter's disease	Whipple's disease
Psoriatic arthritis	Behçet's syndrome.

There are other characteristics linking this group, as shown below:

Absence of subcutaneous nodules

The frequent occurrence of ulceration of skin or mucous membranes (e.g. psoriasis, conjunctivitis, urethral ulceration, ulceration of mouth and gut).

	Seronegative	*Seropositive*
Peripheral arthritis	Asymmetrical	Symmetrical
Spinal involvement	Ankylosis	Cervical subluxation
Cartilaginous joints	Commonly affected (especially S. I. joints)	Rarely affected
Tissue typing	HLA B27-positive	No association known

Eye involvement	Anterior uveitis Conjunctivitis	Scleritis, kerato-conjunctivitis sicca
Skin involvement	"Epidermal dysmaturation", psoriasis, keratoderma blennorrhagica, mucosal ulceration, erythema nodosum	Cutaneous nodules and vasculitis
Heart involvement	Fibrosis of aortic root, aortic regurgitation, conduction defects	Pericarditis
Pulmonary involvement	Chest-wall ankylosis, lung fibrosis	Alveolitis, nodules, pleural effusions
Gastro-intestinal involvement	Bowel ulceration	Rare
Genito-urinary involvement	Frequent	Rare

Ankylosing spondylitis. The sacro-iliac joints are always involved, usually the spine and sometimes the larger peripheral joints of the legs are also affected. The disease is much commoner in men and occurs at an earlier age than rheumatoid arthritis. Presenting symptoms may be low backache, joint pains worse in the morning, and iritis. The clinical criteria for the diagnosis of ankylosing spondylitis are:

Limitation of movement of the lumbar spine in all four directions
Pain in the sacro-iliac joints
Limitation of chest expansion to one inch
Evidence of past or present iridocyclitis.

The diagnosis is easy to miss in the early stages as the symptoms may be non-specific, such as malaise, fever and weight loss. Physical signs which should make one suspicious are: limitation of chest movement, pain in the back on deep breathing, limitation of straight leg raising, pain in the heel and sole of the feet from plantar fascitis, and peripheral joint inflammation. The main complications are:

Aortitis and myocarditis—leading to aortic incompetence and cardiac failure
Iritis in 20–40 per cent of patients
Atlanto-axial subluxation.

Certain accompaniments of rheumatoid arthritis do not occur in ankylosing spondylitis, viz., rheumatoid nodules, rheumatoid factor, arteritis and peripheral neuropathy. There is often a family history of the disease and the incidence of prostatitis is higher than in the general population. There is also a higher incidence of Reiter's disease and psoriasis in the relatives of affected patients.

The sacro-iliac joints are examined by:

Pressing the pelvis backwards by pressing on the anterior superior iliac spines
Pressing the pelvis together by pressing on both iliac crests
Pushing the sacrum forwards when the patient is lying face down.

If sacro-iliac joints are inflamed these manoeuvres will cause pain. In ankylosing spondylitis, pain may also be elicited by pressure on the symphysis pubis, ischial tuberosities and greater trochanters.

Treatment

Phenylbutazone is probably still the drug of first choice, for it seems to relieve the pain better than the other non-steroidal, anti-inflammatory drugs. Only low doses may be required.

Indomethacin may be useful as an alternative to phenylbutazone; both are available as suppositories.

Local irradiation is sometimes indicated if local pain is severe.

Reiter's disease.—This consists of urethritis, conjunctivitis and arthritis. It is rare but not unknown in women; usually it follows an attack of non-gonococcal urethritis due to a mycoplasma, or an attack of bacillary dysentery or non-specific diarrhoea. The first manifestation is usually urethritis followed by arthritis which is characteristically bilateral and involves knees and ankles. The soft tissues surrounding the joint are often excessively tender. The arthritis may last three months and it relapses in 10 per cent of cases. The arthritis is also associated with plantar fascitis and tendonitis—calcification of the plantar fascia gives rise to the calcaneal spur which is virtually diagnostic; iritis and conjunctivitis may not occur in the first attacks. Important diagnostic features are the pain in the feet, low back pain and thickening of the periarticular tissues. The arthritis, which is commonest in the knees and ankles, may relapse and remit. The urethritis may be quite mild. Rarely, keratoderma blennorrhagica, a skin lesion resembling psoriasis, may appear on the palms and soles and involve the nails, it is commoner in the post-dysenteric variety. The incidence of psoriasis and ankylosing spondylitis is higher in the relatives of patients who have Reiter's disease than in the remainder of the population. A shallow ulcerated lesion on the penis known as circinate balanitis involves the glans and is commoner in the venereal variety. The cardiac manifestations are similar to those of ankylosing spondylitis, namely pericarditis, myocarditis and aortitis.

Treatment of Reiter's disease

Tetracycline for urethritis
Bed rest to prevent joint deformity
Phenylbutazone or indomethacin for the arthritis
Iritis should be treated with steroids and atropine eye drops.

Unusual Causes of Arthritis include:

Sickle-cell anaemia and haemophilia
Serum sickness and drug sensitivity
Brucellosis—generally a monoarticular arthritis involving hip or
  knee
Dysentery (amoebic or bacilliary)
Rubella
Mumps
Glandular fever
Behçet's syndrome (stomatitis, genital ulceration, recurrent iritis,
  vasculitis and peripheral neuritis)
Intermittent hydrarthrosis
Meningococcal septicaemia
Sarcoidosis
Whipple's disease (lymphadenopathy, skin pigmentation, stea-
  torrhoea and arthritis)
Familial Mediterranean fever (FMF)
Primary hypercholesterolaemia
Angiokeratoma corporis diffusum
Alkaptonuria
Haemochromatosis
Hyperparathyroidism
Acromegaly
Myxoedema.

OTHER CONNECTIVE TISSUE DISEASES

There is some clinical overlap between the collagen disorders, for
example patients with classical rheumatoid arthritis sometimes develop
polyarteritis or SLE and those with polyarteritis may develop dermatomyositis or rheumatoid arthritis. None the less, the most common
course of each of them is along fairly well-defined, distinct pathways.
It is worthwhile from diagnostic, prognostic and therapeutic points of
view to think of them as distinct clinical entities but to bear in mind
that they may have a common pathogenesis.

Polyarteritis Nodosa

The medium and small arteries are mainly involved and the lesions may be seen in any tissue or organ; however, there are certain clinical features which are useful pointers to the diagnosis. Unlike all the other collagen disorders polyarteritis is commoner in men; the characteristic nodes in relation to the arteries occur in only about a third of patients. Hepatitis B antigen is found in about a third of patients. The antigen, together with C3, is found in the walls of affected areas. As a general rule the collagen disorders are multisystem diseases, but there are exceptions to this rule—one system may be involved in polyarteritis because the lung lesions may present first and prompt diagnosis and treatment with steroids at this stage may prevent the fatal renal lesions developing. The lung lesions consist of transient patchy shadowing in the lung fields which may not be limited by interlobar septa; asthma and a peripheral blood eosinophilia usually accompany the lung shadowing. In polyarteritis there is usually a leucocytosis in the peripheral blood in contrast to SLE, in which there is usually a leucopenia. The leucocytosis is due to an increase in polymorphs unless there are asthmatic features, in which case eosinophilia may contribute to the leucocytosis. Eosinophilia in the absence of asthmatic features is uncommon. Another presentation which should alert one is the presence of hypertension with a slight fever or non-specific abdominal pain which is occasionally severe enough to simulate an acute abdomen. The fever may be accompanied by a tachycardia which is out of all proportion to the height of the temperature. In the eye the usual changes of hypertension may be seen affecting the arteries; in addition nodes are occasionally seen in relation to the arteries. Unlike arteriosclerotic changes the arterial narrowing and irregularity which occurs in polyarteritis may be patchy and involve only one eye. Involvement of the central retinal artery may cause unilateral blindness.

Two other features occur more commonly in polyarteritis than in the other collagen diseases, the first is Raynaud's phenomenon and the second is peripheral neuropathy. The neuropathy tends to be mainly motor and involve individual peripheral nerves, unlike rheumatoid arthritis which is predominantly sensory and has a glove and stocking distribution. Like all the collagen disorders there may be myositis and arthritis. The most suitable sites for biopsy are skin, muscle, artery, testis, liver and kidney. An EMG may be useful in detecting involved muscle and thus indicating the most suitable muscle to biopsy. Renal involvement tends to be of two main types: one in which the larger renal arteries are involved in common with arteries elsewhere in the body, this type of involvement producing systemic hypertension; the other type of renal involvement affects the smaller intrarenal vessels, leading to a clinical picture similar to acute nephritis—in this type of renal involvement the blood pressure may be normal.

Polyarteritis usually runs a course of about a year; at the end of this time the disease either remits or the patient dies, usually from hypertension or chronic renal failure. There is some evidence that steroids promote arterial thrombosis and precipitate malignant hypertension in polyarteritis. There is also some evidence that early treatment with steroids in pulmonary involvement will prevent the renal complications. In the established case steroids should be given in sufficient doses to abolish symptoms; they probably need not be given in doses which completely suppress the disease as this does not improve the long-term prognosis. It is essential to note that before the advent of steroids over half the patients with polyarteritis recovered.

There are four conditions which are variants of polyarteritis:

1. Giant-cell or temporal arteritis
2. Wegener's granulomatosis
3. Senile arteritis (polymyalgia rheumatica)
4. Takayasu's disease.

Temporal Arteritis (Giant-Cell Arteritis)

The term temporal arteritis is a misnomer as the larger medium-sized artery in any organ may be involved, particularly coronary, renal and mesenteric; none the less, the temporal arteries are the most frequently involved. When the temporal artery is inflamed; tender and non-pulsatile the diagnosis is easy but it is important to note that by the time the patient is seen the severe acute signs may have subsided and all that is left is headache and an elevated ESR. It is essential to palpate the whole course of both terminal arteries comparing each side. Pulsation may only be diminished and not abolished; loss of pulsation may only be segmented and may only affect the terminal part of each artery. There may be other systemic manifestations such as fever, anaemia and weight loss. The intracranial arteries may be involved leading to hemiplegia and blindness. Temporal arteritis is a medical emergency and treatment should begin immediately with high doses of corticosteroids until the pain has subsided, and steroids should be continued in moderate doses for six months, as blindness may occur after the acute symptoms have subsided. Steroids should be given in a dose of 40–60 mg per day for 4–6 weeks and then the dose can be halved for a further 6 months. It is worth attempting an alternate-day regime of prednisolone in an attempt to prevent suppression of the adrenal/pituitary axis.

Wegener's Granulomatosis

Wegener's granulomatosis consists of a vasculitis affecting arteries and veins leading to granuloma formation in the upper air passages, lungs and kidneys.

Takayasu's pulseless disease consists of granuloma formation and narrowing of elastic arteries leaving the arch of the aorta and descending aorta, with abnormal vessels in relation to the optic disc which are probably arteriovenous anastomoses. It used to be said that the disease only occurred in young girls but cases have been described in middle-aged men.

Scleroderma (Systemic Sclerosis)

There are two aspects of the pathology of scleroderma which are important; the first is that like polyarteritis there is an arteritis although it tends to affect smaller arteries, and the second is that unlike other collagen diseases there is first an increase and then a degeneration in collagen tissue. This occurs in sites related to the skin and mucous membranes of the gastro-intestinal tract, and results in thickening and oedema of the dermis. The skin lesions consist of a combination of ischaemic atrophy due to the vasculitis, and infiltration and hardening of the skin due to mucinous degeneration of the excess collagen tissue. The degenerating collagen tissue may calcify and the vasculitis result in telangiectasia and Raynaud's[15] phenomenon. The combination of calcinosis of fingers with telangiectasia or purpura around the mouth is known as the CRST syndrome (calcinosis, Raynaud's phenomenon, sclerodactyly and telangiectasia).

As a result of the thickened skin and ischaemia there will be disuse of the affected part and consequent osteoporosis and muscular atrophy. Subcutaneous fibrosis will cause contractures and deformity of joints. This deformity may resemble arthritis, but unlike rheumatoid arthritis there is no joint swelling. Thrombosis of affected vessels may cause gangrene.

The changes of scleroderma may be localised particularly to the neck and the condition is then called morphoea; occasionally it is localised to the fingers and toes and is then known as acrosclerosis. In both these conditions there is usually no evidence of extension or visceral involvement with scleroderma. Acrosclerosis is by far the commonest clinical manifestation of scleroderma. A condition which is rare but may appear similar to the skin manifestation of scleroderma is scleroedema. This is a condition which almost always follows a streptococcal infection and is accompanied by oedema, fibrosis and induration of the skin which may closely resemble scleroderma; however, in scleroedema the hands and feet are spared and the condition is much worse over the face and trunk. It is not accompanied by vasculitis, so that there is no atrophy of the skin or overlying telangiectasia.

In scleroderma visceral involvement may occur in the complete absence of any skin lesions. The commonest is involvement of the lower end of the oesophagus which may cause dysphagia, peptic oesophagitis, oesophageal dilatation and aspiration pneumonia. Loss of proper peristalsis may be demonstrated, before there is demonstrable narrowing of the oesophagus, if a barium swallow is taken with the patient lying down. Any part of the gastro-intestinal tract may be involved and if the small intestine is affected there may be malabsorption.

The respiratory system can be involved in four main ways:

1. Aspiration pneumonia
2. Vasculitis affecting pulmonary arterioles leading to pulmonary hypertension
3. Fibrosis and degeneration of collagen tissue causing interstitial fibrosis and a diffusing defect which involves mainly the lower zones
4. Involvement of skin and diaphragm leading to diminished ventilation of the lungs.

The kidneys and heart are usually involved fairly late in the disease. The renal lesions resemble those of SLE and the main cardiac lesion is a cardiomyopathy possibly complicated by pulmonary hypertension, systemic hypertension and endocardial thickening causing mitral and tricuspid incompetence.

Treatment of scleroderma consists of corticosteroids if the disease is progressing rapidly or is causing discomfort, as it often does. Low-molecular weight dextran (Rheomacrodex) is indicated if arterial lesions are severe. It is given intermittently every 4–6 weeks; it is required more often during the cold weather. There is some evidence that penicillamine prevents excessive formation of collagen and it may be beneficial in scleroderma. Corticosteroids are not thought to prevent progression of the disease.

Dermatomyositis and Polymyositis

From a practical point of view there is no point in distinguishing between these two conditions provided it is appreciated that the skin is not invariably involved—the muscles alone may be affected. The affected muscles are those of the limb girdles and proximal limbs, those of the face and distal limbs are commonly not affected. The affected muscles become weak, atrophic and tender at rest and on palpation. The skin lesions consist of erythema which usually involves the face, chest and arms; involvement of the dorsum of the fingers is very suggestive. The rash is light-sensitive and may closely resemble SLE; however, visceral involvement, arthritis and LE cells are rarely seen in dermatomyositis. In patients over the age of 50 the majority will have an accompanying neoplasm, the common sites being the stomach, breast and ovary. The dermatomyositis may antedate the appearance of the carcinoma or rarely it may develop after the neoplasm has been cured. The response of established dermatomyositis to removal of the tumour is variable but it may be complete. Muscle and skin biopsy are important in diagnosis and estimation of muscle enzymes (phosphocreatine kinase, aldolase and transaminases) are useful indicators of progress. The disease does not usually relapse and remit; the most usual outcome is death after about six months or a slowly progressive downward course. Corticosteroids are usually given in large doses and it is justifiable to continue them for a long time; a careful search should always be made for a primary neoplasm, especially of the lung, ovaries and stomach.

Systemic Lupus Erythematosus

This is the most common and the most catholic of the collagen disorders. Multisystem involvement is the rule rather than the exception. The commonest features are fever, arthritis, and skin and renal involvement. Unlike the skin lesions of dermatomyositis and scleroderma, calcinosis does not occur. The disease is rare in men; a high clinical index of suspicion for SLE is important in a female patient who has a fever and raised ESR, who is being investigated for otherwise unexplained:

Thrombocytopenia and purpura
Haemolytic anaemia
Lymphadenopathy and splenomegaly
False positive WR
Nephrotic syndrome
Peripheral neuropathy
Recent onset of psychosis or epilepsy
Pleural effusions or pericarditis
Patchy shadowing in the lung fields
Hepatitis.

Discoid lupus refers to the occurrence of the skin lesions of SLE in the absence of any systemic manifestations. It is now accepted that many cases of discoid lupus eventually develop SLE.

Management of SLE.—The activity of the disease can be assessed roughly by the level of anti-DNA antibodies. Renal involvement is suggested if the complement levels are low. Corticosteroids are indicated if there is renal involvement, nervous-system involvement, haemolytic anaemia or thrombocytopenia. Treatment is not indicated if the disease is in complete remission. If exacerbations of the disease do not respond to steroids, an immunosuppressive drug such as azathioprine or cyclophosphamide should be added. Antimalarials are indicated for discoid lupus. High titres of DNA antibodies and circulating immune complexes are indications for treatment but high doses of steroids cause a high incidence of avascular bone necrosis.

Polymyalgia Rheumatica

This is defined as pain and stiffness in the muscles with evidence of systemic involvement. It is virtually confined to the elderly and the muscular pains are always accompanied by a high ESR but not other evidence of rheumatoid arthritis. The muscle pain and stiffness are nearly always worse in the early morning and by mid-morning the patient is better. Depression and weight loss are almost inevitable. It is thought to be due to an arteritis similar to giant-cell arteritis. Following the acute onset of muscular pains there is often wasting of the muscles, particularly the proximal groups. The most difficult differential diagnosis of severe cases is from polymyositis.

Weber[16]**-Christian**[17] **disease** (relapsing, febrile, nodular, non-suppurative paniculitis)

The nodules are subcutaneous, the overlying skin is slightly erythematous; the nodules disappear, leaving areas of depressed skin due to underlying fat necrosis. There is sometimes systemic involvement with anaemia, a high ESR and fat necrosis of the viscera and omentum. Occasionally corticosteroids are necessary.

Gout (*L.* Gutta: a drop)

Uric acid and sodium biurate are the end products of purine metabolism. Clinical gout is caused by an increase in the body uric acid pool due to increased purine synthesis and decreased excretion. The arthritis is due to deposition of biurate crystals in the articular cartilages. The first attack of gout occurs in the big toe in 70 per cent of patients but the ankles or wrists are occasionally the site of the first attack. Hyperuricaemia at some time is a prerequisite for the development of gout, although the serum uric acid is often normal at the time of the acute attack; the level of uric acid at which gout occurs varies even in the same patient. A useful clinical rule is that acute gout always affects one joint at a time.

Nearly all patients who have several attacks of gout will develop tophi (*Gk:* volcanic rock), which consists of deposits of urates and an accompanying inflammatory reaction in the soft tissues particularly cartilages, tendons and ligaments. Tophi do not usually calcify and they are responsible for the soft tissue swelling seen in relation to joints affected by gout.

Chronic gouty arthritis refers to joint deformities which develop after frequent acute attacks of gout in those joints; it is usually painless and almost invariably accompanied by tophi. As a general rule gout never occurs in women before the menopause.

Alcohol, salicylates, guanethidine and thiazide diuretics impair the excretion of uric acid by the distal renal tubules; when a factor which diminishes uric acid excretion is combined with increased purine metabolism, which may be familial or racial (as in the Maoris of New Zealand), clinical gout will be produced.

The acute attack of gout is treated with colchicine 0·5 mg two-hourly for four doses or with phenylbutazone 200 mg six-hourly or a combination of both. Following the acute attack there are two ways in which the uric acid pool may be reduced; one is to promote increased excretion of uric acid and the other is to limit its production. The most widely used uricosuric agent is probenecid 100 mg t.d.s.; early in treatment uricosuric agents may precipitate an acute attack of gout, and therefore, some physicians advocate prophylactic colchicine 0·5 mg b.d. for the first few months of treatment with uricosuric drugs.

In long-standing gout, renal impairment may occur, and starts with deposition of urate crystals near the collecting ducts. This leads to tubular damage which manifests itself by inability to concentrate the urine; later, glomerular damage occurs and the blood urea becomes elevated. Urate calculi are common in long-standing gout; they can be prevented and dissolved by a high fluid intake and alkalinising the urine, which increases the solubility of the urates. Uricosuric drugs increase urinary excretion of uric acid and are contra-indicated in gouty nephropathy. Purines are metabolised via xanthine to uric acid; allopurinol is a drug which inhibits the enzyme xanthine oxidase thus preventing the breakdown of xanthine to uric acid. Allopurinol represents a major advance in the treatment of hyperuricaemia because it can be safely used in the presence of renal failure and, because it diminishes the excretion of uric acid, it may also be used to prevent the formation or recurrence of urate calculi. Allopurinol is indicated in secondary hyperuricaemia due to haematological disorders and to malignant disease treated with cytotoxic drugs or radiotherapy. In the absence of renal impairment gouty tophi can be dissolved by a combination of allopurinol and uricosuric drugs. Sometimes an acute attack of gout may be produced when allopurinol is first used.

Chondrocalcinosis or Pseudo-gout

This recently recognised condition is also called calcium gout, and crystal gout. It is characterised by deposition of crystals of calcium pyrophosphate in the articular cartilages, ligaments and tendons. The joints most commonly affected are the knees, hips and wrists, hence these joints are the most suitable for x-raying if the disease is suspected. The disease occurs in acute attacks which are less severe and less sudden in onset than true gout. The condition is more common in women, it may give rise to chronic arthritis which is punctuated by acute attacks. Like gout the overlying skin may be red and tender to touch, and the diagnosis can be confirmed by finding characteristic crystals in the joint fluid or in the synovial membrane. The disease appears to be more common in the presence of diabetes and hyperparathyroidism.

GENERAL REFERENCES

HUGHES, G. R. (1979) *Connective Tissue Diseases*. 2nd edit. Oxford: Blackwell Scientific Publications.

IRVINE, W. T. (1978) *Medical Immunology*. Edinburgh: Teviot Scientific Publications.

SCOTT, J. T. (1978) *Copeman's Textbook of Rheumatic Diseases*. 5th edit. Edinburgh: Churchill Livingstone.

THOMPSON, R. A. (1978) *Practice of Immunology*. 2nd edit. London: E. Arnold.

EPONYMS

1. LOUIS PASTEUR (1822–1895)

Pasteur trained as a chemist, and although he made fundamental discoveries in microbiology, the lack of a medical qualification was a handicap. He discovered optical isomerism and noted the biological activity of the dextrorotatory isomer of tartaric acid. At Lille he investigated faulty fermentation in the local wine and conceived that fermentation was a biological and not chemical process and that putrefaction was due to anaerobic organisms. It was then an easy step to develop the concept that some infectious diseases were due to putrefaction in the living, and therefore possibly due to micro-organisms. The process of "Pasteurisation" was originally related to wine—heating the wine destroyed those organisms which resulted in contamination. He discovered attenuation of virulent organisms in chicken cholera and later applied the principle to the production of a rabies vaccine. By 1886 350 patients had been treated for rabies with only one death, in what had previously been a uniformly fatal disease. Pasteur also solved many of the problems of anthrax by insisting on the burial of infected carcasses in chalky soil in which earthworms could not disseminate the infected material.

2. GEORGES FERNAND ISIDORE WIDAL (1862–1929)

Widal was born in Algeria; he qualified in Paris where he became Professor first of Pathology and then of Medicine. He developed the agglutination test in 1896.

3. ELIE METCHNIKOFF (1845–1916)

Metchnikoff succeeded Pasteur as director of the Pasteur Institute. He shared the 1908 Nobel Prize with Ehrlich. He was the first to conceive cellular immunity, that leucocytes were "the policemen of the blood" and that they destroyed bacteria—it had previously been thought that leucocytes provided sustenance for invading bacteria (hence their presence in inflammation). The humoral and cellular concepts of immunity and inflammation became partially reconciled with the work of Sir Almroth Wright, who found that leucocytes may also produce a humoral antibody.

4. KARL ALBERT LUDWIG ASCHOFF (1866–1942)

Aschoff studied with von Recklinghausen in Strasbourg, and became Director of Pathology in Freiburg. He had close links with Japan, and with a Japanese student, Tawara, he described the atrioventricular node. He also described (after Rokitansky) the Rokitansky-Aschoff sinuses in the gall bladder. Using supravital stains he investigated and named the reticulo-endothelial system. He was not in sympathy with the Nazi suppression during the nineteen thirties, which resulted in the enforced departure from Germany of so many academics.

5. SIR JAMES PAGET (1814–1899)

Surgeon at St Bartholomew's Hospital. Paget was quick to see the potential of the then recent introduction of both anaesthesia and antisepsis. He chaired the great London Medical Congress of 1881 which was attended by Virchow, Lister, Pasteur, Osler, Huxley, Koch and Volkmann.

6. HEINRICH ERNST ALBERS-SCHÖNBERG (1865–1921)

A friend of Röntgen, Albers-Schönberg became Professor of Röntgenology in the University of Hamburg. He recognised earlier than most the possibilities of x-rays being used for treatment as well as diagnosis, and also the importance of protecting workers exposed to radiation hazards.

7. LOUIS ARTHUR MILKMAN (1895–1951)
Milkman qualified in Philadelphia, specialised in radiology and worked in Scranton, Pennsylvania.

8. EMIL LOOSER (1877–1936)
Looser was born in Constantinople and qualified and worked in Zürich. He trained at first as an engineer, but eventually became Professor of Surgery at Zürich. Because of his engineering leanings he was always interested in bone pathology.

9. FRIEDRICH DANIEL VON RECKLINGHAUSEN (1833–1910)
Von Recklinghausen qualified in Berlin, worked with Virchow and eventually became Professor of Pathology at Strasbourg.

10. CHRISTIAN GEORG SCHMORL (1861–1932)
Schmorl was born and qualified in Leipzig and became Professor of Pathology in Dresden. He died of a wound infection sustained while dissecting a specimen of spinal cord.

11. JEAN MARTIN CHARCOT (1825–1893)
Born in Paris Charcot became physician at Salpetriere, where over 5000 inmates had neurological diseases. He described clearly for the first time several diseases outside the nervous system (for example, rheumatoid arthritis is still sometimes known on the Continent as Charcot's arthritis). He clearly delineated or described for the first time: multiple sclerosis, which was previously confused with Parkinson's disease; tabes dorsalis (and Charcot's joints); peroneal muscular atrophy; amyotrophic lateral sclerosis; multiple cerebral aneurysms (with Bouchard); hysteria; and ankle clonus.

12. HENRIK SAMUEL CONRAD SJÖGREN (b. 1899)
Sjögren was a Swedish ophthalmologist. He qualified in Stockholm and wrote his thesis on the sicca syndrome in 1933. Sjögren's syndrome is an auto-immune disorder and is often associated with auto-immune features in other organs. Mikulicz (1850–1905) syndrome refers to enlargement of the salivary and lachrymal glands from many causes including sarcoidosis.

13. AUGUSTUS ROI FELTY (b. 1895)
Connecticut physician.

14. HANS CONRAD REITER (1881–1969)
Reiter described the clinical association of arthritis, conjunctivitis and urethritis while in the German Army during the First World War. Earlier, he had identified the causative organism of Weil's disease. After the War he worked with August von Wasserman and developed a technique for culturing *Treponema pallidum*; from this "Reiter strain" a specific antigen was produced, resulting in the Reiter Protein Complement Fixation Test for syphilis. In 1932 Hans Reiter signed the oath of allegiance to Hitler and became involved in the infamous studies on eugenics. He was briefly interned in an American prison camp in 1945.

15. MAURICE RAYNAUD (1834–1881)
Raynaud was to have addressed the great Medical Congress held in London and chaired by Sir James Paget in 1881. Lister, Koch, Pasteur, Virchow and Osler were all there, but they had to hear Raynaud's paper read by someone else, Raynaud having died of a coronary the month before. He was very religious and this probably prevented his achieving professorial status. His description of "local asphyxia and gangrene" was published in 1862.

16. FREDERICK PARKES WEBER (1863–1962)
London physician.

17. HENRY ASBURY CHRISTIAN (1876–1951)
Boston physician. As Professor of Medicine at Harvard he was much involved in modernising the medical teaching in the United States. He later edited Osler's textbook of medicine.

6

NEUROLOGY

In neurology as in the other specialised branches of medicine there are clinical concepts which are reasonably straightforward and simple. These clear concepts are the cornerstone of more detailed knowledge and expertise. In neurology, the situation tends to become confused for the non-expert because of the rarity with which he has to apply the simple concepts and because the complicated anatomy can vary the clinical features so much. Nevertheless, it is possible to define, understand and remember enough of the essential concepts for practical purposes.

Internal Capsule

All motor and sensory fibres which begin or end in the cerebral cortex pass through the internal capsule. The internal capsule is part of the cerebral hemispheres; its middle part is occupied by motor fibres, behind these are sensory, visual and auditory fibres. As a working rule all motor and sensory fibres in one internal capsule serve the opposite side of the body; the exception is a collection of motor fibres that do not cross which supply muscles innervated bilaterally from both cerebral cortices. These muscles are mainly those of the trunk, neck and limb girdles. As well as motor and sensory fibres, the internal capsule also transmits autonomic and extrapyramidal fibres. Internal capsular lesions often involve the autonomic fibres leading to vasomotor and sweating disturbances in the weak limbs. Involvement of the extrapyramidal fibres accounts for the increased tone and spasticity of the weak muscles; this increased tone affects the extensor muscles of the limbs much more than the flexor muscles. In contrast in hemiplegias or paraplegias due to lesions in the spinal cord, the tone is increased in the flexor muscles, leading to paraplegia-in-flexion and painful flexor spasms. The fibres subserving movements of the head and eyes lie close together, and both are usually involved together. Lesions of the internal capsule cause weakness of muscles *of* the opposite (contralateral) side, and weakness of movements *to* the contralateral side. Thus, following a lesion in one internal capsule, there is weakness of the opposite side of the body, and deviation of the head and eyes away from the weak (contralateral) side. In many cases this effect is transitory because many of the trunk, neck and eye muscles have bilateral innervation.

The Brain Stem (Fig. 28)

From the internal capsule all the fibres pass to the cerebral peduncle and thence to the brain stem. A simple concept, often confused, is that the brain stem joins the cerebral peduncles to the spinal cord. The brain stem consists of three principal parts:

1. Midbrain
2. Pons
3. Medulla.

The pons is so-called because there is a thick band of fibres passing anterior to it which "bridges" between the two cerebellar hemispheres. As well as transmitting nerve fibres from cerebral peduncles to spinal cord, the brain stem contains the nuclei of the cranial nerves and their interconnections.

The Spinal Cord

The overall structure of the spinal cord is similar throughout its length (Fig. 29), and there are only minor modifications due to increase in number of nerve fibres. Most motor and sensory nerve fibres decussate at some point in the nervous system. The main exceptions to this are a small number of motor fibres carried in the anterior corticospinal tract which generally serve bilaterally innervated muscles.

Nerve fibres subserving the various sensory modalities are carried in tracts which decussate at different levels and have a different destination in the brain stem. The principal sensory tracts, their site of decussation and the sensory impulses which they convey are shown in Table XI. All sensory impulses enter the spinal cord by the posterior nerve roots and are, therefore, situated posteriorly for at least part of their journey to the brain. Hence, any posteriorly situated lesion in the spinal cord will generally affect some form of sensation first.

The signs of damage to the posterior columns are:

1. Loss of proprioception and vibration sense, leading to ataxia, because increased movements have to be performed in order to produce proprioceptive impulses, and wrong movements are not appreciated and corrected quickly.

2. Loss of "deep" pain (loss of tenderness of the tendo Achillis).

3. Positive Rombergism.[1] Ataxia occurs with the eyes closed, but not when they are open because lack of proprioception may be corrected by looking at the position the limbs are in.

4. Hypotonicity due to the fact that many spinocerebellar fibres travel in the posterior columns before entering the spinocerebellar tract.

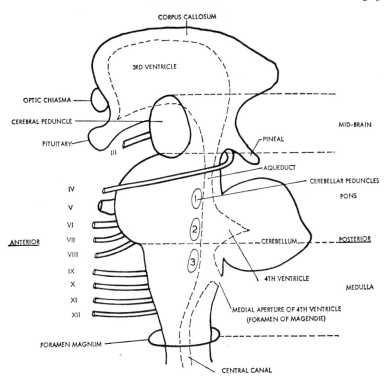

FIG. 28.—The brain stem showing the midbrain, pons and medulla and the origin of the cranial nerves.

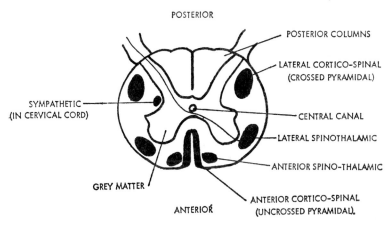

FIG. 29.—Cross-section of the spinal cord showing the position of the important tracts.

TABLE XI

Tract	Sensory Impulses	Site of Decussation
Posterior columns	Proprioception Vibration Deep pain Some light touch	In the medulla, after forming medial lemniscus
Anterior spinothalamic	Light touch	In the spinal cord several segments above their entry
Lateral spinothalamic	Superficial pain Temperature Tickle	In the spinal cord immediately above entry
Spinocerebellar	Concerned with muscle tone and co-ordination	Probably do not cross

5. Diminished tendon reflexes. The sensory stimulus for the deep reflexes is a stretch (hence proprioceptive) reflex, hence diminished proprioception will diminish the tendon reflexes.

It is important to note that not all the above signs need be present to diagnose a posterior column lesion, the two most important causes of which are tabes dorsalis and subacute combined degeneration of the cord.

Loss of proprioception can be quickly tested by the examiner's placing the limbs and fingers of one side of the patient in a certain position and then getting the patient with his eyes closed to place the limbs and fingers of the other side in the same position.

Detailed Consideration of the Brain Stem (Fig. 28)

The motor and sensory fibres of the cranial nerves join their counterparts from the spinal cord. *It is essential to note that all the motor fibres of the cranial nerves are derived from the opposite cerebral cortex in the same way as are the motor fibres of the spinal nerves.* The motor fibres of the spinal nerves (corticospinal or pyramidal fibres) decussate in the upper part of the medulla just below the pons. They continue on the opposite side to the spinal cord, where they become the pyramidal or lateral corticospinal tract. Most of the cranial nerves leave the brain stem higher than the decussation of the pyramids, hence the motor fibres of the cranial nerves must cross higher in the brain stem—they do not form distinct recognisable pathways before they reach their nuclei from which the lower motor neurones are derived. The fact that the upper motor neurones of the cranial nerves decussate at a higher level than the decussation of the pyramids explains the phenomenon of crossed hemiplegia, i.e. weakness of the opposite side of the body with weakness of the cranial nerve muscles on the same side. A lesion which damages the cranial nerve *after* it has decussated, and which also damages the pyramidal tract *before* it has decussated, will cause a crossed hemiplegia. The best known examples of crossed hemiplegias are:

Weber's[2] syndrome: ipsilateral lower motor neurone lesion of the oculomotor nerve with contralateral hemiplegia.

Millard[3]-Gubler[4] syndrome: lower motor neurone lesion of the abducens nerve which supplies the lateral rectus and contralateral hemiplegia.

Foville's[5] syndrome, in which there is a hemiplegia with paralysis of conjugate deviation towards the side of the lesion, i.e. the eyes are fixed *towards* the weak side; in a hemiplegia due to a lesion in the internal capsule, the eyes tend to be fixed *away* from the weak wide.

Hemiplegia on one side with weakness of muscles supplied by the lower cranial nerves (IX–XII) on the opposite side.

Most sensory fibres end in the thalamus, cerebellum or cerebral cortex. Like the motor fibres, all the sensory fibres decussate at various levels (except those going to the cerebellum via the spinocerebellar tracts). The thalamus is the main destination of sensory impulses; from it, selected impulses are relayed to the cerebral cortex on the same side. The cerebral cortex is concerned with discriminatory functions at a conscious level. The main ways of testing this clinically are:

Two-point discrimination.

Assessment of size, weight, texture and purpose of objects (stereognosis), e.g. naming the value of a coin.

Ability to recognise symbols written on the skin (graphaesthesia).

Naming correctly which part of the body the examiner is touching.

Position sense (provided, of course, that the posterior columns are intact).

In the brain stem, the tracts of the spinal cord end as follows (Fig. 30):

The posterior columns, containing uncrossed fibres, form the medial lemnisci which decussate in the medulla.

The anterior spinothalamic (light touch), which forms the reticular substance in the medulla and then joins the medial lemniscus in the pons.

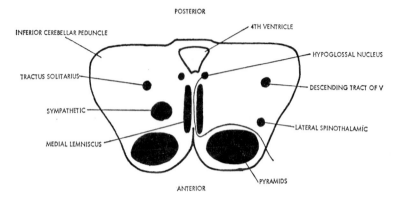

Fig. 30.—Cross-section of the medulla showing the position of the important tracts.

The lateral spinothalamic (pain and temperature), which continues through the medulla as the lateral spinothalamic tract and then also joins the medial lemniscus in the pons.

The medial lemniscus, which terminates in the thalamus.

Other clinically important structures which are seen in the brain stem are:

Medial longitudinal bundle, which interconnects the nuclei of the cranial nerves and is concerned with co-ordination of face and eye movements.

Ascending tract of the trigeminal nerve, which contains proprioceptive and touch fibres, corresponding to the posterior columns. The fibres immediately cross the midline and join the medial lemniscus.

Descending tract of the trigeminal nerve, which carries pain and temperature impulses corresponding to the lateral spinothalamic tract. This tract descends to the level of C.2 on the same side as it enters, and then crosses the midline and joins the lateral spinothalamic tract.

Tractus solitarius, which contains fibres conveying taste.

Corticospinal tracts.

Nuclei of the cranial nerves. These occur as follows: Midbrain: oculomotor and trochlear. The oculomotor nerve emerges from the midbrain close to the cerebral peduncle, so that a lesion in this area gives rise to a lower motor neurone oculomotor palsy on the same side and a hemiplegia on the opposite side (Weber's syndrome). Pons: abducens, trigeminal, facial and auditory. Medulla: glossopharyngeal, vagus, accessory and hypoglossal.

The basilar artery runs along the anterior surface of the brain stem as far as the upper border of the pons, and is its main blood supply (Fig. 31). The three portions of the brain stem are also supplied by various other arteries. The most important are the posterior cerebral, supplying the midbrain (including the cerebral peduncles), the anterior inferior cerebellar artery, supplying the pons and posterior inferior

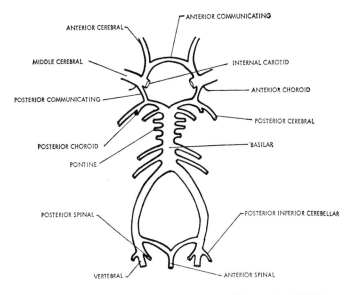

FIG. 31.—The arteries at the base of the brain and the circle of Willis.[6]

cerebellar artery supplying the medulla. The posterior inferior cerebellar arteries are derived from the vertebrals and in practice, narrowing of one vertebral artery may result in ischaemia of the medulla. Ischaemia of the midbrain, if severe and bilateral, will result in a quadriplegia, because both cerebral peduncles are involved. The nuclei of the cranial nerves and their connections in this region of the midbrain will be involved (III and IV), resulting in lower motor neurone oculomotor and trochlear palsies and impairment of conjugate eye movements, as the nuclei subserving conjugate movements are in the same region. In lesser degrees of unilateral midbrain ischaemia, there will be a crossed hemiplegia caused by involvement of the corticospinal tract and third nerve. Particular features of midbrain ischaemia which are sometimes present are:

Hemiballismus, due to involvement of part of the thalamus.
Thalamic syndrome.

Akinetic mutism (coma vigil), in which the patient appears to be
almost awake, with the eyes open, and yet in a coma.

Lesions near the pineal. These result in impairment of upward
movement of the eyes, due to the proximity of the nucleus
concerned with upward conjugate deviation.

From a consideration of the structures of the pons, the probable
consequences of partial ischaemia can be deduced. The important
considerations are firstly the cranial nerve nuclei dealing with the
conjugate lateral deviation and secondly the fact that in the pons the
medial lemniscus is joined by the lateral spinothalamic tracts and the
anterior spinothalamic fibres via the reticular formation; thus, the
possible consequences are:

Lower motor neurone lesions of the cranial nerves arising from
the area, i.e. abducent, trigeminal, facial and auditory nerves.

Impairment of lateral conjugate deviation.

Variable loss of sensation of one side of the body, depending on
whether the medial lemniscus is involved before or after it has
been joined by fibres from the anterior and lateral spinothalamic tracts.

Contralateral hemiplegia due to involvement of the corticospinal
tracts.

Other considerations are the presence of fibres of the sympathetic
nervous system which, if affected, will give rise to Horner's syndrome
and the cerebellar tracts which, if affected, may cause cerebellar signs.
Particular features of pontine lesions include pin-point pupils and
hyperventilation.

Ischaemic lesions of the medulla are commoner than either midbrain
or pontine lesions. From Fig. 30, the possible consequences of lesions
in the medulla can be deduced. They are:

Involvement of the cranial nerves of the area: the glossopharyngeal and vagus, leading to dysarthria, dysphagia, and vocal
cord paralysis (bulbar palsy). Involvement of the vestibular
branches of the eighth nerve causes vertigo and nausea.

Involvement of the corticospinal tract leads to a contralateral
hemiplegia.

Involvement of the medial lemniscus leads to loss of proprioception and vibration sense on the opposite side of the body.

Involvement of the cerebellar peduncle may lead to unilateral
cerebellar signs.

From Fig. 30, it will be seen that if the lesion is mainly of the lateral
side of the medulla, the descending tract of the trigeminal, the lateral
spinothalamic and the sympathetic tract will be involved. This leads

to contralateral loss of pain and temperature over the body and an ipsilateral loss over the face because the descending tract of the trigeminal is involved before it has decussated (which is does in the cervical spine), whereas the lateral spinothalamic fibres decussate soon after they enter the cord; in addition there will be an ipsilateral Horner's syndrome (lateral medullary syndrome). If the medial part of the medulla is mainly involved the above will be absent, but instead, the medial lemniscus and the hypoglossal nucleus will be involved and there will be unilateral atrophy of the tongue, which will be absent in the lateral medullary syndrome.

LOCALISING FEATURES OF MOTOR LESIONS

Site

Cerebral cortex — Flaccid weakness. Flexors and extensors equally affected ("global weakness")
Cortical sensory loss may be present

Internal capsule — Spastic weakness
Extensors more affected than flexors
Distal limb muscles more affected than proximal muscles
Paralysis of head and eye movements so that patient looks away from the weak *limbs*

Brain stem — Crossed hemiplegia, i.e. ipsilateral cranial nerve palsy with contralateral limb palsy

Cord lesion — Flaccid
Flexors more affected than extensors

Root and peripheral nerve — Lower motor neurone lesion
Peripheral nerve lesions usually affect both motor and sensory function in muscles and skin supplied by the nerve. The following is a *rough* guide to the muscles supplied by clinically important motor nerve roots:

C 5, 6	Biceps and deltoid	L 2, 3	Adductors
C 7, 8	Triceps	L 3, 4	Quadriceps
C 7	Finger extensors	L 4, 5	Dorsiflexors
C 8	Finger flexors	L 5, S 1	Hamstrings
T 1	Small muscles of the hand	S 1, 2	Plantar flexors and small muscles of the feet

The Plantar Reflex (Babinski's[7] Sign)

One of the perennial discussions in which non-neurologists indulge is the significance of the plantar response and the correct means of eliciting it. It is now generally accepted that the *extensor* response is part of the general *flexor* response of the limbs reacting to injury and that the extensor hallucis longus is in fact physiologically a flexor muscle because its contraction results in shortening of the limb.

The reflex is best elicited by firm, slightly painful stroking of the lateral border of the sole. The normal response when the nervous system is intact is a downward movement of the big toe and slight downward movement of the remaining toes, as if the foot were relaxing itself to receive a painful stimulus. When the plantar response is elicited the important movement of the big toe is the early movement; the later movements particularly when the ball of the foot is stroked may develop into a general "flexor" movement of the limb (i.e. dorsiflexion) as part of the withdrawal reaction.

It is helpful to consider the movements of the foot and leg which occur in normal people when different parts of the foot are stimulated. All the reflex movements of the limb are designed to reduce the effects of harmful stimuli affecting the sole of the foot, bearing in mind that the human foot has been modified for the erect posture. It has been shown that all the movements are co-ordinated (i.e. there is reflex inhibition of opposing muscles). Stimulation of the ball of the foot *in normals* results in dorsiflexion of the toes, flexion of ankle and knee. Stimulation of the hollow of the foot results in plantar flexion of the toes, flexion of the ankle, etc. Stimulation of the plantar surface of the heel results in plantar flexion of the toes and extension of the heel, flexion of the knees, *extension* of the hips (i.e. the heel is raised off the ground). Thus the ball of the foot is the only area of the sole where *dorsiflexion* is the *normal* response.

The distinction between a normal response and patients with upper motor neurone lesions is that the pathological "extensor" plantar response (dorsiflexion) can be elicited from a much wider receptive field, i.e. the area from which dorsiflexion can normally be elicited (the balls of the feet) extends over a wider area of the sole. The reason why the outside of the foot is stimulated is that it is a *less* sensitive area than the inside of the sole—stimulation of the inside of the sole with a minor pyramidal lesion may still produce a normal plantar flexor downward response.

CEREBRAL CORTEX

The surfaces of the cerebral hemispheres are divided by certain fissures which are constant. These are the lateral fissure (Sylvian[8] fissure) and the central sulcus (Rolandic[9] fissure). In front of the

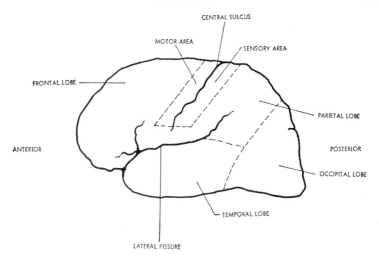

FIG. 32.—The cerebral cortex showing the position of the lobes and the motor and sensory areas.

central sulcus is the motor area and behind it is the sensory area. The lobes of the cerebral cortex are not clearly defined by any internal arrangement, but are merely areas of the surface of the cortex which are in contact with the bones of the skull of the same name. However, it is usually convenient to consider the functions of the different areas of the cortex in terms of the named lobes (Fig. 32).

The area in front of the central sulcus (known as the precentral gyrus) is concerned with motor functions of the opposite side of the body. The part of the motor area concerned with movements of the feet is at the top and the part concerned with movements of the head is at the bottom, i.e. the body image is represented upside down. The area behind the central sulcus (the postcentral gyrus) is concerned with appreciation of sensation and this is represented in precisely the same way as in the motor area, i.e. feet at the top and head at the bottom.

The Speech Centres (Broca's[10] area)

The centre concerned with the reception of information which will lead to speech is situated in the sensory cortex; and the centre concerned with the motor side of speaking is situated in the motor area. As a rule, only the dominant cerebral hemisphere contains the speech centre. In a right-handed person, this is the left cerebral hemisphere. Lesions of one or other of the two speech centres give rise to motor or sensory dysphasia. In motor dysphasia, the patient knows what he wants to say, but cannot say it. It is best tested for by asking the patient to obey a command (such as "close your eyes" or "open your mouth"), to write down his reply to a question or to ask him to nod when you supply him with the correct answer to a question you have given him.

The two ways in which the sensory speech area is stimulated are either by the patient reading or hearing a question or command. Thus, sensory dysphasia can be due to inability to comprehend the spoken word (auditory dysphasia) or the written word (visual dysphasia). In their pure forms, auditory and visual dysphasia are very rare. The more common occurrence is for auditory and visual aphasia to be mixed; under these circumstances, the patient may be able to speak, but the words are often unrecognisable or completely irrelevant to the question. Although he is able to talk, he is unable to name common objects although he may still be able to use them for their correct purposes (e.g. a comb or a glass of water). Thus, a rough way of assessing dysphasia is to ask the patient a simple question and, if he is unable to reply, he probably has either motor aphasia or has not understood the question (auditory sensory aphasia). In order to establish whether he understands he is asked to perform a simple movement. If he obeys the command this will confirm that he has motor dysphasia. If he does not do a simple movement in response to a verbal order he may do it in response to a written order. This will confirm that he has a combined motor and auditory dysphasia. If the patient replies in an incomprehensible way, then he probably has a sensory dysphasia. Aphasia is usually accompanied by an inability to calculate (acalculia) or to write (agraphia).

Dysarthria refers to difficulty with the mechanical act of producing spoken words and is due to disorder of the muscles of articulation, which include the tongue and facial and laryngeal muscles. Various phrases are traditionally used when testing for dysarthria—these particular phrases are used because they test all the groups of muscles involved in speaking (labials, linguals, palatal and laryngeal). The traditional phrases are: "British constitution", "baby hippopotamus", "West Register Street" and "Methodist Episcopal Church".

The important causes of dysarthria are:

> Lesions of the cranial nerves serving the muscles of articulation, which include the facial, glossopharyngeal, vagus and hypoglossal nerves. A lower motor neurone lesion of the nerves gives rise to a "bulbar palsy".
> Disorders of the co-ordination of movement, seen particularly in cerebellar lesions.
> Disease or weakness of the muscles of articulation, e.g. myopathies and myasthenia gravis.

The muscles of articulation are innervated from both cerebral cortices, hence a lesion of one internal capsule will not produce dysarthria, but if both internal capsules are affected, dysarthria will follow—"pseudo-bulbar palsy".

The Visual Pathways

The visual areas of the cerebral cortices are in the posterior part of the occipital lobes. The macular region of each eye is represented in both occipital lobes, furthermore, the macular area of each occipital lobe has a dual blood supply via the middle and posterior cerebral

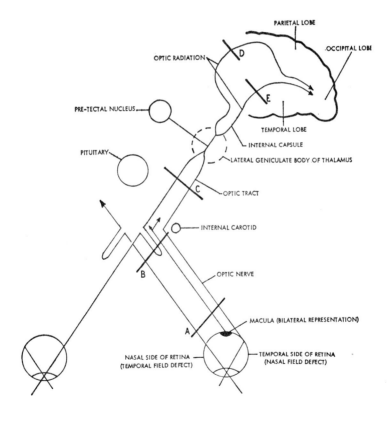

FIG. 33.—The visual pathways. Note the pituitary in relation to nasal fibres from both retinae, the optic radiation, the internal carotid artery and the muscular fibres passing to both optic tracts.

arteries. Figure 33 shows the visual pathways. Defects of vision of one-half of the visual field are hemianopias; because of the effects of the lens of the eye a temporal hemianopia is due to a lesion of the nerve fibres supplying the nasal side of the retina, and vice versa. A field defect which affects the corresponding field of vision of both eyes, i.e. the nasal field of one eye and the temporal field of the other, is a homonymous hemianopia. If only a quarter of the visual field is involved it is a quadrantanopia, and if only a small portion of the field is involved, it is a scotoma. The macula is concerned with fixation of vision and is the area of maximum visual acuity.

From Fig. 33 it will be seen that a lesion of the optic nerve at (A) will lead to complete blindness in one eye. A lesion at (B) will lead to complete blindness in one eye and a temporal hemianopia in the other eye, due to the fact that fibres from the nasal side of the retina loop into the optic nerve of the opposite eye. Enlargement of the pituitary from below is almost always asymmetrical, it compresses fibres from the lower nasal side of one eye first and hence causes an upper temporal field defect. Later, the defect may involve the lower temporal field and become equal in both eyes (bitemporal hemianopia). The optic chiasma may also be involved by a meninigioma or by fibrosis following meningitis (meningococcal, tuberculous or syphilitic). The internal carotid arteries lie on the lateral side of the chiasm; excessive atheroma or an aneurysm of the internal carotid may press on the temporal fibres from the eye on that side, causing a nasal hemianopia. The optic tract carries fibres backwards to the lateral geniculate body, and in the optic tract the fibres from each eye remain fairly distinct, hence any lesion affecting the tract (C) does not affect the congruous fields of both eyes to the same extent; the hemianopia or scotoma is therefore not congruous. The commonest lesions affecting the optic tracts are meningitis, pituitary tumours, temporal lobe lesions and aneurysms of the posterior communicating or internal carotid arteries.

The optic fibres pass from the lateral geniculate body through the internal capsule, and fan out, before converging again to reach the occipital cortex. Fibres from the upper part of the retina (lower field of vision) pursue a long course and are related to the parietal lobe, whereas fibres from the lower part of the retina (upper field of vision) pursue a shorter course and are related to the temporal lobe. Hence, a lesion of the parietal lobe (at D) will produce a lower homonymous quadrantanopia, whereas a lesion of the temporal lobe (at E) will produce an upper homonymous quadrantanopia. In the optic radiation, fibres from both eyes serving congruous areas of both retinae lie very close together, unlike in the optic tract where fibres of congruous areas are separated. This difference is the main way of distinguishing lesions of the optic tract from those of the optic radiation. Tract lesions will cause non-congruous hemianopias or scotomata, but radiation lesions will produce congruous hemianopias or scotomata.

Damage to one occipital lobe will produce a homonymous hemianopia, but the macula will be spared because it has bilateral representation. Damage to both occipital cortices occurs if both posterior cerebral arteries are damaged or if the basilar artery is occluded because both the posterior cerebral arteries arise from the basilar. Bilateral occipital cortical infarction leads to cortical blindness, in which the patient is totally blind but the pupillary light and accommodation reflexes remain intact. In all other forms of neurological bilateral blindness, either the optic nerves or tracts have to be involved and the afferent fibres for the pupillary light reflex will be damaged, leading to loss of the pupillary light reflex. In cortical blindness the optic nerves and tracts are intact and the damage is distal to the point where the pupillary afferent fibres leave the visual fibres to go to the pretectal nucleus of the midbrain.

DISTURBANCES OF FUNCTION OF THE LOBES OF THE CEREBRAL CORTEX

Frontal Lobes

The frontal lobes are concerned with intellectual functions as well as containing the motor area within the precentral gyrus. Damage to the frontal lobes leads to forgetfulness, dementia, and incontinence with indifference. If the lesion involves the motor area, there may be Jacksonian[11] focal epilepsy and weakness of the corresponding area of the body. Motor aphasia will occur if the dominant hemisphere is involved. The frontal lobes lie directly over the olfactory tracts, which may be compressed, leading to anosmia; alternatively, a meningioma, arising from the olfactory groove, may compress the frontal lobes. A parasagittal meningioma (one occurring in the midline in the sagittal or antero-posterior plane) above the cerebral hemisphere will press on the top of the frontal lobes, leading to loss of motor function at the top of the motor area (i.e. affecting the legs). The frontal lobe may press on the optic nerves, giving rise to optic atrophy on that side, if the tumour enlarges and causes a raised intracranial pressure there may be papilloedema in the opposite eye. The occurrence of papilloedema in one eye and optic atrophy in the other is known as the Foster Kennedy[12] syndrome. A physical sign believed to be pathognomonic of frontal lobe tumours is the grasp reflex, which affects the limbs of the opposite side of the body and is similar to the physiological grasp reflex of babies.

Parietal Lobes

The parietal lobes are mainly concerned with sensory recognition and orientation of the body image. Lesions which involve the postcentral gyrus will cause cortical sensory loss in the corresponding part of the body. The important tests of cortical sensation are stereognosis, two-point discrimination, localisation of a stimulus to the correct part of the body, and recognition of letters or figures drawn on the skin. Parietal lobe lesions may cause a lower homonymous quadrantanopia. If the dominant lobe is involved, there will be sensory aphasia accompanied by inability to calculate (acalculia), inability to read (alexia) and inability to write (agraphia). Lesions of the non-dominant parietal lobe (usually the right lobe) cause inattention and inability to recognise the left half of the body. This can be tested by touching both sides of the body at the same time, the patient will always say that the right side only has been touched. The combination of confusion of right and left, inability to identify the fingers and acalculia, is known as Gerstmann's[13] syndrome. A curious feature of parietal lobe lesions is that the signs vary from day to day.

Temporal Lobe

The upper homonymous quadrantanopia of temporal lobe lesions has already been mentioned; other features are hallucinations of taste and smell, often accompanied by excessive lip smacking. Patients who have temporal lobe epilepsy often have auditory hallucinations and a dazed look. The best known temporal lobe symptom is an excessive number of déjà-vu phenomena (a feeling of having been in the same situation before).

Epilepsy

The drug treatment of epilepsy has moved away from giving mixtures of several drugs to giving single drugs in the dose necessary to control fits. This has led to a more rational and safe use of drugs, particularly as several of the older drugs were converted in the body into the same metabolites. The use of single drugs allows earlier recognition of the known side-effects of each drug. Furthermore, the monitoring of drug blood levels allows the dose to be adjusted for each patient. The drugs of choice are shown in Table XII (from Laidlaw and Richens, 1976).

TABLE XII
DRUGS OF CHOICE IN VARIOUS TYPES OF EPILEPSY

Type of epilepsy	EEG correlates	Drugs of first choice	Drugs of second choice
Grand mal, motor and sensory	Spike-and-wave, focal spike and sharp waves	Phenytoin Carbamazepine Phenobarbitone	Methoin Pheneturide Sodium valproate
Psychomotor	Temporal spikes and sharp waves	Phenytoin Carbamazepine Primidone	Methoin Sodium valproate Methsuximide
Minor myoclonic and akinetic	Polyspike-and-wave; 2 per second spike-and-wave	Nitrazepam Clonazepam	Ethosuximide Sodium valproate
Petit mal absences	3 per second spike-and-wave	Ethosuximide Phensuximide	Sodium valproate Clonazepam Troxidone

The dosage details of these drugs are shown in Table XIII (from Laidlaw and Richens, 1976).

TABLE XIII

Drug (tablet/ capsule size in mg)	Dose frequency (doses/day)	Starting dose (mg/day)	Range of maintenance doses (mg/day)
Phenytoin (50, 100)	1	200	150–600
Methoin (100)	1	100	100–600
Carbamazepine (100, 200)	2–3	400	600–1600
Phenobarbitone (15, 30, 60, 100)	1	60	60–240
Primidone (250)	1	500	500–1500
Pheneturide (200)	2	200	400–1000
Sodium valproate (200)	2–3	400	1000–2400
Ethosuximide (250)	1	500	750–1500
Methsuximide (300)	1	300	600–1200
Phensuximide (250, 500)	3–4	1000	1000–3000
Troxidone (300)	2	600	900–2100
Nitrazepam (5)	2	5	5–20
Clonazepam (0·5, 2)	2	1	4–10

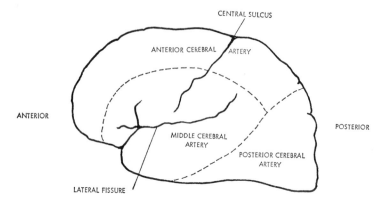

FIG. 34.—The cerebral cortex showing the distribution of the cerebral arteries.

Blood Supply of the Cerebral Cortex (Fig. 34)

Anterior cerebral artery.—This artery supplies the frontal lobes and the superior portion of the cerebral cortex (leg area). A large branch of the anterior cerebral, Heubner's[14] artery (medial striate artery) supplies the anterior portion of the internal capsule which carries fibres supplying the upper part of the body. Occlusion of the artery beyond the origin of Heubner's artery gives rise to:

Motor dysphasia (on dominant side) because of involvement of precental gyrus of the frontal lobe

Cortical (flaccid) weakness of opposite leg

Cortical sensory loss in opposite leg because of involvement of superior surface of cerebral cortex

Frontal lobe involvement, possibly causing a grasp reflex, incontinence and intellectual deterioration.

Occlusion of Heubner's artery affecting the anterior limb of the internal capsule and extrapyramidal nuclei leads to contralateral weakness in the upper body—the weakness is accompanied by spasticity.

Middle cerebral artery.—This artery supplies the majority of the internal capsule (via the lateral striate arteries), the cortical speech areas, and the part of the motor and sensory cortex concerned with the upper part of the body as well as the larger part of frontal, temporal and parietal lobes. Obstruction of the lateral striate branches of the middle cerebral artery results in:

Contralateral spastic weakness

Hemianopia (involvement of visual fibres in internal capsule).

Obstruction of frontal branches leads to flaccid (cortical) weakness and cortical sensory loss of the upper part of the body. Interruption of branches to the parietal and temporal lobes results in parietal and temporal lobe signs (see p. 338).

Posterior cerebral artery.—This supplies the occipital lobe and has a branch to the thalamus and midbrain. Occlusion distal to the thalamic branch produces an homonymous hemianopia with sparing of the macula; occlusion proximal to the thalamic branch will produce the thalamic syndrome in addition. The thalamic syndrome consists of increased sensitivity to stimuli from one-half of the body with a feeling of severe pain in various parts.

If both posterior cerebral arteries are occluded "cortical blindness" results. The patient is blind but all the pupillary reflexes are intact; the patient is completely unaware when a light is shone into the eyes. The fundal appearances are normal. In other forms of blindness due to lesions of the retina, optic nerve or optic tracts, the pupillary reflexes are usually affected, there are changes seen in the fundus and the patient is usually aware of the fact that a light is being shone into the eyes. A curious feature of "cortical blindness" is that the patient may be unaware of or deny his inability to see.

Transient Ischaemic Attacks

These are brief episodes of neurological symptoms and signs which recur and are thought to be due to temporary arterial insufficiency. The intervals between recurrences vary widely from a few minutes to several months. Their occurrence almost invariably means that there is *widespread* although not necessarily *severe* cerebral arteriosclerosis. They are precipitated by a variety of causes:

Haemodynamic disturbances—hypotension and fall in cardiac output, or dysrhythmias which are often transient.

Anaemia and polycythaemia.

Emboli—from any stenotic or atheromatous lesion within the arteries supplying the circle of Willis, from the left atrium, left ventricle or aortic valve.

Temporary obstruction to arteries supplying the circle of Willis, particularly compression of the vertebral arteries in cervical spondylosis. The carotid arteries may occasionally be compressed by the transverse process of the atlas when the head is rotated.

Subclavian steal syndrome in which blood flows from one subclavian artery to the other via the vertebrals and basilar artery because of occlusion of one subclavian artery at its origin; this diverts blood from the circle of Willis.

Hypertensive crises.

Rarely, cerebral tumour and cerebral aneurysms.

The clinical features of transient ischaemic attacks vary widely but they can be roughly grouped into ischaemia of the carotid and middle cerebral artery territories and ischaemia in the region supplied by the basilar artery—this includes the posterior cerebral arteries into which the basilar artery drains.

Carotid and middle cerebral features are:

Transient monocular blindness due to interruption of flow in one retinal artery
Confusion due to frontal-lobe ischaemia
Hemiplegia ⎱
Hemianopia ⎰ due to internal capsular ischaemia
Horner's syndrome
Stuttering hemiplegia.

Basilar and posterior cerebral features are:

Vertigo ⎫
Dysarthria ⎪
Dysphagia ⎬ Pontine and medullary signs
Facial pain ⎪
Hemiplegia ⎭
Altitudinal or hemianopic visual-field disturbances due to ischaemia of optic radiation or occipital lobe (posterior cerebral artery)
Drop attacks, believed to be due to ischaemia of the reticular formation.
Rarely, temporal-lobe symptoms.

Management.—The known aetiological factors should be excluded or treated (e.g. anaemia, polycythaemia, hypertension, emboli arising from the heart).

Carotid and vertebral artery angiography (four-vessel angiography) should probably be performed:

In young patients (say those under 55)
If the clinical features suggest carotid artery or middle cerebral ischaemia
If there is a carotid artery bruit or diminished pulsation on one side. (It is important to try to palpate the internal carotid artery in the tonsillar fossa)
If signs and symptoms are unequivocally related to moving the head and neck
To exclude a tumour or cerebral aneurysm as the cause
If the patient is normotensive.

If a definite stenosis of the extracranial vessels is found surgery (disobliteration) should be considered together with anticoagulants.

If no stenotic lesion is found anticoagulants alone are used if the usual contra-indications are absent. Anticoagulants are usually given empirically *for one year* and then gradually withdrawn *provided* symptoms do not recur.

Apart from transient ischaemic attacks and extracranial artery stenosis the main indications for anticoagulants for vascular disorders affecting the brain are:

Cerebral embolism
"Stroke in evolution."

Features suggesting embolic infarction are:

Signs are complete at the onset
The signs are usually attributable to occlusion of a single artery
Headache is often present, due to compensatory vasodilatation.

The prognosis is poor if recovery is not rapid because there is usually no pre-existing atherosclerosis of the cerebral arteries to encourage collaterals.

The main indication for carotid and cerebral angiography following a completed stroke are (Marshall, 1968):

Young patients
Cardiovascular accident preceded by transient ischaemic attacks
    suggesting a lesion in one of the extracranial vessels
Skull or arterial bruit
Possibility of preceding trauma
Possibility of a cerebral tumour.

One difficult problem particularly for the non-expert is the decision about further radiology in the management of patients with transient ischaemic attacks. Kendall and Marshall (1974) suggest that practically all normotensive patients with carotid transient ischaemic attacks should be investigated because these attacks are ten times more likely to progress to a completed stroke than vertebrobasilar ischaemic attacks. In these patients angiography is indicated to answer two questions:

1. Has the patient a lesion relevant to his symptoms?
2. If so, is it surgically correctable?

In the case of vertebrobasilar transient ischaemic attacks the situation is different because firstly they are much less likely to progress to a completed stroke and secondly the scope of surgery is much more limited. There are two main situations in which angiography is indicated; firstly when there is a supraclavicular bruit or inequality of brachial blood pressures, indicating a subclavian steal situation, and secondly when the attacks are clearly related to neck movements in which case simple surgery may be effective in removing an offending osteophyte.

CRANIAL NERVES

Optic Nerves

The optic nerve is surrounded by the meninges and the subarachnoid space. The dura fuses with the sclera and the optic nerve pierces the sclera through a series of holes known as the lamina cribrosa. The central artery and vein of the retina also pierce the lamina cribrosa and travel in the optic nerve for a short distance before leaving it, crossing the subarachnoid space and joining the ophthalmic vessels. The practical importance of this crossing of the subarachnoid space by the vein is that any change in pressure in the subarachnoid space can easily compress the vein, leading to congestion of the veins in the retina.

The fibres from the macular area occupy the central portion of the optic nerve; they are not so vulnerable to changes of pressure in the subarachnoid space surrounding the optic nerves, but are more prone to damage by inflammatory lesions of the optic nerves. Hence, retrobulbar neuritis gives rise at an early stage to severe disturbance of vision, with a central scotoma involving the blind spot and fixation spot (macula), whereas in papilloedema, due to raised intracranial pressure, vision is little disturbed until the papilloedema has been present for some time. When visual disturbances do occur in papilloedema, they consist of some enlargement of the blind spot, which is due to oedema increasing the size of the nerve head in the eye, and constriction of peripheral fields of vision. The fixation point is not affected. This difference in visual disturbance is the main distinguishing feature between papilloedema and retrobulbar neuritis.

The optic disc consists of the fibres of the optic nerve entering the back of the eye, turning at right angles and being distributed to the retina. Because all the fibres turn outwards and individual fibres are transparent, there will be a funnel-shaped hole in the centre of the disc (the optic cup); in the bottom of the hole a few fibres of the nerve pierce the sclera, and although the nerve fibres cannot be seen, the holes in the sclera through which they travel are seen as the lamina cribrosa. It is sometimes helpful in understanding the anatomy of the optic disc to use an analogy—imagine a hollow pipe opening flush onto a flat surface; emerging from the pipe are many pieces of string which are distributed in all directions over the flat surface. Provided there are many pieces of string they will obviously have to be heaped on top of each other as they turn at right angles after leaving the pipe. Furthermore, as they all turn outwards there will be a funnel-shaped hole in the centre.

The contour of the optic disc is sharply defined: it consists of the layers of the retina coming to an end as the optic nerve emerges through the sclera. As the fibres of the optic nerve turn outwards over the inside of the eye, they tend to become heaped up between the optic cup and the edge of the disc. In the normal, the optic nerve protrudes about 2 mm above the surface of the retina. The optic disc is normally slightly paler on the temporal than on the nasal side; it is important to be aware of this normal temporal pallor because increased temporal pallor is a sign of disseminated sclerosis, but it takes considerable experience to say whether the temporal pallor is more than normal. Another important normal feature of the optic disc is blurring of its nasal margins. The contour of the disc should normally only be blurred on the nasal side: similar blurring of the contour elsewhere indicates papilloedema.

Papilloedema

The earliest sign of papilloedema is swelling of the veins, which normally are approximately twice the thickness of the arteries; they are swollen if they are more than twice the thickness. The next step in the development of papilloedema is blurring of the disc margins, and then the disc becomes more red than usual. Normally, the optic disc is much paler than the surrounding retina, and one which is the same colour as the retina is almost certainly abnormal. The oedema of the optic nerve causes the funnel-shaped hole in the centre of the nerve (the optic cup) to become filled with fluid, so that the lamina cribrosa cannot be seen. As oedema and congestion continue, small veins rupture, leading to haemorrhages in the layers of the retina. All the nerve fibres in the retina radiate outwards from the optic disc, so that haemorrhage between the nerve fibres will tend to be linear (or sometimes flame-shaped). This radial arrangement of the nerve fibres also applies to the macular area, so that any oedema which collects near the macula appears to radiate from it—this is called the "macular star", and it occurs in severe papilloedema.

If the raised intracranial pressure is not relieved, the congestion of the disc remains. The continued pressure on the optic nerve causes the fibres to atrophy and become white. This makes the optic disc appear very pale. The increased pressure tends to involve the central retinal artery, which may become narrowed causing attenuation of the arteries of the retina, and the veins usually remain congested. Because of the accompanying oedema, the disc margin remains blurred, the optic cup remains filled with fluid and therefore indistinct, and the lamina cribosa cannot be seen. This is the appearance of secondary optic atrophy because it occurs secondary to papilloedema. Primary optic atrophy is atrophy of the optic nerve, due to external pressure or inflammation—there is no interference with the venous drainage or arterial supply of the eye. The disc in primary optic atrophy will appear paler than usual but because there is no oedema, the contour, the optic cup, and the lamina cribrosa will be easily seen. The arteries and veins of the retina are normal. Consecutive optic atrophy refers to atrophy of the optic nerve due to disease within the eye, damaging the nerves of the retina after they have left the optic nerve. The appearances of the optic nerve are the same as those of primary optic atrophy, but in addition, the cause of the optic atrophy can also be seen within the eye. The two commonest causes are glaucoma and choroiditis. When the optic disc is inspected, the following should be noted: circulation (arteries and veins), colour, contour, cup, cribriform plate and the complete retina.

Some conditions cause inflammation of the optic nerve; if the nerve is only affected behind the eyeball the condition is called retrobulbar neuritis. In the early stages of retrobulbar neuritis there are no abnormalities to be seen in the optic disc, although vision may be severely affected. Later primary optic atrophy follows. Optic neuritis refers to inflammation of the optic nerve where the nerve can be seen with the ophthalmoscope within the eye, the appearances are those of papilloedema. The causes of optic neuritis and retrobulbar neuritis are the same, namely:

Disseminated sclerosis
Tabes dorsalis
Vitamin B_1 and B_{12} deficiency
Toxic causes such as tobacco, alcohol (particularly methyl alcohol), quinine and lead.

The pupillary reaction in retrobulbar neuritis may be helpful: the pupil reacts briskly to accommodation and consensual light reaction, but slowly to the direct light reaction because the afferent light pathway has been interrupted by the damage to the optic nerve. Conditions which may be associated with papilloedema are:

1. Intracranial tumours. Papilloedema is usually more severe with tumours arising in the posterior fossa.
2. Malignant hypertension. This probably causes papilloedema by raising the intracranial pressure, although local spasm of arterioles may lead to local ischaemia and oedema and thickened arteries may press on veins, causing venous congestion.

3. Venous obstruction affecting the central vein of the retina. Causes include: orbital neoplasms, cavernous sinus thrombosis, superior vena cava obstruction and thrombosis of the central retinal vein.
4. Unusual causes, such as severe anaemia, polycythaemia and raised blood CO_2.

Once primary optic atrophy has occurred, the changes are permanent, so that, should raised intracranial pressure arise later, papilloedema will not occur. In a tumour of a frontal lobe which presses on one optic nerve, optic atrophy occurs on that side; later as the tumour grows, the intracranial pressure rises, leading to papilloedema in the opposite eye—this is known as the Foster Kennedy syndrome.

Thrombosis of the central artery of the retina results in extreme pallor of the retina, with narrowing of the retinal arteries and a "cherry-red" spot at the macula. There is, of course, sudden complete blindness. Thrombosis of the central vein of the retina results in papilloedema and oedema of the rest of the retina with grossly congested veins and numerous haemorrhages. Unlike papilloedema the condition is usually unilateral, the retinal oedema extends to the periphery of the retina and visual acuity is affected. In papilloedema visual acuity usually remains normal until the late stages. Following retinal vein thrombosis anastomotic vessels may develop or the retinal appearances may return to normal. Vision may be severely affected even though the retinal appearances have returned to normal.

Following subarachnoid haemorrhage, a subhyaloid haemorrhage may be seen in the eye, situated between the retina and the vitreous humour. In this position it takes up the shape of the eye and has a curved lower margin, its upper border is horizontal. The exact cause is not known, as the subarachnoid space is not in continuity with the subhyaloid space in the eye; it may result from a sudden increase in venous pressure in the central retinal vein due to a sudden outpouring of blood into the subarachnoid space.

The appearances of choroiditis are of white, opaque areas of any size, surrounded by a black, pigmented margin. The retinal vessels are always seen superficial to an area of choroiditis. In glaucoma, the increased intra-ocular pressure causes an increase in size of the optic cup which is the weakest part of the sclera. The cup may become so large that its base is wider than its apex, so that it shelves under the emerging fibres of the optic nerve. Continued pressure may lead to atrophy of the nerve fibres and a pale disc. If a small vessel is followed from the retina onto the disc it suddenly disappears as it enters the optic cup, whose walls are sloping outwards towards its base. The small vessel will reappear again as it crosses the floor of the optic cup to enter the lamina cribrosa.

At the optic disc, two physiological conditions may cause confusion. The first is the myopic crescent which occurs in severe myopia; it merely consists of an opaque crescent lying against one margin of the disc; the other is opaque medullated nerve fibres which radiate out from the disc; these are white and may simulate optic atrophy.

The walls of the retinal arteries are normally not visible. All that is seen is the column of blood within the artery and the reflection of light from the curved surface of the artery. Normally this light reflex is of constant thickness along the length of the vessel; when atheromatous plaques are deposited on the intima, the visible column of blood appears indented, and, therefore, the artery appears to have increased in tortuosity. Deposition of atheroma in the intima of the arteries leads to a small lumen and a thinner column of blood which appears as arterial narrowing. The thickening and infiltration of the wall of the artery with atheroma leads to the wall becoming white and visible, the artery will now appear as a column of blood on either side of which is a white margin. This is known as "silver wiring". Because the arterial wall is thickened and irregular, the light reflex will vary in thickness and appear interrupted. At the stage of silver wiring, veins will be compressed by the thickened arterial wall, leading to the appearance of arteriovenous nipping. All the changes mentioned may be seen in severe atheroma in the absence of hypertension. However, in the presence of long-standing hypertension, the same changes may be seen—they are due to atheroma which has been accelerated by the hypertension. Hypertension alone will produce a change in the retinal arteries: this consists of irregular spasm of the arteries, and consequently an irregularity of the light reflex in narrowed arteries. The retinal artery appearances of hypertension may, of course, be superimposed on those due to accelerated atheroma.

Accelerated hypertension may go on to produce haemorrhages and "soft" exudates—these are poorly demarcated and are probably caused by resolving small retinal infarcts as a result of the arterial narrowing. "Hard" exudates have a well-defined border and are due to degeneration of part of the retina. They are also seen in hypertension but are more common in diabetes. In malignant hypertension there is always papilloedema. These changes in the retinal arteries and retina form the basis for a graded classification of the severity of the retinal changes in hypertension.

Grade I Indicates mild changes in the retinal arteries.
Grade II Indicates arteriovenous nipping.
Grade III Indicates haemorrhages and exudates.
Grade IV Indicates papilloedema.

From the previous discussion it will be seen that Grades I and II may indicate atheroma and not always hypertension. For this reason it is probably better to qualify the grades by a description of the changes in the retinal arteries.

Movements of the Eye

Voluntary eye movements in all directions are controlled bilaterally by centres in the frontal cortices. In the midbrain, there are the nuclei for oculomotor and trochlear nerves and nuclei dealing with conjugate deviation of the eyes upwards and downwards. In the pons, there is the nucleus of the sixth nerve and a centre dealing with lateral conjugate deviation. All the nuclei are interconnected by the medial longitudinal bundle.

The abducens nerve (VI) supplies the lateral rectus, the trochlear (IV) supplies the superior oblique and the oculomotor nerve (III) supplies the remainder of the ocular muscles. The lateral and medial recti move the eye outwards and inwards, the superior and inferior recti elevate and depress the eyes when they are turned outwards, and the superior and inferior obliques depress and elevate respectively when the eye is turned inwards.

The third nerve emerges from the midbrain close to the cerebral peduncles, passes between the posterior cerebral and superior cerebellar arteries and then passes through the cavernous sinus where it is very close to the fourth and sixth nerves and the ophthalmic division of the fifth nerve.

The third nerve also supplies the levator palpebrae superioris and the constrictor muscle of the pupils. If the nerve is paralysed there is ptosis due to drooping of the levator palpebrae superioris, a dilated pupil due to the unopposed action of the sympathetic impulses, and paralysis of all eye muscles except the lateral rectus and superior oblique. Thus, the eye is rotated outwards (by the lateral rectus) and downwards (by the superior oblique).

The fourth nerve arises from the dorsum of the midbrain, passes between the posterior cerebral and superior cerebellar arteries and enters the cavernous sinus.

The sixth nerve arises from the pons and its nucleus is very close to that of the seventh nerve. It has a very long intracranial course before entering the cavernous sinus. It passes with the seventh nerve through the cerebellopontine angle over the petrous bone where it lies close to the fifth nerve. Because of their long intracranial courses, the third, fourth and sixth nerves are subject to a large number of lesions, some of which are common to them all. The three nerves have their origins in the brain stem; midbrain lesions will affect the third and fourth, while pontine lesions will affect the sixth. Within the brain stem, they are subject to vascular lesions, neoplasms, encephalitis and disseminated sclerosis.

They all lie on the meninges and are therefore prone to damage in meningitis, syphilis, meningioma and carcinoma of the meninges.

They have a common pathway in the cavernous sinus and through the superior orbital fissure, and can be damaged in:

Cavernous sinus thrombosis
Aneurysm of the internal carotid artery
Lesions within the orbit.

Like all nerves they may be victims to polyneuritis and myasthenia gravis.

The third nerve passes near the posterior cerebral and posterior communicating arteries, and may be pressed by aneurysms of these arteries. It may also be damaged by a raised intracranial pressure: the nerve is fixed where it pierces the dura to enter the cavernous sinus, but the brain stem may be pushed downwards by cerebral tumours towards the foramen magnum, causing excessive stretching of the nerve. The same applies to the sixth nerve, but the fourth nerve is not usually affected. The only lesion which usually damages the fourth nerve alone is an aneurysm of the posterior cerebral artery. The sixth nerve is more vulnerable than the third to a rise in intracranial pressure and may be damaged by the transient rise of intracranial pressure that occurs following a subarachnoid haemorrhage.

The sixth nerve crosses the cerebellopontine angle, where it may be involved in an acoustic neuroma (in which the eighth, seventh and fifth nerves may also be affected). As the nerve passes forwards, it crosses the apex of the petrous temporal bone, and lies near the fifth nerve: in this situation it may be involved in periostitis of the petrous temporal bone which results from otitis media, usually in childhood. The combination of sixth nerve palsy with pain in the distribution of the trigeminal nerve is known as Gradenigo's[15] syndrome.

The main symptom from any ocular palsy is diplopia, and the main signs are strabismus (or squint) and inability to move the eyes in certain directions. The eyes should be tested one at a time by moving the finger in all directions to see in which directions the eye will not move. There are three basic rules with regard to the assessment of diplopias:

1. Diplopia is present when the eye is moving in the direction of the paralysed muscle.
2. Diplopia is maximal when the eye is looking in the direction of pull of the paralysed muscle.
3. The most peripheral image of the two is from the eye with the weak muscle so that covering one eye at a time will distinguish which eye has the weak muscle.

Strabismus

Some conditions cause deviation in the direction of the optical axis of each eye which remains constant irrespective of which direction the eyes are looking: this is known as concomitant strabismus. It occurs if there is slight asymmetry of strength of corresponding muscles of each eye—it is a common occurrence in children and often follows an attack of measles. A paralytic or divergent strabismus is a squint due to paralysis of ocular muscles and it will only be present when an attempt is made to move the eye in the direction of the paralysed muscles; in other positions the optical axes of both eyes will be parallel.

In a concomitant strabismus, the range of movements of each eye is normal, and the deviation in the direction in which both eyes are looking is constant in all positions; furthermore, it is present at rest. In a paralytic strabismus the squint is not usually present at rest and is worse on looking in the direction of pull of the paralysed muscle. A fundamental difference between paralytic and concomitant strabismus is that there is no diplopia in a concomitant strabismus because the image from one eye is suppressed. It is usually found that one eye has a severe refractive error and the image from this eye is the one that is usually suppressed, although the eye can be used if the other is covered.

The centres concerned with voluntary conjugate movement of the eyes are situated in the frontal lobes; however, in addition, there are, in the brain stem, the centres concerned with involuntary conjugate movements: the centres in the brain stem are near the nuclei of the corresponding cranial nerves. It is possible to have lesions between the voluntary centre and the reflex centres for conjugate movements. Such lesions will abolish conjugate eye movements when the patient is asked to look in a particular direction or to follow a moving finger; however, conjugate movements will be intact if the patient is asked to look at a fixed object and his head is slowly rotated. The lesions responsible for such supranuclear ocular palsies are always bilateral.

The Pupils

The constrictor pupillary muscle is controlled by parasympathetic fibres, travelling via the third nerve and ciliary ganglion. The dilator pupillary muscle is supplied by fibres from the cervical sympathetic chain, the fibres travelling both via ciliary ganglion and via the ophthalmic division of the trigeminal nerve. The pupillary light reflex is stimulated by afferents travelling in the optic nerve to the lateral geniculate body and thence to the bilateral nuclei in the midbrain concerned with pupillary constriction: this nucleus lies very close to that of the third nerve, through which the motor side of the reflex is mediated.

The reaction to accommodation is complex: it involves convergence of the eyes, using both medial recti, contraction of ciliary muscle rendering the lens of the eye more globular and constriction of the pupils. The afferent side of the reflex probably arises from the frontal cortex; the motor side is mediated by the third nerve; however, there is some evidence that the fibres concerned with the accommodation reaction do not pass through the ciliary ganglion, unlike those concerned with the pupillary light reflex.

The essential features of the Argyll Robertson[16] pupil is that it reacts to accommodation but not to light. The most likely position for a lesion which interferes with the light but not the accommodation reflex is in the ciliary ganglion because it is believed that the fibres of the oculomotor nerve carrying accommodation reflex impulses do not pass through the ganglion. The other possible position for such a lesion is in the midbrain near the aqueduct where the light-reflex fibres decussate on their way to the third nerve nuclei of the two sides. Other features of the Argyll Robertson pupil are that it is irregular, that it is contracted and that there is depigmentation of the iris. The fact that contraction is a cardinal feature of the Argyll Robertson pupil means that the lesion does not only involve the oculomotor nerve fibres, otherwise the pupil would be dilated. This suggests that the sympathetic innervation is also impaired, which is added evidence for the lesion being in the ciliary ganglion, because some sympathetic pupillary fibres travel to the eye via the ciliary ganglion. The Argyll Robertson pupil occurs with conditions other than syphilis, including diabetes, postencephalitic Parkinsonism and polyneuritis, as well as vascular and neoplastic lesions involving the midbrain.

The Holmes[17]-Adie[18] pupil is quite distinct from the Argyll Robertson pupil. It is larger than normal, does not react to light, but may react to accommodation very slowly. The condition is virtually always unilateral, confined to women and associated with diminished tendon jerks.

Ptosis

The upper lid is elevated by the levator palpebrae superioris, which is supplied by the sympathetic and by the third nerve. The sympathetic supply is mainly responsible for maintaining the tone of the muscle at rest; if the sympathetic supply is interrupted but the third nerve is intact, the upper lid will appear ptosed at rest, but can be raised normally when the patient is asked to look upwards: this is the situation in Horner's syndrome. In ptosis due to paralysis of the third nerve, the levator palpebrae superioris is paralysed and the upper lid can only be raised by overaction of the frontalis muscle which is seen as excessive wrinkling of the forehead. Despite the overaction of the frontalis, the upper lid cannot be raised as much as normally when the patient looks upwards.

The important causes of ptosis are:

> *Horner's syndrome* due to interruption of the sympathetic system anywhere from the upper thorax to the ciliary ganglion. The main conditions causing this are enlarged cervical lymph glands, syringobulbia and syringomyelia, and vascular lesions of the medulla.
>
> *Tabes dorsalis* and lesions of the third nerve.
>
> *Mild bilateral congenital ptosis.*
>
> *Hysteria*, in which case the ptosis is always unilateral.

Trigeminal Nerve

The motor and sensory divisions arise from nuclei in the pons. When the sensory division enters the brain stem the fibres subserving pain and temperature descend on the same side to the level of the third cervical segment, cross the midline and ascend in the lateral spinothalamic tract. The fibres of this descending tract which reach the lowest level are those derived from the upper part of the face. This explains why syringomyelia which affects the middle of the cervical cord may cause loss of pain and temperature of the upper part of the face. The sensory fibres of the trigeminal nerve carrying touch and proprioceptive impulses cross the midline as soon as they enter the brain stem and ascend to the thalamus and cerebral cortex by way of the medial lemniscus.

The sensory and motor roots leave the pons and cross the cerebello-pontine angle; the sensory root relays in a large ganglion which lies near the sixth nerve at the apex of the petrous temporal bone, where it may be involved in spread of infection from otitis media. From this ganglion the ophthalmic division travels in the cavernous sinus with the three ophthalmic nerves; hence, any lesion within the cavernous sinus (internal carotid artery aneurysm or thrombosis of the cavernous sinus) generally involves the three ophthalmic nerves and the ophthalmic division of the fifth nerve.

The ophthalmic division conveys sensation from the cornea and remainder of the eye; it is the afferent part of the corneal reflex, the motor part being the facial nerve which innervates the orbicularis oculi. Stimulation of the cornea of one eye results in bilateral contraction of the orbicularis oculi, so that even in the presence of a lower motor neurone facial nerve weakness on one side the corneal reflex can still be tested. Loss of the corneal reflex is an early sign of a tumour in the cerebellopontine angle.

The ophthalmic division of the trigeminal nerve is more frequently affected by herpes zoster than the other two sensory branches. Involvement of the ophthalmic division may lead to anaesthesia of the cornea and subsequent ulceration, keratitis and blindness. The fifth nerve supplies sensation to the whole of the face, pharynx and nose except for taste sensation. Taste sensation from the anterior two-thirds of the tongue is carried for a short distance in the lingual nerve which is a branch of the mandibular division of the fifth nerve; taste fibres then leave the lingual nerve to join the chorda tympani of the facial nerve in the facial canal. Thus, a peripheral lesion of the mandibular nerve may affect taste over the anterior two-thirds of the tongue, although such lesions are very rare.

Because of the extensive distribution of branches of the trigeminal nerve, pain may be referred to an area remote from its origin. The most important examples of this clinically are pain in the ear and temples in the case of an apical tooth abscess or carcinoma of the maxillary antrum. Pain from the eye (as in glaucoma) may be referred to the temples or to the dura mater (causing severe headache). The exclusion of referred pain is important in the diagnosis of trigeminal neuralgia. The drug carbamazepine (Tegretol) has considerably improved the treatment of trigeminal neuralgia; it does not relieve referred pain. The motor branch of the fifth nerve supplies the muscles of mastication.

Seventh Nerve

The facial nerve is purely motor, its nucleus is situated in the pons and as the nerve emerges from the brain stem it is closely associated with the nucleus of the sixth nerve. It crosses the cerebellopontine angle, passes into the internal auditory meatus and then into its own bony canal. In the bony canal it gives off a branch to the stapedius muscle, then forms the geniculate ganglion which receives taste fibres via the chorda tympani from the anterior two-thirds of the tongue. The facial nerve emerges from the skull via the stylomastoid foramen and is then distributed to the facial muscles which include the platysma of the neck.

Lower motor neurone lesions beyond the nucleus of the facial nerve cause complete paralysis of all the facial muscles on one side. The nucleus of the facial nerve in the pons receives two sets of upper motor neurone fibres which run together; one set derived only from the opposite cerebral cortex is concerned with movements of the lower facial muscles and the other set derived from both cerebral cortices is concerned with movements of the upper facial muscles. Thus, an upper motor neurone lesion of the facial nerve will cause total paralysis of the lower facial muscles, but the upper facial muscles can still be moved because the part of the facial nucleus on each side concerned with the upper facial muscles is supplied by both cerebral cortices. An internal capsular lesion which causes a facial weakness will only affect the lower face on one side whereas a Bell's palsy will affect the whole of the face on one side. The principal sites of damage to the facial nerve are:

1. *Pons.*—Lesions here will be associated with a lateral rectus palsy, damage to the fifth nerve (both descending and immediately decussating parts), spinothalamic tract and pyramids (before they have decussated).

2. *Cerebellopontine angle.*—The commonest tumour is an acoustic neuroma. If the facial nerve is damaged in this situation there will be loss of taste over the anterior two-thirds of the tongue and hyperacusis because the nerve to the stapedius muscle will be paralysed. In the cerebellopontine angle the fifth, sixth and eighth nerves are also affected.

3. *The facial canal.*—The nerves will be affected by suppuration from the middle ear; taste from the anterior two-thirds of the tongue will be lost.

4. *In the face.*—Here the commonest lesion is Bell's[19] palsy, although it may also be affected in neoplasms of the parotid gland.

Although loss of taste and hyperacusis are unusual in a Bell's palsy they do sometimes occur, indicating that the lesion is sometimes within the facial canal. The cause of the condition is not known. There are several controlled trials which show that prednisolone given soon after the onset of Bell's palsy accelerates recovery, which is also more complete than in untreated cases. It is worth giving corticosteroid therapy up to 7 days after the onset of palsy. The usual dose regimen is prednisolone 80 mg daily for 5 days followed by 60, 40, 20, 10 mg for one day each.

As a rule if there is some *recovery* of voluntary function after one week, full functional recovery of the nerve will occur. Ideally the management of cases of Bell's palsy should include nerve excitability tests; these are extremely simple to perform and involve no discomfort for the patient. Small electric currents are passed via electrodes applied to the skin over the stylomastoid foramen, the lowest current which stimulates the facial nerve, producing a twitch of the corner of the mouth, is recorded. Nerve excitability tests should be done 7, 14 and 21 days after the facial palsy has developed; by 14 days electrical recovery should have started (i.e. the current needed to excite the nerve should be less than on day 7). If recovery has not started by day 21 decompression of the facial nerve *may* be indicated although the results of decompression are difficult to evaluate.

EIGHTH NERVE

The cochlear portion of the nerve is concerned with hearing and the vestibular part with balance and position sense. Both parts arise from the pons, cross the cerebellopontine angle close to the seventh, fifth and sixth nerves, enter the internal auditory meatus and terminate in the cochlear and vestibular apparatus in the inner ear. In the pons the cochlear fibres pass up both lateral lemnisci to the temporal cortices. Whereas vestibular fibres join the medial longitudinal bundle which co-ordinates the nuclei of the cranial nerves concerned with movements of the face and eyes, some vestibular fibres terminate in the cerebral cortex, and these are concerned with the appreciation of vertigo.

Deafness

Deafness is caused by lesions of the middle ear, cochlea, auditory nerve or its central connections. Damage to the middle ear leads to conduction deafness; this can be distinguished from nerve deafness by Weber's[20] and Rinne's[21] tests: bone conduction of sounds is better than air conduction if there is middle ear disease, i.e. a conduction deafness.

The important causes of middle-ear deafness are otitis media and otosclerosis; the important causes of cochlear destruction are mumps, Menière's[22] disease and idiosyncrasy or overdose of quinine, salicylates and streptomycin; the important causes of auditory nerve deafness are acoustic neuroma, Paget's disease and meningitis (usually syphilitic). Cochlear deafness can be distinguished from nerve deafness in audiometric tests by the fact that in cochlear deafness once a sound can be heard at all it appears louder than it should (loudness recruitment).

Nystagmus

Nystagmus generally consists of two phases, one rapid and the other slow. There are three groups of causes of nystagmus each of which has distinguishing features. They are:

1. Lesions of the eye in which the nystagmus is associated with defective vision and consists of two phases which are equal in speed.
2. Lesions of the vestibular system (labyrinth and vestibular nerve). These are usually accompanied by damage to the auditory apparatus or auditory branch of the eighth nerve, with frequently coexisting

deafness and tinnitus. Vestibular nystagmus is always accompanied by vertigo and usually lasts only a few weeks because central compensation occurs.

The direction in which nystagmus is greatest is sometimes helpful in establishing its cause. The simple rule is that in vestibular nystagmus the slow phase is towards the diseased side and the excursions are greatest when looking in the direction of the quick phase. This means that vestibular nystagmus is constant in the direction of its slow and fast phases and is maximal in its excursion when the patient is looking *away* from the affected labyrinth or nerve. The commonest causes of vestibular nystagmus are Menière's disease and middle ear infections.

3. Central lesions (usually brain stem and cerebellum). There is usually no vertigo, deafness or tinnitus, unlike vestibular nystagmus. The slow phase is always directed to the rest position of the eyes so that the direction of the slow and fast phases changes with full excursion of the eyes. The commonest causes of central nystagmus are disseminated sclerosis, cerebellar lesions, hereditary ataxias and syringomyelia.

Other points of useful significance in elucidating nystagmus are:

1. Peripheral causes of nystagmus (which include lesions of the vestibular apparatus and acoustic nerve) produce nystagmus which does not usually persist more than a few weeks. Prolonged testing for nystagmus itself may lead to a reduction in the nystagmus.

2. Fixation of the eye ahead abolishes peripheral nystagmus but may enhance central nystagmus.

3. Peripheral nystagmus of labyrinthine origin is usually worse in particular positions of the head (but this may also occur with nystagmus due to disorders of the vestibular nuclei in the brain stem).

4. Nystagmus may occur with incomplete movement of one eye; in the case of ocular muscle weakness the nystagmus is greater in the affected eye; in the case of "ataxic" nystagmus due to brain-stem pathology (usually MS or Wernicke's encephalopathy) the nystagmus is greater in the abducting eye.

5. The direction of the fast and slow components of the nystagmus may change, this always indicates a central brain-stem lesion.

6. The amplitude of the nystagmus may also vary with the direction of gaze; nystagmus which is pronounced on looking in one direction is usually due to a cerebellar cause, provided ataxic nystagmus and ocular muscle weakness have been excluded.

Caloric tests are of limited value in elucidating the cause of nystagmus and vertigo. The principle on which they are based is simple but their interpretation is often difficult. The principle is that when hot and then cold water is run into one ear each induces nystagmus in opposite directions; normally the nystagmus lasts for about two minutes. In diseases of the vestibular apparatus or vestibular nerve (e.g. Menière's disease or acoustic neuroma) the nystagmus in both directions from the affected ear is shorter than normal (canal paresis). In disease of the central connections the nystagmus in one direction from stimulation of both ears (hot in one and cold in the other) is increased (directional preponderance).

Ninth Nerve (Glossopharyngeal)

This supplies the muscles of the pharynx, taste from the posterior third of the tongue and sensation from the inside of the mouth.

Tenth Nerve (Vagus)

The motor branch supplies the soft palate in addition to the muscles of the pharynx and larynx.

Eleventh Nerve (Accessory)

This is entirely motor and is joined by a branch from the upper cervical spine; together they supply the trapezius and sternomastoid muscles.

Twelfth Nerve (Hypoglossal)

This is the motor nerve of the tongue. A lower motor neurone lesion causes atrophy of one-half of the tongue—this is a very dramatic physical sign, it occurs within days and is always severe and unmistakable; the tongue deviates from the weak side as it lies in the mouth but protrudes from the mouth *towards* the weak side. In bulbar palsy there is bilateral wasting of the tongue; in pseudobulbar palsy the tongue is not wasted but it can only be protruded with difficulty because it is stiff and spastic (in keeping with the fact that pseudobulbar palsy is due to bilateral upper motor neurone lesions).

The ninth, tenth, eleventh and twelfth cranial nerves are usually involved together in lesions within the posterior fossa (syndrome of the jugular foramen).

Raised Intracranial Pressure

The cerebrospinal fluid is produced by the choroid plexuses of the lateral ventricles deep in the cerebral hemispheres; it passes to the third ventricle of the midbrain, through the narrow aqueduct into the fourth ventricle of the medulla (Fig. 28). Note that so far the fluid has been *inside* the substance of the brain and brain stem. It leaves the fourth ventricle by three holes, the two foramina of Luschka[23] laterally and the median foramen of Magendie,[24] and for the first time the fluid finds itself in the subarachnoid space surrounding brain and spinal cord. The fluid is absorbed by the arachnoid granulations on the surface of the brain.

A point often overlooked is that wherever the obstruction to flow of the CSF occurs there is *always* enlargement of the ventricular system of the brain and it is the increased pressure in the ventricular system which causes enlargement of the cerebral hemispheres. It is this enlargement of the cerebral hemispheres which gives rise to the increased pressure in the subarachnoid space. Another factor which contributes to the later increase in pressure of CSF is that a small rise in intracranial pressure causes obstruction of the venous drainage of the arachnoid granulations, leading to decreased absorption of CSF. A cerebral tumour causes back-pressure dilatation of the ventricular system by pushing the cerebral hemispheres downward and blocking the hole between the free edges of the tentorium. Meningitis causes enlargement of the ventricular system by obstructing the flow in the subarachnoid space over the surface of the cerebral hemispheres.

Classification of hydrocephalus into communicating and obstructive is of no value clinically because the pathogenesis of the increased pressure in both cases is the same, namely, increase in size of the ventricular system causing swelling of the cerebral hemispheres. Obstructive hydrocephalus refers to obstruction to the flow of CSF before it has left the ventricular system—it will occur in ependymomas of the third ventricle, pineal and midbrain tumours, congenital stenosis of the aqueduct between third and fourth ventricles, and obstruction to outflow from the fourth ventricle such as may occur in the Arnold-Chiari malformation or basilar impression. Communicating hydrocephalus refers only to the fact that there is free communication between the ventricular system and subarachnoid space; in the case of a communicating hydrocephalus the block is within the subarachnoid space, usually at the hiatus of the tentorium. Raised intracranial pressure develops much more quickly with tumours in the posterior fossa than in other sites because they readily obstruct the openings in the roof of the fourth ventricle.

The clinical features of raised intracranial pressure are:

Papilloedema due to obstruction of retinal veins
Headache, vomiting and epilepsy
Mental changes
Pressure-cone features and false localising signs.

There are two positions where the brain and brain stem can attempt to expand if there is a rise in intracranial pressure. The midbrain passes between the two free edges of the tentorium; increased pressure above the tentorium, as in cerebral tumours, will force part of the temporal lobes through the hiatus compressing any structures in contact with the tentorium—these are the midbrain, the cerebral peduncles, the third and sixth nerves and the posterior cerebral arteries. The features of a tentorial pressure cone are therefore:

> Contralateral hemiplegia due to pressure on the cerebral peduncle on the side of the tumour. Occasionally the brain is displaced laterally, compressing the opposite cerebral peduncle, in which case the hemiplegia is on the side of the lesion—hence the description "false localising sign".
> Ipsilateral third nerve palsy leading to a fixed dilated pupil.
> Ipsilateral lateral rectus palsy (sixth nerve).
> Occlusion of one posterior cerebral artery leading to homonymous hemianopia.
> Midbrain infarction.

If the increased pressure occurs in the posterior fossa, part of the cerebellum is forced through the foramen magnum and the medulla will be compressed at its anterior and posterior parts as well as being pushed downwards. This is the foramen magnum pressure cone. It leads to:

> Compression of the nuclei of the posterior columns, leading to loss of proprioception.
> Compression of pyramidal tracts anteriorly.
> Acute angulation of the lower cranial nerves, leading to a bulbar palsy. The nerves are fixed by the foramina through which they emerge from the skull, hence, if the medulla is pushed downwards the nerves will be unduly stretched.
> Severe pain in the occipital region and the neck.
> Occasionally, cerebellar signs.

The same clinical features as in the foramen magnum pressure cone may be seen in abnormalities of the base of the skull. The most important of these are:

> Arnold[25]-Chiari[26] malformation, in which herniation through the foramen magnum occurs as a congenital anomaly. The condition may present as hydrocephalus if the outflow of the CSF from the fourth ventricle is obstructed. The condition is often associated with syringomyelia and meningocele.
> Congenital fusion of cervical vertebrae (Klippel[27]-Feil[28] deformity).

Basilar impression and platybasia in which the upper cervical spine is invaginated into the base of the skull. It may occur as a congenital anomaly or be due to bone disease such as Paget's disease or osteomalacia.

Benign intracranial hypertension.—This is a rare condition in which the intracranial pressure is raised in the absence of a tumour but the ventricles are often normal in size. Papilloedema and a sixth-nerve palsy may occur; the condition is usually self limiting but the papilloedema may damage vision permanently. The exact cause of the raised intracranial pressure is not known but it is commonly associated with certain conditions:

Sudden reduction or increase in corticosteroid dosage
Addison's disease
Hypoparathyroidism
Pregnancy, obesity and the menarche
Previous head injury
Chlortetracycline administration
Sagittal sinus thrombosis (otitic hydrocephalus)
Anaemia
Polycythaemia
Nalidixic acid administration
Ingestion of oral contraceptives.

Normal Pressure Hydrocephalus

Another relatively common condition is normal-pressure hydrocephalus, in which there is enlargement of the ventricles associated with cerebral atrophy and neuropsychiatric manifestations, particularly unsteadiness of gait and urinary incontinence, but in which the CSF pressure is normal. It is believed that the flow of CSF from the ventricles is disturbed possibly by arachnoid adhesions over the surface of the brain, preventing absorption of CSF by the arachnoid granulations in the superior longitudinal sinus. Adhesions may follow previous meningitis or subarachnoid haemorrhage.

Blood Supply of the Brain and Spinal Cord

Figure 31 shows the principal arteries supplying the brain. The basilar artery runs on the undersurface of the brain stem, supplying branches to the medulla and pons. The midbrain is supplied by the posterior cerebral arteries. Occlusion of one of the vessels feeding the circle of Willis may give rise to symptoms even though the remainder of the circle is patent. The converse is also true, namely that ischaemic symptoms may not be present even if there is total occlusion of one, two or even three of the main vessels feeding the circle of Willis. It is important to remember that all the cerebral arteries leaving the circle are end-arteries and there is no collateral circulation.

The middle cerebral artery is more or less a continuation of the internal carotid artery, hence occlusion of the internal carotid will usually cause the features of middle cerebral artery occlusion. However, an aneurysm of the internal carotid may involve the optic chiasma or optic tracts, leading to a nasal or homonymous hemianopia respectively; or an aneurysm of the internal carotid may occur in the cavernous sinus leading to damage to the third, fourth, sixth or ophthalmic division of the fifth nerve. Obstruction of the internal carotid may involve a small branch of the artery before it joins the circle of Willis; this is the anterior choroidal artery which supplies part of the optic radiation near the internal capsule, leading to a homonymous congruous scotoma or hemianopia.

As it leaves the midbrain the third nerve lies close to the posterior cerebral and posterior communicating arteries so that an aneurysm on either may lead to an isolated third-nerve palsy. The posterior cerebral artery supplies the occipital visual cortex, so that complete occlusion causes a complete homonymous hemianopia, but the macula is spared. However, small branches of the posterior cerebral supply the lower part of the optic radiation (which contains fibres from the lower part of the retinae), hence partial occlusion or a transient fall in blood flow in the posterior cerebral will cause an upper homonymous quadrantanopia. This explains why patients with vertebrobasilar insufficiency may complain of a defect of vision which is "like a curtain coming down".

The upper part of the optic radiation is supplied by the middle cerebral artery, hence ischaemia due to narrowing of the middle cerebral (or internal carotid) may cause a field defect in the lower part of the visual fields.

Aneurysms on the anterior cerebral or anterior communicating artery may compress the optic nerves, leading to optic atrophy, or they may compress the frontal lobes, leading to frontal lobe symptoms.

Subarachnoid Haemorrhage

Oculomotor palsies are the commonest single manifestation of unruptured aneurysms. The pupillary fibres within the oculomotor nerve are superficially situated and are usually affected before the remainder of the nerve, so that dilatation of one pupil usually precedes ptosis and complete oculomotor palsy. Less commonly the aneurysm is on the internal carotid artery. These are usually classified as supraclinoid of infraclinoid but it is more convenient to think of them in terms of whether they are:

Within the cavernous sinus (infraclinoid) where they may compress other structures, e.g. III, IV, V and VI nerves (dilated pupil, facial pain, variable loss of facial sensation).

Above the cavernous sinus (supraclinoid) where they most frequently compress the oculomotor nerve, optic tracts and chiasm, and may extend into the frontal lobes.

Aneurysms arising from the bifurcation of the basilar artery and posterior cerebral artery are likely to compress the cerebral peduncles, oculomotor nerve, the hypothalamus and aqueduct of the IVth ventricle, causing internal hydrocephalus and dementia. They may extend into the temporal lobe causing hemianopia and temporal lobe features. Aneurysms of the basilar and cerebellar arteries are likely to cause brain stem compression and features of an acoustic neuroma. Aneurysms of the middle cerebral artery are liable to involve the cerebral peduncle and internal capsule, leading to hemianopia, hemianaesthesia and hemiplegia.

The commonest cause of blood in the subarachnoid space is rupture of any aneurysm of one of the cerebral arteries; however, blood may occur in the CSF in a number of other conditions which it is important to recognise. Bleeding may not necessarily be arterial, and in severe encephalitis capillaries may be damaged and lead to oozing of blood into the CSF; severe meningitis and pyaemias may cause venous damage and venous bleeding. Other causes of blood in the CSF include:

Intracerebral haemorrhage
Bleeding into cerebral tumours
Haemorrhagic diathesis (including anticoagulants)
Bleeding from angiomas
Bleeding from arteriovenous malformations.

Arterial aneurysms always occur at the junction of two blood vessels, and are probably due to congenital weakness of the wall of the blood vessels which becomes critical when associated hypertensive or arteriosclerotic changes are present. At least two-thirds of ruptured aneurysms occur in women and half these are hypertensive. Anterior and middle cerebral aneurysms are considerably more common than posterior cerebral or posterior communicating aneurysms.

The diagnosis of a ruptured cerebral aneurysm is confirmed by finding blood in the CSF, but one very important practical point is that lumbar puncture should be delayed at least six hours after the ictus as it may take this time for blood to pass down into the spinal subarachnoid space; occasionally, it takes very much longer.

The mortality from rupture of a cerebral aneurysm is about 50 per cent. About one-third of those that die will do so within 48 hours from the effects of the first haemorrhage. Of the other two-thirds that die, most will succumb within six weeks from a second bleed—the greatest risk is in the second week after the first bleed. Of the patients who survive, one-fifth will have severe neurological damage. Broken down, the approximate percentages are:

	Per cent
Survival without severe impairment	40
Survival but with severe impairment	10
Die within 48 hours	15
Die within 6 weeks having survived 48 hours	25
Die after 6 weeks	10

Management of Subarachnoid Haemorrhage

Patients who are comatose are managed conservatively once the diagnosis has been made, but virtually all will die. This somewhat nihilistic view is accepted by the majority of neurosurgeons and it may be the only practical policy; however, some neurosurgeons believe that early cerebral angiography is indicated in younger patients in case the intracerebral haematoma is readily accessible and removable. Patients who do not have evidence of severe neurological damage or severe coincidental disease should have bilateral carotid and vertebral angiography as soon as practicable. If no aneurysm is found the prognosis is considerably better.

In a few patients repeat angiography after all cerebral artery spasm has subsided may reveal an aneurysm which was not apparent on the earlier angiogram.

Microsurgical techniques have improved the results of operations on cerebral aneurysms although the mortality is still high in patients who are operated on early and in those who are comatose. Medical management of ruptured cerebral aneurysm includes:

Absolute bed rest
Hypotensive therapy
Anticonvulsant therapy
Reduction of raised intracranial pressure using steroids
Repeated lumbar punctures to remove blood and vasoactive factors
Antifibrinolytic therapy to encourage clot formation around aneurysms, using aminocaproic acid (Epsikapron).

Subarachnoid haemorrhage due to leakage of blood directly into the spinal subarachnoid space is almost invariably due to an angioma. At the time of the bleed the patient has severe pain in the back which comes on so suddenly that it feels as if he has just been kicked in the back.

Thrombosis in the venous sinuses of the brain is rare, but when it occurs it is usually as a result of sepsis or trauma. Thrombosis in the cavernous sinus will cause damage to the third, fourth and sixth nerves and the ophthalmic division of the fifth nerve, as well as exophthalmos and papilloedema due to congestion of the veins behind the eye. The other important sinus which may be affected is the sagittal sinus which runs anteroposteriorly in the midline. It runs over the frontal and parietal lobes of both cerebral cortices in the top of the falx cerebri. Thrombosis of the sagittal sinus will cause damage to the top of both cerebral cortices and, therefore, produce loss of sensation and movement in the legs—crural dominance. Other conditions which cause crural dominance are thrombosis of the anterior cerebral arteries, parasagittal meningioma or subdural haematoma.

Blood Supply of the Spinal Cord

The anterior spinal artery (Fig. 31) arises from both vertebral arteries at the level of the medulla, passes down the anterior border of the spinal cord, and sends branches to the lower medulla; occlusion of the anterior spinal artery at its origin will give rise to the medial medullary syndrome (involvement of corticospinal tracts, medial lemniscus and hypoglossal nerve). There are two small posterior spinal arteries which also arise from the vertebral arteries. The spinal arteries receive additional blood from the segmental arteries, although the extent to which segmental arteries contribute to the arterial supply of the cord varies. There are two very important and fairly constant segmental arteries: one arises from the costocervical trunk and enters the lower cervical cord and the other arises from one of the lower thoracic or upper lumbar segmental arteries usually on the left side and is known as the artery of Adamkiewicz.[29] It is believed that blood from the artery entering the lower cervical region flows mainly downwards and that the cervical cord above this region is supplied either by the anterior spinal or segmental arteries. Blood entering via the artery of Adamkiewicz flows both up and down the cord. The amount of anastomosis between the segmental arteries and the longitudinal spinal arteries is variable. If the anastomosis is poor it is easy to see how localised disease in one segment which occludes a vital artery can damage the tract of the spinal cord, even though the blood supply of the remainder of the cord is adequate. From the site and distribution of the main segmental boosters to the arterial supply it will be appreciated that there are two zones of the spinal cord which are particularly vulnerable to ischaemia; the first is the lower cervical region just above the segment that the artery from the costocervical branch enters, as blood from the artery is believed to flow mainly downwards. The second zone vulnerable to ischaemia is the mid-thoracic region between the area of the cord supplied by the costocervical booster and that supplied by upward flow from the artery of Adamkiewicz.

Damage to the blood supply of the cord is particularly likely to occur due to damage to the artery of Adamkiewicz as in dissection of the aorta, left lower thoracotomies and lower left intercostal nerve blocks. The distribution of the blood supply to the spinal cord explains some of the anomalies of severe neurological damage with relatively minor lesions in certain areas, such as mild cervical spondylosis in the absence of evidence of cord compression. Damage to the arterial supply of the cord may occur following neck injuries, particularly "whip-lash" injuries.

MENINGITIS

The cardinal signs of inflammation of the meninges are neck stiffness due to reflex spasm of extensors of the neck when the head is flexed, and Kernig's[30] sign which is spasm of the hamstring muscles when the knee is extended with the hips fully flexed. Meningism is the occurrence of neck stiffness in the absence of meningeal infection; it occurs particularly in subarachnoid haemorrhage and acute febrile illness in children. In meningism the pressure in the CSF is usually increased, the chloride is low but the protein and cell content are normal. Fibrosis of the meninges may occur following meningitis, resulting in isolated cranial nerve palsies, hydrocephalus or epilepsy. Meningococcal meningitis is the commonest form of meningitis in children and young adults and usually occurs as a result of overcrowding. Asymptomatic carriers may carry the organism in their throats for 2–3 weeks, but widespread treatment with sulphonamides of a population at risk will eliminate organisms carried by these asymptomatic carriers and will usually bring an epidemic to an end. There is often an erythematous or purpuric skin rash; another notorious feature is the syndrome of acute adrenal insufficiency or the Waterhouse[31]-Friderichsen[32] syndrome. *Neisseria*[33] *meningitidis* (the meningococcus) is always sensitive to the sulphonamides in this country although resistant strains have been reported from the United States. Sulphonamides are usually combined with penicillin in case the pneumococcus is responsible for the meningitis. The most suitable sulphonamide is probably sulphadiazine rather than sulphadimidine. Sulphadiazine is not as strongly bound to the plasma proteins and reaches the CSF in higher concentrations than sulphadimidine; however, sulphadiazine is more likely to produce crystalluria.

In cases of meningitis in which the infecting organism is not known, many physicians use a combination of sulphonamide, penicillin and chloramphenicol to cover the meningococcus, the pneumococcus and

H. influenzae. Pneumococcal meningitis usually occurs as a result of spread from the nose or sinuses which harbour the organisms—this type of meningitis is particularly liable to occur following fractures of the skull which involve the nasal sinuses.

Meningitis due to *H. influenzae* is fairly common and may present in an interesting way: the meningitis may not be acute and it may cause a localised collection of fluid which behaves in the same way as subdural haematoma. Chloramphenicol is the drug of choice in treatment.

As a rule all forms of meningitis are accompanied by some inflammation of the brain and spinal cord (encephalitis and myelitis) and conversely all forms of encephalitis have some degree of meningeal irritation and meningism—this is particularly true of the viral infections of the nervous system. Non-viral causes of meningo-encephalitis are:

Tuberculosis
Syphilis
Malaria
Trypanosomiasis
Brucellosis[35]
Leptospirosis (Weil's disease and canicola fever)
Toxoplasmosis
Behçet's disease (possibly due to a virus)
Sarcoidosis
Torulosis (cryptococcosis)
Typhoid and typhus (*Gk.* typhos, mist; referring to mental and visual mistiness)
Carcinomatosis.

Viral Causes of Meningo-encephalitis

The diagnosis of virus infection can be substantiated by:

Clinical features
Leucopenia and lymphocytosis
Demonstration of the virus by electron microscopy
Circumstantial evidence by observing a particular cytopathogenic effect of the virus on certain cells in the laboratory, or producing an illness in animals which previous experience has shown to be due to a known virus.
Demonstration of serum antibodies.

There are two main ways of demonstrating antibodies:

Complement fixation tests.—When antibody-antigen reactions take place, complement (which is a globulin) is used up. Various dilutions of sera are incubated with a known quantity of virus antigen. In those dilutions in which an antibody reaction has taken place complement will be used up (or fixed). Any complement remaining means that not enough antibody from the patient is present to react with the known amount of virus antigen. Complement is detected by observing haemolysis of red cells when they are mixed with haemolysin. Haemolysis of the cells will not occur unless complement is present.

Neutralisation tests.—Serial dilutions of the patient's serum (containing antibody) are mixed with a known quantity of virus and inoculated into tissue cultures; the viruses not neutralised by antibody will grow. The dilution from which no growth on the tissue culture occurs indicates the titre of viral antibody present.

Complement fixation tests are better for the diagnosis of acute infections because the rise in antibody occurs quickly and subsides quickly and the test is quicker and easier to perform. Neutralisation tests are more time-consuming and the antibody titre may not fall even years after an infection. The main snag of serological tests for virus infections is that in many cases the virus has to be available for the tests to be performed. In the case of Coxsackie and ECHO viruses there are so many groups that may cause infection that it is not practicable to test for antibodies against the 30 odd members of each group. In order to perform the serological tests the virus has to be grown from the patient, usually from the stools but sometimes from throat swabs or CSF. The antibody titre against any virus grown is tested and if the titre is rising then this is presumptive evidence that the infection has been recently acquired. In some infections the virus has never been grown so that it is impossible to test for an antibody against it, e.g. infective hepatitis.

The main virus infections of the nervous system are:

Acute lymphocytic meningitis
Acute aseptic meningitis. (Both of these may be due to Coxsackie and ECHO viruses)
Poliomyelitis
Arbor virus encephalitides
Nervous sytem secondarily involved, as in:
    Mumps
    Glandular fever
    Herpes simplex
    Herpes zoster
    Exanthemata
    Psittacosis
    Infective hepatitis
    Rickettsial diseases
    Royal Free disease
    Epidemic vomiting, vertigo and cervical myalgia.

Acute lymphocytic meningitis and aseptic meningitis refer to the occurrence of meningeal irritation with a predominance of lympho-cytes in the one case and a normal cell count in the other. The commonest causes of these two forms of meningitis are Coxsackie and ECHO virus infections; however, both forms of meningitis may occur in any of the other virus infections of the nervous system. When due to Coxsackie or ECHO virus infections the disease has a good prognosis. The diagnosis can be confirmed by growing the virus from the faeces or CSF, demonstrating a rising titre of neutralising antibodies and excluding other causes of lymphocytes in the CSF such as tuberculosis, poliomyelitis, glandular fever and herpes infections.

The arborviruses are a group that are always spread by insect vectors and which cause three main types of illness:

1. Short, prostrating fevers, e.g. dengue and sandfly fever.
2. Haemorrhagic tendencies, e.g. yellow fever and various hae-morrhagic fevers.
3. Encephalitis, e.g. St. Louis encephalitis, Japanese B en-cephalitis and Russian Spring fever.

Diseases caused by arborviruses should not be confused with those caused by rickettsiae, which are organisms larger than viruses, but can exist free from animal cells. There is, however, one important similarity between arborviruses and rickettsiae—they are both exclusively spread by insect vectors. The main rickettsial diseases are typhus, Q fever and scrub typhus (tsutsugamushi disease).

SYPHILIS

The primary chancre usually occurs within 2–3 weeks of infection, it is associated with regional lymphadenopathy and always with blood dissemination of spirochaetes. The primary chancre usually heals within six weeks. Secondary syphilis consists of the visible manifesta-tions of blood-borne spread of the spirochaetes. The most important manifestations of secondary syphilis are mucous and cutaneous; it is vitally important to realise that the lesions of secondary syphilis may recur in crops and that the lesions are highly infectious. It has been found by experience that after a period of 2–4 years the lesions of secondary syphilis no longer recur. However, despite the fact that skin and mucous lesions will not recur the spirochaetes may still persist in the nervous and cardiovascular systems and can cause structural damage. Any stage of syphilis following the primary chancre, in which there is no evidence of structural damage, is known as latent syphilis. The stage of secondary syphilis before the mucocutaneous crops stop recurring is known as early latent syphilis, and after the period 2–4 years when crops of lesions will no longer occur, is known as late latent syphilis. It is worth emphasising that latent syphilis can only be diagnosed if syphilitic infection can be proved to have occurred by positive serology, but there must be no evidence whatsoever of any structural lesion in the nervous or cardiovascular systems. Should the CSF be abnormal in any way, then structural change in the nervous system must have occurred and the syphilis cannot be latent even if the structural lesion cannot be found—this state is called asymptomatic neurosyphilis. The changes in the CSF which indicate neurosyphilis are an increase in lymphocytes, the presence of a positive WR in the CSF, the presence of globulin (normally globulin does not occur in the CSF; it is tested for by Pandy's[36] test) and alteration of the Lange[37] colloidal gold test. It is worth noting at this point that if the patient has received anti-syphilitic treatment, the blood WR may be negative even though asymptomatic neurosyphilis is present.

Beside the mucocutaneous manifestations of secondary (or early latent) syphilis there may be an iritis, retinitis or alopecia areata. Following early latent syphilis or late latent syphilis, structural changes may occur and the two parts of the nervous system involved are the meninges and the blood vessels—this is the stage of meningovascular neurosyphilis or tertiary syphilis. Later the spirochaetes may directly involve parenchymatous nerve tissue leading to so-called quaternary syphilis: the manifestations of this are general paresis of the insane (GPI), in which the parenchymatous tissue of the cerebral hemispheres is affected, and tabes dorsalis, in which the posterior nerve roots are involved.

Serological Tests for Syphilis

There are two main types:

1. Non-specific, which can develop after other infections such as yaws and leprosy and which usually become negative after treatment of early syphilis; they can therefore be used to indicate successful treatment. The Wassermann[38] reaction (WR) is a complement fixation test for non-specific antibody; this test is no longer widely used and has been replaced by a modification of the Kahn[39] test, which is a flocculation test known as the VDRL test (Venereal Disease Reference Laboratory). There are other non-specific tests such as the Rapid Plasma Reagin Test (RPRT) and Automated Reagin Test (ART).

2. Specific. These are specific for treponemal infections (not necessarily specific for syphilis). Once they have become positive these tests usually remain positive for many years, and hence are of no value in assessing response to treatment.

The main specific tests are:

Reiter protein complement fixation test (RPCF).—This is a complement fixation test and is relatively simple and inexpensive, but false positives occasionally occur.

Fluorescent treponemal antibody test (FTA).—This test becomes positive early, and false positives are rare.

Treponema pallidum haemagglutination test (TPHA).—This is simpler to perform than the FTA but takes longer to become positive.

Treponema pallidum immobilisation test (TPI).—This is more complicated and uses live pathogenic *Treponema pallidum*, is therefore potentially dangerous, and is absolutely specific.

The non-specific VDRL test usually becomes positive about two weeks after the primary chancre has developed. It is almost always positive in secondary, early latent, late latent and tertiary syphilis, but eventually it becomes negative even without treatment. After treatment it should become negative after 6 months and should always be negative after 12 months; however in late syphilis it usually remains positive, even after treatment.

False positive tests are much less common with the VDRL test than the WR but may occur with acute and chronic infection and connective tissue disorders.

Following the primary chancre the reagin tests become positive after about two weeks while the TPI usually becomes positive after about two months. As a general rule the RPCF test remains positive for life even following adequate treatment. In untreated patients the reagin tests will become negative in about a quarter of the patients— "biological cures". Following adequate treatment of primary or secondary (early latent) syphilis the reagin tests will become negative after about six months in 90 per cent of the patients. In the remainder, the titre of reagin may drop but not reach zero; it may remain low or it may later rise again (sero-relapse). Rarely, following adequate treatment, the reagin titre does not fall at all. Sero-relapse is generally followed by clinical relapse, and it is impossible to establish whether relapse has really occurred or whether there has been a fresh infection. It is very important to detect sero-relapse because there is evidence that the clinical manifestations will be more severe than those of relapse in the untreated patient.

Neurosyphilis may develop with a negative blood WR; hence it is essential to examine the CSF one year after a primary lesion has been treated even if the blood WR is negative; if the CSF is normal the patient is followed for a further year or two to ensure that there is no sero-relapse. If the patient presents with late latent syphilis, i.e. more than 2–4 years after the primary chancre, positive blood WR, no clinical features and a normal CSF, he should be treated because in the absence of previous treatment it is possible that he may develop the cardiovascular complications even though his CSF is normal. The patient who presents in the stage of *early* latent syphilis, i.e. *less* than 2–4 years following the primary infection, positive WR, no clinical features and negative CSF, is also treated, and provided the CSF is normal after one year he is followed for a further year or so in case sero-relapse occurs. It is important to note that a patient is only discharged if his blood WR is negative or if the titre is very low; normally patients should be followed for 2–5 years after treatment.

The treatment at the primary stage consists of ten days penicillin, to which *Treponema pallidum* is always sensitive. The type of penicillin used varies; the main ones are:

Procaine penicillin; daily injection of 2 ml (600 000 units).
Delayed released procaine penicillin combined with aluminium monostearate (PAM) every second or third day.
Benzathine penicillin; one injection only.

Following the first dose of penicillin there may be adverse effects from a sudden release of toxic material from killed organisms—Jarisch[40]-Herxheimer[41] reaction. This may be important if there is a lesion situated near the opening of the coronary arteries or the origin of one of the spinal arteries. It is important to note that this type of reaction will only occur following the first dose of penicillin; any reactions which occur after the first dose of penicillin are likely to be due to hypersensitivity to penicillin, in which case tetracycline may be used instead. These reactions are common and usually consist only of pyrexia and malaise which lasts a few hours. The patient should be warned to expect it, otherwise he may cease to attend. These reactions do not occur following bismuth injections, hence bismuth is often given first when late untreated syphilis is being treated for the first time. In patients who have cardiovascular or nervous system involvement a Jarisch-Herxheimer reaction could be serious if it involved a spinal, cerebral or coronary artery.

In the treatment of late latent syphilis, or neuro- or cardiovascular syphilis, 2–3 weeks of penicillin are given. The CSF should be examined before and after treatment; further treatment is indicated if the CSF continues to be abnormal after six months or if there is a progression of signs.

Neurological Manifestations of Syphilis

It cannot be emphasised enough that syphilis may simulate any known lesion in the nervous system by the following mechanisms:

Syphilitic endarteritis may affect any blood vessel, e.g. cerebral arteries, anterior spinal artery and branches.

Meningeal involvement may cause meningitis.

Cerebral tumours may be simulated by gummata.

Meningioma may be simulated by local collections of fluid as a result of local meningitis—meningitis serosa circumscripta. These may also simulate a subdural haematoma and if very localised may be responsible for individual cranial or spinal nerve palsies and epilepsy.

Posterior column lesions occur in tabes dorsalis.

Parenchymatous involvement of the nervous system occurs in GPI.

Tabes Dorsalis (*L*. tabes: wasting)

The name refers to the wasting of the posterior columns; the old name of locomotor ataxia reflected the predominant symptom of ataxia as a result of loss of proprioception. The reason why only the posterior columns are affected is not known; the explanation that the posterior nerve roots are constricted by local thickening of the arachnoid is probably untrue because the sensory loss is selective. Optic atrophy occurs almost always and is due to:

Constriction of the optic nerves by arachnoiditis.

Degeneration of the retina due to a retinitis during the secondary stage.

Direct damage to the fibres of the optic nerves by the organisms —this is, therefore, one form of retrobulbar neuritis.

Tabes dorsalis is very rare in women. The main features of tabes are:

Argyll Robertson pupils and ptosis

Optic atrophy

Charcot joints

Loss of ankle and knee jerks

Loss of deep pain sensation

Posterior column loss leading to lack of position sense, ataxia and positive Romberg's test and loss of vibration sense

Delayed appreciation of pinprick

Perforating ulcers of the feet and painful tabetic crises.

The WR in the blood and CSF are positive in about 60 per cent of patients, but are negative in about 20 per cent; following treatment the CSF abnormalities and blood WR may revert to normal.

SYRINGOMYELIA

The syrinx (*Gk*. pipe) is situated in the cervical region of the cord or brain stem (syringobulbia). It occurs anterior to the central canal in relation to the decussation of the fibres of the lateral spinothalamic tracts. It is also near the anterior horn of the grey matter, through which the motor root enters the cord, and it is near the pyramidal tracts. Thus, the characteristic features of syringomyelia in a segment of the cervical cord are:

> Loss of pain and temperature sensation in skin supplied by that segment or the one below.
> Lower motor neurone lesions in the motor nerve of that segment due to involvement of the anterior horn of the grey matter.
> Upper motor neurone lesions below the affected segments due to involvement of the pyramidal tracts.

The commonest segment to be affected initially is the first thoracic, hence wasting of the small muscles of the hand with loss of pain and temperature sensation in the hands is the characteristic presenting feature. If the gliosis surrounding the syrinx or the syrinx itself spreads, the lateral spinothalamic tracts as well as the decussation of some lateral spinothalamic fibres may be compressed, leading to loss of pain and temperature in dermatomes below the lesion. Syringobulbia produces similar changes in relation to the medulla.

Three signs which occur in the cranial nerves when the disease is still limited to the cervical cord are Horner's syndrome, nystagmus, and loss of pain and temperature in the lower part of the face. The Horner's syndrome is due to involvement of the sympathetic pathway in the cervical cord, the nystagmus is due to involvement of fibres of the vestibulospinal tracts and the loss of pain and temperature in the lower face is due to involvement of the descending tract of the trigeminal nerve as it descends into the cervical cord.

MOTOR NEURONE DISEASE

The pathological changes in motor neurone diseases are situated in and anterior horn cells, the pyramidal tracts and the motor cranial nerve nuclei in the medulla and pons. The position of the lesions causes the three dominant clinical features, namely; progressive muscular atrophy (lower motor neurone), amyotrophic lateral sclerosis (pyramidal tracts) and progressive bulbar palsy (motor cranial nerve nuclei). Certain clinical features of the disease are characteristic: it never begins before the age of 40, there are never any sensory disturbances or pain, the sphincters are never affected and the course of the disease is never more than seven years.

The disease most frequently starts with lower motor neurone lesions in the hands with wasting and fasciculation of muscles and diminished reflexes. Later, there are pyramidal signs which also begin in the cervical spine, and these lead to upper motor neurone signs in the legs with weakness, no wasting, extensor plantar responses and exaggerated reflexes. The upper motor neurone signs may then affect the arms leading to further weakness but no further wasting, thus the weakness of the arms may be more severe than the wasting would suggest. Eventually lower motor neurone signs may develop in the legs leading to abolition of the reflexes. The effect of the disease on the reflexes is variable depending on whether lower or upper motor neurone signs predominate.

Lower motor neurone lesions affecting the lower cranial nerves lead to progressive bulbar palsy. Upper motor neurone signs may be present in the lower cranial nerves leading to pseudobulbar palsy which is associated with spasticity of the muscles, stiffness but not wasting of the tongue and an exaggerated jaw jerk.

The main differential diagnosis is myelopathy due to cervical spondylosis, syringomyelia and bilateral cervical ribs; however, sensory changes are present in all these and the presence of a bulbar or pseudobulbar palsy will exclude lesions in the cervical spine.

PERONEAL MUSCULAR ATROPHY

This misnamed condition is not all that uncommon and has a very characteristic appearance. Muscle wasting occurs in the legs but the wasting has a definite upper margin above which all the muscles are normal—thus the wasting may affect the leg below the mid-thigh or below the mid-calf. There are sometimes mild posterior column signs. The disease is familial and usually begins in the teens. The arms are only rarely affected.

ABNORMAL INVOLUNTARY MOVEMENTS

The important types of abnormal involuntary movements are:

Tremor—in which one single movement is continually repeated rapidly. Common causes are old age, Parkinsonism, cerebellar disease, thyrotoxicosis, familial tremor, hysteria and alcoholism (delirium tremens).

Athetosis—in which the movements are writhing in nature and are completely purposeless. Common causes are familial, psychogenic, and vascular lesions of the basal ganglia.

Chorea—in which the movements are often semi-purposeful, like continually clutching for the bed-clothes or more complicated like continually opening and closing the eyes. Common causes are pregnancy (chorea gravidarum), rheumatic fever (Sydenham's chorea), old age, psychogenic causes and Huntington's[42] chorea.

Myoclonus.—Sudden quick contractions of whole muscles.

Tic.—Repeated complicated movements.

Tonic-clonic contractions (convulsions).
Jacksonian epilepsy.

Parkinsonism[43].—It is essential to realise that nowadays Parkinsonism is regarded as a collection of common clinical features which have a variety of causes:

> Idiopathic degeneration of the basal ganglia—paralysis agitans or Parkinson's disease.
> Arteriosclerotic degeneration of the basal ganglia.
> Encephalitis lethargica.
> Toxic, e.g. phenothiazines, manganese and carbon monoxide poisoning.

There are some helpful distinguishing features: Parkinson's disease usually comes on earlier than arteriosclerotic Parkinsonism. In Parkinson's disease the mental state is normal and there are no upper motor neurone signs. Arteriosclerotic Parkinsonism comes on at a later age, is often associated with a history of transient weakness of the limbs, and there are usually bilateral upper motor neurone signs due to ischaemia of the internal capsules so that the reflexes are increased and the plantar responses are extensor; the reflexes in Parkinson's disease are normal. There may be evidence of a pseudobulbar palsy if there is bilateral softening of the internal capsules in arteriosclerosis; other arteriosclerotic manifestations such as dementia or epilepsy may occur. Post-encephalitic Parkinsonism comes at an earlier age than Parkinson's disease and like Parkinsonism associated with phenothiazine administration is usually accompanied by oculogyric crises.

The two important features of Parkinsonism are tremor and rigidity, and it is worth emphasising that each feature may occur alone; it is easy to miss mild Parkinsonism in an old person in whom the only feature is slowness of facial expression.

The main pathological feature of idiopathic Parkinsonism is loss of pigmentation in the substantia nigra. There is loss of the neurotransmitter dopamine which is normally antagonised by acetylcholine leading to an alteration in the relative amounts of each.

The tremor affects the distal muscles first and is worse at rest. The rigidity is accompanied by increased tone—this can often be demonstrated by passively flexing the other arm. Hypokinesia is often the most difficult of the features to recognise. Parkinsonism can present in unusual ways; for example, unexpected falling or ankle oedema due to relative immobility of the feet. There are two main approaches to pharmacological treatment, the first is to attempt to increase the concentration of dopamine in the brain and the second is to inhibit the action of acetylcholine with anticholinergic drugs. The concentration of dopamine can be increased by giving levodopa which is a precursor of dopamine. Unfortunately levodopa does not cross the blood-brain barrier in high concentrations. The concentrations of levodopa can be increased by giving a drug, carbidopa, which prevents the breakdown of levodopa to dopamine outside the CNS. However, although carbidopa does not cross the blood-brain barrier the increased concentrations of levodopa which do cross the barrier in small amounts will be available to the brain to be converted into dopamine.

When confronted with a patient whose face appears slightly abnormal there are five common conditions which should be considered:

Parkinsonism   Acromegaly
Myxoedema   Paget's disease.
Mild pseudobulbar palsy

ENTRAPMENT SYNDROMES

This rather graphic name refers to those conditions caused by mechanical constriction of nerve roots or spinal cord. The commonest causes of entrapment are cervical spondylosis, herniation of a lumbar intervertebral disc and cervical ribs.

A number of simple anatomical points are worth making. The intervertebral discs are anterior to the spinal cord. Herniation of the discs occurs, laterally compressing the nerve roots as they leave the spinal canal between the vertebra. Herniation and osteophyte formation can occur on the posterior part of the disc compressing the cord from before backwards. For some reason, in the cervical region compression of the nerves in the intervertebral foramen affects the sensory root more than the motor. Sensory disturbances are, therefore, much commoner than motor disturbances in cervical spondylosis. In the cervical region, as the disc protrudes backwards, the anterior part of the cord will be compressed first; this is the part where the pyramidal tracts are located, hence cervical spondylosis severe enough to compress the cord as well as nerve roots may lead to upper motor neurone signs in the legs. The anterior spinal artery may be directly compressed in this situation, leading to more extensive damage to the anterior part of the cord, particularly the pyramidal tracts.

An interesting sign of spinal cord compression in the cervical region is inversion of the biceps and triceps reflexes—tapping the biceps tendon leads to contraction of the triceps. The biceps muscle is supplied by C5 and 6 and the triceps by C6 and 7; if there is compression at the level of C6 there will be upper motor neurone signs below this level which will include C7, the main nerve supply of the triceps muscle. Thus, there will be a lower motor neurone lesion of the biceps muscle and an upper motor neurone lesion of the triceps; because they have one nerve in common which can carry the afferent impulse from stimulation of the biceps tendon, the triceps will contract in the manner of an upper motor neurone lesion, i.e. briskly. Disc protrusion and calcification, osteophyte formation and osteoarthritis all contribute to the pathogensis of spondylosis. The osteophyte formation will cause narrowing of the canal carrying the vertebral artery, possibly leading to vertebrobasilar insufficiency.

Prolapsed Intervertebral Disc

Approximately 60 per cent of disc protrusions affect the L5–S1 disc (S1 nerve root), 30 per cent affect the L4–L5 disc (L5 nerve root) and combined lesions occur in about 10 per cent. The lumbar pain which occurs in acute disc protrusion is probably related to tearing of the annulus fibrosis and protrusion of the nucleus pulposus. The *lumbar* pain of long-standing disc protrusion is probably due to stretching of the posterior longitudinal ligament of the spine and reflex protective spasm of the erector spinae muscle. Disc protrusion which results in pressure on the nerve root results in pain along the course of the nerve root, tenderness of the nerve and pain of myotome distribution, i.e. in the *muscles* supplied by the nerve. This accounts for the well-known symptom of pain radiating down the back of the thigh (in the course of the sciatic nerve and in the region of the biceps femoris), and down the back of the lower leg in the region of gastrocnemius (S1) or anterolateral part of the leg in the region of the tibialis anterior (L5).

Note that the *pain* does not radiate in the cutaneous distribution of the affected nerve root, i.e. lateral part of the lower leg and medial side of the foot (L5) and sole and lateral side of the foot (S1). However, compression of the nerve root may result in *paraesthesiae* and/or *numbness* in the appropriate *cutaneous* distribution. Further nerve root compression will result in a lower motor neurone palsy of the muscles by the affected nerve root. These are:

L5 and S1:   (1) Glutei (extension of thigh—G. maximus; abductors—G. medius and minimus).
    (2) Biceps femoris (flexion of the knee).
    (3) Peronei (eversion of the foot).

L5 (with L4): Dorsiflexors of the foot ("extensor" muscles and tibialis anterior).

S1 (with S2): (1) Plantar flexors of the foot (gastrocnemius and soleus).
    (2) Small muscles of the foot (patient is asked to "make the sole of the foot into a cup").

Note that the dorsiflexors of the foot are supplied by the lateral popliteal nerve. Lesions of this nerve may result in foot drop—this may also occur with lesions affecting the nerve roots; however, if the lateral popliteal nerve is involved peripherally there is no involvement of the glutei. Gluteus medius is best tested by asking the patient to abduct the thigh against resistance. Gluteus maximus extends the thigh; this can be tested either with the patient lying prone or in the supine position by passing one's arm behind the lower end of the thigh, raising the leg 3–4 inches off the bed and then asking the patient to "push my arm into the bed".

Other evidence of lower motor neurone weakness will be loss or diminution of deep reflexes (loss of ankle jerk in lesions of S1; note that L5 lesions do not affect either the knee or the ankle jerk—the knee jerk is mediated through roots L3 and L4). Other signs of prolapsed intervertebral disc which should be carefully sought are:

Restricted movements of the lumbar spine
Loss of normal lumbar lordosis
Lumbar scoliosis (the direction of the scoliosis is no guide to the side of the disc protrusion)
Tenderness on palpation of the lumbar spine
"Sagging" of the glutei on one side
Tenderness with "percussion" over the sciatic nerve
Restriction of straight leg raising (Lasègue's [44] sign).

Occasionally lumbar disc protrusion may be painless, or a disc other than L4–L5 and L5–S1 may protrude. L3–L4 disc lesions result in loss of the knee jerk. It is usually the posterolateral part of the intervertebral disc which is the site of herniation of the nucleus pulposus, rarely the posterior part of the disc is the site of herniation. This central protrusion may cause bilateral symptoms and signs and may compress the cauda equina. The cauda equina consists of all the nerve roots below L2 at which level the spinal cord ends; for this reason prolapse of the L4–L5 or L5–S1 discs can never produce *upper* motor neurone signs. Compression of the cauda equina whether by central disc protrusion or tumour produces a flaccid paraplegia with numbness and sphincter disturbance which, in the case of the bladder, causes hesitancy, urgency and then retention of urine. Space-occupying lesions in the cauda equina are more likely to produce compression of the lower sacral nerves because these nerves travel the whole distance of the lumbar sac from the point where the cord ends to their emergence from the spinal column; the lowest sacral nerves, therefore, have a longer course than the other nerve roots constituting the cauda equina. Nerve roots which occur in the upper part of the cauda equina will not, of course, be compressed by tumours arising below their points of exit from the spine. Muscles supplied by the affected nerve roots are always weak and wasted, there is usually pain of sciatic distribution; pain is nearly always an early symptom of cauda equina lesions. Impotence, urinary symptoms, numbness and lower motor neurone weakness occur later. Rectal examination is mandatory particuarly as it may reveal a patulous anal sphincter which is sometimes an early sign of cauda equina compression. Sacral, anal and perianal anaesthesia are nearly always present.

Evidence of cauda equinal compression is a medical emergency: unless the pressure of the nerve roots is relieved permanent paralysis will result; the nerves of the bladder are particularly sensitive in this respect. A myelogram is generally performed before proceeding to laminectomy.

Claudication of the cauda equina.—In 1961 Blau and Logue described a syndrome which most clinicians have been able to confirm. The syndrome consists of bilateral pain and paraesthesiae brought on by exercise and relieved by rest; the peripheral arterial pulses are normal and neurological examination may show weakness of the foot dorsiflexors and reflex changes. It is suggested that the cause of the syndrome is intermittent claudications of the cauda equina.

It is important to note that lumbar disc protrusion may cause a marked elevation of the protein in the cerebrospinal fluid.

Cervical rib (scalenus anterior) syndrome.—The syndrome is caused by the subclavian artery and first thoracic nerve being damaged either by acute angulation over a cervical rib (or radiotranslucent fibrous band representing the cervical rib) or compression between first rib and insertion of scalenus anterior (on the first rib). Symptoms usually begin in middle age and may be precipitated by carrying heavy loads, shoulder bags or anything which causes the shoulder to sag. The syndrome is commoner in women than men. Vascular symptoms are much commoner than nerve pressure symptoms and consist of pallor, coldness and cyanosis of the fingers. The radial pulse may be weak, especially if palpated with the arm held downwards; if narrowing of the artery occurs there may be post-stenotic dilatation, thrombus formation and recurrent peripheral emboli. A murmur may be heard over the narrowed artery, the radial pulse may become weaker if the patient turns his head towards the side of the lesion and takes a deep inspiration—this will tense the scalenus anterior which is one of the accessory muscles of respiration. The costoclavicular syndrome is much rarer than the cervical rib syndrome. The subclavian artery and, rarely, the first thoracic nerve are compressed between the first rib and clavicle. The radial pulse will become obliterated if the patient pulls his shoulders (and clavicles) backwards as in standing to attention. Both the cervical rib and costoclavicular syndromes may closely resemble Raynaud's disease.

Peripheral Neuropathy

Peripheral neuropathy is defined as bilateral symmetrical muscle weakness usually accompanied by sensory disturbances due to dysfunction of several peripheral nerves simultaneously. The principal causes are:

Toxins, e.g. alcohol, lead, arsenic, isoniazid, nitrofurantoin, gold, aniline, and benzene derivatives

Deficiency of vitamins B_1 and B_{12}

Metabolic disorders, e.g. diabetes, uraemia, porphyria and amyloid disease

Carcinoma

Collagen disorders: polyarteritis, SLE, rheumatoid arthritis

Allergy, e.g. serum sickness

Infections (almost any infection from typhoid to tubercle may be complicated by a peripheral neuropathy)

Acute infective polyneuropathy or Guillain-Barré syndrome.

The cause of polyneuropathy in an individual case is often not found. Occasionally, an industrial, geographical, dietary, social or family history is helpful. One rather surprising problem in clinical practice is to distinguish between a polyneuropathy and myopathy. The presence of sensory impairment will indicate neuropathy, but if sensation is normal it may be difficult, because in both there is muscle wasting and tenderness, with diminished reflexes. In some cases of peripheral neuropathy both the nerves and the myoneural junction may be involved, as in many cases of carcinoma—hence the use of the term carcinomatous neuromyopathy.

An electromyogram will indicate reduced interference pattern in a myopathy, and nerve conduction times will be slowed in a polyneuropathy. In a difficult case, nerve biopsy is performed.

As well as an aetiological classification the peripheral neuropathies can be classified on a pathological basis. This has a closer relationship to the natural history and physiological changes which occur in the peripheral neuropathies. As a very general rule neuropathies associated with loss of the nerve axon (or neurone) recover slowly while those associated with demyelination may recover rapidly; loss of the myelin sheath (and Schwann's[45] cell) may be patchy but conduction time in the nerve is usually slow. Infiltrations and ischaemia of the peripheral nerves form separate groups.

Pathological Classification of Peripheral Neuropathies

Axonal or neuronal damage

Toxic causes —alcohol
     porphyria
     uraemia
     isoniazid
     lead
     acrylamide
Deficiencies —vitamin
Hereditary —peroneal muscular atrophy
     hereditary sensory neuropathy
Others   —carcinomatous sensory neuropathy

Proximal segmental demyelination
Guillain-Barré neuropathy
Diabetes

Distal segmental demyelination
Carcinomatous mixed neuropathy
Diabetes
Myeloma neuropathy

Ischaemia
Polyarteritis
Diabetes
Entrapment neuropathies

Infiltrations
Reticulosis
Amyloidosis
Sarcoidosis
Refsum's syndrome

Acute Infective Polyneuropathy

This usually starts with a fever, headache and sore throat, with gradual onset of weakness in the distal muscles of the legs some days later. The weakness gradually spreads upwards to the trunk, arms and sometimes the cranial nerves. The muscles are usually very tender. Severe paraesthesiae occur at this stage, even if there is no objective sensory loss. In severe cases, there is a bulbar palsy, paralysis of respiratory muscles, sphincter disturbances and an encephalitis.

The pathological changes are not restricted to the peripheral nerves. There may be a myelitis, arachnoiditis, encephalitis and occasionally inflammatory changes in the liver and kidneys. The cerebrospinal fluid usually shows a marked increase in protein with either a normal or only slightly increased cell count. This is often called the Guillain[46]-Barré[47] syndrome.

Some confusion exists about the eponyms Guillain-Barré syndrome, Froin's[48] syndrome and Landry's[49] paralysis. Guillain and Barré described cases of infective polyneuropathy with the "dissociation albumino-cytologique". Froin described a high protein content in the CSF associated with xanthochromia due to obstruction of the spinal subarachnoid space. Since then Froin's syndrome has come to mean a high CSF protein content due to any cause, including meningitis, blockage of the subarachnoid space and acute infective polyneuropathy. Landry described a clinical syndrome consisting of weakness, beginning in the lower limbs and spreading upwards, called acute ascending paralysis, and it is now accepted that this one way in which any of the polyneuropathies may present—Landry's paralysis is not a specific disease entity. One further important fact to note is that "dissociation albumino-cytologique" is not specific for acute infective polyneuropathy. It may occur with nearly all the causes of polyneuropathy. But in acute infective polyneuropathy the level of protein in the CSF is usually higher than that found in other types of neuropathy.

With regard to the diagnosis of acute infective polyneuropathy, it is obviously essential to exclude as far as possible the other causes of polyneuropathy, the most important ones being the metabolic causes, such as diabetes, uraemia and porphyria. It is important to note that the neurological complications of diabetes may appear before the diabetes causes other symptoms, so it is essential to exclude diabetes by a formal glucose tolerance test. A polyneuropathy may complicate any severe infection including septicaemia, and it will improve as the infection is controlled.

The prognosis of acute infective polyneuropathy is variable; as a general rule, sporadic cases have a favourable prognosis. In the epidemic form, some epidemics are associated with a mild disease, and others with a more severe form. The place of corticosteroids has not been clearly established; however, one thing is certain: severe cases may sometimes respond dramatically and unexpectedly to steroids (Miller, 1966). For this reason, high doses are usually given in the first week, and moderate doses given for a further month.

Autonomic Neuropathy

Many causes of peripheral neuropathy, particularly diabetes, may cause damage to the autonomic nervous system. The sites at which lesions may produce autonomic dysfunction are in the afferent, central and efferent part of the reflex. The afferent side is best demonstrated by testing the automatic compensatory changes in the cardiovascular system in response to alterations in cardiac output, and the two easiest ways of doing this are to observe the blood pressure in response to changes of posture or the Valsalva manoeuvre. The central pathways can be tested by observing the rise in blood pressure in response to mental arithmetic or in the ability of the patient to sweat in response to heat. The efferent autonomic pathways are rather easier to test: the parasympathetic efferents in the vagus can be tested by blocking the vagus with atropine and observing an increase in heart rate. If the vagus is already damaged there will be no response to atropine. The ability of the vagus to stimulate the production of gastric acid can be tested by an insulin test meal. Sympathetic efferent pathways can be tested by infusing noradrenaline and demonstrating a rise in blood pressure, indicating that the blood vessels are able to respond; or acetylcholine can be locally injected into the skin and if the post-ganglionic fibres of the sympathetic are intact, piloerection will follow. Symptoms which should suggest the possibility of an autonomic neuropathy are postural hypotension, diarrhoea, impotence and loss of sweating.

As well as peripheral neuropathies which may damage either the afferent or efferent pathways of the autonomic reflexes, some central lesions may impair autonomic function. The most important of these is damage to the sympathetic pathways in the spinal cord, or medulla, as a result of syringomyelia, vascular or neoplastic lesions. The hypothalamus is the co-ordinating centre of autonomic activity and damage to the hypothalamus results in disturbances of sleep rhythm, temperature regulation, appetite regulation, glucose metabolism, and diabetes insipidus.

Treatment of an autonomic neuropathy is often difficult; if postural hypotension is a problem, the patient should wear thick, tight elastic stockings on the legs and should only stand up slowly. It sometimes helps for a patient to sleep feet-down so that blood is already pooled within the legs, and therefore, when he stands up, postural hypotension is minimised. The sympathetic system may be stimulated by sympathomimetic drugs such as ephedrine or, if cardiovascular symptoms are severe, a salt-retaining drug which increases the plasma volume may help (e.g. fludrocortisone).

Psychopharmacology

Behaviour or mood is influenced by three main "structures" in the central nervous system:

1. Reticular activating system in the midbrain concerned with arousal and anxiety, sleep patterns and modulation of reflex autonomic functions.

2. The limbic system, which consists of at least three integrated systems:
  (a) thalamus, which integrates emotional state with motor activity and is involved with sensory attention
  (b) basal ganglia or extrapyramidal system (caudate nucleus, putamen and globus pallidus), concerned with integration of muscle tone and fine movements
  (c) hippocampus, concerned with recent memory
3. Hypothalmus, concerned with some autonomic functions particularly those mediated via the pituitary.

Unlike the peripheral nervous system, in which there are only two neurotransmitters, acetylcholine and noradrenaline, the central nervous system contains many, among which are:

Noradrenaline
Dopamine
Serotonin (5HT)
Histamine
Enkephalins
Gamma-aminobutyrate (GABA) and probably several other amino acids.

The cause of many psychiatric diseases can be deduced by:

An awareness of the main actions of those drugs known to improve the psychiatric condition
Studying the distribution and quantity of neurotransmitters in the brains of patients.

The situation is complicated by the fact that many of the patients will have been treated by psychotropic drugs and therefore it may be difficult to disentangle the effects on neurotransmitters of the drug and the disease; furthermore, there is no certainty that neurotransmitter excess or depletion is the basic cause of the disease.

Schizophrenia.—There is increased dopamine activity in the limbic system; this may be due to increased sensitivity or increased number of synaptic dopamine receptors. Phenothiazines (which structurally resemble antihistamines) are competitive antagonists of dopamine. Dopaminergic drugs like alphamethyldopa (Aldomet) make schizophrenia worse. Dopaminergic neurones also exist in the extrapyramidal system (now often called the striatonigral system) and in the hypothalmus. Dopaminergic neurones have a widespread distribution. Phenothiazines also have a number of actions other than being dopamine antagonists (they have some cholinergic activity, and Largactil was so called because it has such a large number of actions). Where there are dopaminergic-induced activities, phenothiazines have an effect, e.g. on the hypothalmus, causing prolactin release. Unfortunately, blocking dopaminergic neurones has a number of side-effects:

(a) Parkinsonism.—This is due to a deficiency of dopamine and unopposed activity of cholinergic neurones in the extrapyramidal system. If the Parkinsonism is drug induced, it is logical to give anticholinergics rather than dopamine agonists. Hence L dopa is not used in drug-induced Parkinsonism; it will either not work or will counteract most of the effects of the chlorpromazine.

(b) Tardive dyskinesia.—This is a condition which occurs 2–3 years after phenothiazines have been started and consists of involuntary choreoathetoid movements. The phenothiazines reduce dopaminergic transmission but this leads to increased dopamine sensitivity by two postulated mechanisms:

1. A failure of a feedback mechanism in the presynaptic neurone leading to increased dopamine production (which may only be counteracted by *increasing* the phenothiazine dose)
2. A growth of dopamine receptors in the postsynaptic neurone leading to impulses occurring with a much lower dopamine stimulus.

In patients with tardive dyskinesia the neuroleptic must not be withdrawn suddenly, or the condition may get worse; furthermore, anticholinergic drugs, by reducing cholinergic balance may also make dyskinesia worse. The rational therapy for tardive dyskinesia may involve:

Increasing the neuroleptic
Withdrawing the neuroleptic very slowly
Attempting to reduce the dopamine stores by tetrabenazine or reserpine
Stopping anticholinergics
Giving acetylcholine precursors such as deanol or choline
Giving neuroleptics intermittently ("drug holidays").

Depression.—The effects of a variety of drugs give some insight into pathogenesis:

1. Amphetamines, which may improve depression, release noradrenaline stores and prevent its re-uptake in the proximal neurone by inhibiting the "amine pump"
2. Iproniazid, first discovered as a result of isoniazid influencing mood in tuberculous patients; iproniazid inhibits monoamine oxidase

3. Reserpine causes depression and is known to reduce stores of noradrenaline.

Thus depression was linked with amine depletion and monoamine oxidase inhibitors should result in repletion of noradrenaline, which is then able to pass back into the proximal neurone and be available for neurotransmission ("amine pump mechanism")

Action of other psychotropic drugs.
1. Lithium, used in mania, enhances the destruction of noradrenaline and reduces the sensitivity of the postsynaptic neurone to normal amounts of amines
2. Benzodiazepines act on the reticular system (reducing sensory input), on the limbic systems (influencing affect), and affect the increase of GABA, an inhibitory neurotransmitter which may be in excess in anxiety states.

TABLE XIV(A)

ACTIONS OF PSYCHOTROPIC DRUGS

Psychotropic drug	Disease symptoms improved	Main action	Implied causation of disease
Cholinergics or anticholinesterase (e.g. physostigmine)	Alzheimer's disease	Increase acetylcholine	Deficiency of choline
Phenothiazines	Schizophrenia	Dopamine receptor blockade	Overaction of dopaminergic system
Monoamine oxidase inhibitors	Depression	Decreased destruction of amine	Decreased monoamine function
Tricyclics	Depression	Inhibition of presynaptic re-uptake of amines— (inhibition of "amine pump")	Decreased monoamine function
Lithium	Mania	Increases 5HT	Disturbance of 5HT function

TABLE XIV(B)

SIDE-EFFECTS OF PSYCHOTROPIC DRUGS

Psychotropic drug	Side-effect	Main action	Implied causation
Reserpine	Depression	Depletion of monoamines	Decreased monoamines
Phenothiazines alpha methyldopa	Parkinsonism	Depletion of dopamine	Deficiency of dopamine
LSD	Hallucinations	Blocks 5HT	
H2 receptor		Blocks histamine	
beta blockers	Hyperactivity syndrome	Blocks 5HT	Excess 5HT

ORGANIC PSYCHOSES

It is of great practical importance to be aware of the organic causes of mental symptoms. Many causes of mental symptoms are reversible if treated promptly. As a working hypothesis it is convenient to divide the organic psychoses into those which present acutely with a short illness and those with a more long-standing illness. In general the acute mental symptoms are those of delirium and the chronic mental symptoms those of dementia. Delirium refers to a sudden onset of confusion, restlessness and disorientation. Dementia refers to a gradual onset of diminished intellect, memory, assimilation of new ideas, social awareness together with inattention and confusion. There is often no change of mood (called by the psychiatrists "affect") although this depends on the previous personality of the patient.

The main disorders of affect (mood) are depression, anxiety and mania; in a mild form depression and mania are called apathy and excitement. These disorders of affect may be part of well-recognised psychiatric disorders which are as well defined as most organic disease. The four most important psychiatric diseases of affect are endogenous and reactive depression, involutional melancholia and manic-depressive psychosis.

The important causes of delirium are:

Infection.—The delirium resulting from infections remote from the nervous system may be surprisingly severe, sometimes, necessitating admission to a mental hospital before the correct diagnosis is made. Infections of the nervous system such as malaria and meningitis may also present as delirium.

Injury, either directly to the head or, rarely, to the long bones, resulting in a fat embolus.

Intoxications, the most important of which are alcohol, Wernicke's[50] encephalopathy, barbiturates, cocaine and heroin. Withdrawal of addictive drugs may also cause delirium.

Metabolic, such as hypoglycaemia, uraemia, hypocalcaemia, hypernatraemia, hypoxia and hepatic failure.

Cerebrovascular accidents.

Miscellaneous such as Korsakoff's[51] psychosis, puerperal psychosis and postepileptic confusion states.

The important headings to remember when assessing dementia are:

Ability to reason and to form valid judgements
Memory for recent events
Alteration of affect and emotional reactions
Presence of delusions
Loss of personal care and hygiene.

Mild dementia is surprisingly common in general medical out-patients. If one does not detect four to five new and unsuspected cases a year one is probably missing a few. Besides the usual careful history, examination and routine investigations, the following investigations should always be performed in a suspicious case:

T4 and T3 levels
Plasma B_{12}
STS
Blood urea
Liver function tests
Serum calcium
Skull x-ray
EEG.

Alzheimer's[52] Disease

This is the commonest cause of dementia and is responsible for about half the cases; multi-infarct dementia accounts for a further 20 per cent. Other causes include:

Alcoholism
Normal-pressure hydrocephalus
Cortical atrophy
Huntington's chorea
Chronic epilepsy
Head injury
Folate and B_{12} deficiency
Myxoedema
Hypocalcaemia.

The main feature of Alzheimer's disease is short-term memory loss but with preservation of the personality. There are characteristic histological appearances of senile plaques with amyloid neurofibrillary tangles and angiopathy. There are also disturbances of transmission in cholinergic fibres, which may be reduced in number.

Disorders of Muscle

Persistent complaints of "weakness", "cramps after exercise", "tiredness and heaviness in the legs" in teenagers and young adults are among the most difficult which physicians have to evaluate. When there are obviously physical signs such as wasting or skeletal deformities the problem is relatively simple but often unequivocal physical signs are absent. The first questions to be considered in such cases are:

Are the symptoms genuine?
If so is it a disease of muscles or of the nervous system?
Are there any associated clinical features to suggest that the symptoms are secondary to a generalised disease?

The main features which suggest that the disorder is due to disease of the nervous system are the presence of muscle wasting, fasciculation, sensory changes and associated clinical features. The muscle wasting which occurs secondary to neurological disease is usually referred to as "amyotrophy"; the term myopathy refers to muscle changes due to disorders of the muscles alone.

Aspects of the history which are essential to establish a differential diagnosis are:

The age of the patient
The speed of onset and progression of the weakness
The family history
Preceding history of febrile illness
Drug or toxin exposure
History of trauma or nerve entrapment
Nutritional history.

By now one should be able to select the most probable diagnosis from the following:

Motor neurone disease in older patients
Developmental abnormalities such as syringomyelia, hereditary ataxias, peripheral neuropathy, myasthenia gravis, secondary muscle disorders such as polymyositis or endocrine myopathy, or primary muscle disorder.

The primary muscle disorders are:

Muscular dystrophy
Glycogen storage diseases
Periodic paralysis
Congenital myopathy
Myotonia.

Other investigations which may be necessary to elucidate problems of muscle weakness are:

Serum muscle enzyme levels, e.g. aldolase and creatine kinase. These are almost always elevated in muscular dystrophies and inflammatory disorders of muscles (myositis).

Muscle biopsy, which may show features of one of the muscular dystrophies, one of the congenital myopathies or glycogen deposits.

Muscular Dystrophies

The most important clinically are:

X-linked
Severe (Duchenne[53])
Benign (Becker)
Autosomal recessive
Limb-girdle type
Childhood type
Facioscapulohumeral
Distal
Ocular
Oculopharyngeal

X-linked.—The severe type invariably occurs in young boys, there is always cardiac involvement and pseudohypertrophy, and the life span is reduced. It usually begins in the upper legs and spreads to the pelvis and lower legs. In the benign type cardiac involvement is absent, the onset is later, often during adolescence, and the life span normal. The disease is confirmed and carrier states detected by finding raised levels of serum creatine kinase and aldolase. EMG and muscle biopsy may also be helpful.

Autosomal recessive.—This limb-girdle type occurs in either sex, begins in the 20s or 30s and is slowly progressive. The childhood type begins in adolescence and has a worse prognosis than the limb-girdle type; clinically it may come to resemble the Duchenne type.

Other types (distal, ocular, oculopharyngeal).—The distal type usually begins in the hands and spreads to the feet; it is distinguished from peroneal muscular atrophy by the complete absence of any sensory signs (particularly vibration sense which is usually lost in peroneal muscular atrophy).

Glycogen Storage Diseases

These diseases are rare and most of them occur in childhood; they are associated with glycogen deposition in liver and spleen resulting in severe hepatosplenomegaly. There are many enzyme deficiencies which end up with excessive storage of glycogen. The characteristic features are hypoglycaemia and failure to produce lactate and pyruvate from glycogen (failure of glycogenolysis); this is tested by demonstrating a failure of venous pyruvate or lactate to rise in an occluded limb following exercise. Only two types of glycogen storage disease affecting muscles are of concern to general physicians; these are Type III, in which the deficient enzyme is amylo-1, 6-glucosidase, and Type V or McArdle's[54] disease in which muscle phosphorylase is deficient. Both these conditions *usually* begin in childhood and cause muscle pain and fatigue on exercise, the fingers may not be able to be extended after prolonged forced flexion and there may be myoglobinuria after exercise.

Periodic Paralysis

These conditions are almost invariably associated with either a high or low serum potassium level. In both types the symptoms may be mild and localised or severe and generalised; the paralysis may last 2 or 3 days. Attacks are much more likely after a large meal or heavy exercise.

Congenital Myopathies

This is a rare group of disorders occurring in children, due to degenerative changes in muscle fibres, and which can only be classified by histochemical means.

From a clinical point of view it is often necessary to distinguish muscle weakness due to a disease of the muscle itself from disease of the peripheral nerves. This can be done fairly simply by recording the electrical potentials of a muscle at rest and on contraction with a needle electrode placed in the muscle (electromyogram or EMG). In the normal there is no activity at rest, on voluntary contraction individual motor units will be recorded and on maximum contraction so many motor units are occurring at the same time that no individual motor unit potential will be seen (interference pattern). A motor unit consists of many muscle fibres supplied by one nerve fibre.

In a myopathy in which there is a patchy involvement of muscle fibres within one motor unit, the motor unit potentials recorded on slight exertion will be smaller than normal because there are fewer muscle fibres contracting, also the interference pattern will be at a lower voltage than normal because of damage to some fibres of each motor unit. In complete denervation the degenerating nerve (Wallerian[55] degeneration) occasionally fires off impulses spontaneously, and denervated muscle fibres also may contract spontaneously, which results in occasional discharges at rest. Some of these resemble normal motor unit potentials while others are of a lower voltage. There is no activity with attempted contraction of the muscle. In the normal muscle at rest there are never any spontaneous motor unit potentials. If the nerve is recovering, on voluntary contraction a few motor unit potentials will be seen but not as many as normal, hence there will be less of an interference pattern, although the height of the interference pattern is normal, in contrast to a myopathy in which the height of the interference pattern is reduced.

Diseases Characterised by Myotonia

In these conditions the muscles contract and relax more slowly than normal, but this tends to improve with exercise and as the patient gets older. As a result of the slower muscular contraction there may be difficulty in balance and if the muscles are tapped a local dimple forms which lasts for several seconds. A curious feature is that the tendon reflexes are always normal.

Myotonia congenita (Thomsen's[56] disease). This is always present from birth and tends to improve as the patient gets older; the muscles are always well developed. Variants of the condition are myotonia paradoxa in which the myotonia gets worse after exercise, and paramyotonia in which the myotonia is worse on exposure to cold.

Dystrophia myotonica.—As its name suggests, this is a combination of muscular dystrophy and myotonia, and the combination is pathognomonic of the condition, which usually begins in adult life. The dystrophic or wasted muscles are those of the face, neck and distal parts of the limbs. Other features which may be present are cataract, testicular and ovarian atrophy and frontal baldness.

Diphenylhydantoin, procainamide and corticosteroids may each relieve the symptoms of myotonia, but do not affect the progress of dystrophia myotonica.

REFERENCES

BLAU, J. N. and LOGUE, V. (1961) *Lancet*, **1**, 1081.
KENDALL, B. E. and MARSHALL, J. (1974) *J. roy. Coll. Phycns. Lond.*, **9**, 30.
LAIDLAW, J. and RICHENS, A. (1976) *A Textbook of Epilepsy*. Edinburgh: Churchill Livingstone.
MILLER, H. (1966) *Brit. med. J.*, **2**, 1219.
TAVERNER, S. (1971) *Brit. med. J.*, **4**, 20.

GENERAL REFERENCES

PATTEN, J. (1977) *Neurological Differential Diagnosis*. London: Harold Starke.
WALTON, J. N. (1977) *Brain's Diseases of the Nervous System*. 8th edit. Oxford: Oxford University Press.

EPONYMS

1. MORITZ HEINRICH ROMBERG (1795–1873)
Romberg qualified in Berlin. He remained at his hospital post during the Berlin cholera epidemics of 1831 and 1837. His influential textbook of neurology was significant because of its attempt to classify neurological disorders according to physiological principles.

2. SIR HERMAN WEBER (1823–1918)
London physician.

3. AUGUSTE LOUIS JULES MILLARD (1830–1915)
Paris physician.

4. ADOLPHE MARIE GUBLER (1821–1879)
Paris physician.

5. ACHILLE LOUIS FRANÇOIS FOVILLE (1799–1878)
Paris neurologist.

6. THOMAS WILLIS (1621–1675)
Willis qualified in Oxford where he frequently met with Boyle, Wren, Hooke and Sydenham. With the Restoration of Charles II many of Willis' colleagues moved to London, but he remained in Oxford. His work on the brain, the drawings for which were done by Christopher Wren, was published in 1664. After the Plague, Willis went to London and set up a large and lucrative practice.

7. JOSEF FRANÇOIS FÉLIX BABINSKI (1857–1932)
Born in Paris of Polish parents, Babinski studied under Charcot at Salpetriere. During the First World War he was successful in dealing with shell-shocked soldiers suffering from hysteria and neuroses. He was responsible for localising the first spinal-cord tumour to be successfully removed in France, and was more proud of this accomplishment than of his eponymous sign. So frequent was hysteria that the discovery of a sign which was never present in hysterics was of great practical value, which was the reason that Babinski's sign became so rapidly accepted.

8. FRANCISCUS SYLVIUS (1614–1672)
Sylvius qualified in Basle but became Professor of Medicine in Leyden. He recognised the significance of Harvey's discovery of the circulation of the blood; his ideas on chemical changes in the body as the causes of diseases were propagated in Britain by Thomas Willis. Sylvius was the first to recognise that tubercles were the prime pathological feature of tuberculosis.

9. LUIGI ROLANDO (1773–1831)
Turin anatomist.

10. PIERRE PAUL BROCA (1824–1880)

Broca trained and practised as a surgeon, and while at La Pitie he attended the wounded from the siege of Paris during the 1870 Franco-Prussian war. He married the daughter of the wealthy Parisian physician J. G. A. Lugol (1786–1851). Broca's greatest achievements were in the field of anthropology, and his suggestion of cerebral localisation was first made at a meeting of the French Anthropological Society in 1861. The concept of a specific speech area was based on a patient nicknamed Tan (this being the only word he could say). At the post-mortem on Tan a lesion in the left third frontal convolution was found. Broca called the speech defect "aphemia" (no voice); it was Armand Trousseau who introduced the term "asphasia". The post-mortem on Tan was later re-examined by Pierre Marie (1853–1940) who showed that Tan had many more defects than the one involving the third left frontal convolution, and that speech may not therefore have the cerebral localisation ascribed to it.

11. JOHN HUGHLINGS JACKSON (1835–1911)

Jackson was a Yorkshireman, and studied at the York School of Medicine. He knew Hutchinson and also Brown-Séquard when the National Hospital for Nervous Diseases, Queen Square was founded. Like Hutchinson he was involved with Moorfields Hospital and the London Hospital.

12. FOSTER KENNEDY (1884–1952)

New York neurologist.

13. JOSEF GERSTMANN (1887–1969)

Vienna neurologist.

14. JOHANN OTTO LEONHARD HEUBNER (1843–1926)

Heubner qualified in Leipzig, where he became Professor of Paediatrics, before proceeding to the chair of Paediatrics in Berlin (where he succeeded Henoch). He described syphilitic endarteritis in the cerebral arteries in 1860. He was one of the first paediatricians to use lumbar puncture and he successfully used von Behring's diphtheria antitoxin.

15. GIUSEPPE GRADENIGO (1859–1926)

Naples otologist.

16. DOUGLAS ARGYLL ROBERTSON (1837–1909)

Argyll Robertson qualified in Edinburgh, studied ophthalmology under von Graefe in Berlin and eventually, like his father, became President of the Royal College of Surgeons of Edinburgh. His interest in the pupillary reaction was stimulated by the pharmacological properties (due to physostigmine) of the Calabar bean from Zanzibar, then recently brought to Edinburgh by one of Livingstone's companions.

17. SIR GORDON MORGAN HOLMES (1876–1965)

Holmes qualified from Trinity College Dublin. He studied in Frankfurt under Edinger and Weigert and was appointed to the staff of the National Hospital for Nervous Diseases, Queen Square. His influence on British neurology is unquestioned, and in recognition of his contribution he was made a Fellow of the Royal Society in 1933.

18. WILLIAM JOHN ADIE (1886–1935)

Adie was born in Australia but qualified in Edinburgh. He was on the staff of the National Hospital for Nervous Diseases, Queen Square, and was one of the few to survive the retreat from Mons.

19. SIR CHARLES BELL (1774–1842)

Although qualifying in Edinburgh, local jealousies at the success of his brother John's anatomy classes compelled him to go to London, where he became a partner in the Great Windmill Street School of Anatomy founded earlier by John and William Hunter (also Scots). Bell eventually became involved in the formation of the Middlesex Hospital and Medical School. He attended the wounded from the battles of Corunna and Waterloo, and returned in some triumph to Edinburgh as Professor of Surgery in 1836, having been knighted in 1831. Bell devised the experimental method of cutting nerves and stimulating the cut ends electrically to study the function. He and Magendie separately discovered that the anterior and posterior spinal nerve roots were motor and sensory respectively.

20. FRIEDRICH EUGEN WEBER-LIEL (1832–1891)

Berlin and Jena otologist.

21. HEINRICH ADOLF RINNE (1819–1868)

Rinne qualified in Munich. He described his test in 1855, but died of dysentery shortly after being appointed to Hildesheim Mental Hospital.

22. PROSPER MENIÈRE (1799–1862)

Menière worked with Dupuytren and during the 1830 Revolution they both had extensive experience with war-wounded patients. Dupuytren is said to have used Menière's treatise as his own. Menière was decorated by Louis Philippe for combating a cholera epidemic, and was also involved in confirming the pregnancy of the Duchesse de Berry. After this Menière wisely devoted his working life to being an ENT specialist.

23. HUBERT VON LUSCHKA (1820–1875)

Luschka qualified in Freiburg. In 1857 he edited *Die Brust organe des Menschen in ihrer Lage* (The human breasts and their position).

24. FRANÇOIS MAGENDIE (1783–1855)

Magendie was born in Bordeaux; his father, a surgeon, was politically involved with the Revolution and was an ardent believer in the philosophy of Rousseau; Magendie could not even read by the age of 10. However, he eventually persuaded his father to have him educated. He qualified in 1808 and was at first a physician and then in 1814 became the physiologist responsible for the teaching and indoctrination of the great Claude Bernard. He published in 1816 his famous text book of physiology—*The Precis*. It went to several editions and was translated into German and English.

25. JULIUS ARNOLD (1835–1915)

Arnold qualified in Heidelberg contemporaneously with Bunsen (of the burner) and Helmholtz (of the ophthalmoscope). His father was an anatomist and the young Arnold studied in his father's department. He worked briefly with Virchow and then established the department of Pathology in Heidelberg.

26. HANS CHIARI (1851–1916)

Prague and Strasbourg pathologist.

27. MAURICE KLIPPEL (1858–1942)

Klippel published papers covering medicine, psychiatry, pathology and congenital malformations; he also wrote several novels, works of poetry and philosophy. His most significant contributions was probably to confirm the neuropathology of many psychiatric diseases and infections affecting the brain. He was one of the first to recognise the dominance of one cerebral hemisphere.

28. ANDRÉ FEIL (1884–1956)
Paris neurologist. Feil was Medical Adviser to the Renault factories and head of Hygiene and Occupational Medicine in Paris.

29. ALBERT ADAMKIEWICZ (1850–1921)
Adamkiewicz took part in the Franco-Prussian war. He worked with Heidenhain, von Recklinghausen, and in Westphal's neurological department in Berlin before moving first to Cracow and then Vienna. He did a great deal of original work.

30. VLADIMIR MIKHAILOVICH KERNIG (1840–1917)
St Petersburg physician.

31. RUPERT WATERHOUSE (1873–1958)
Waterhouse qualified at St Bartholomew's Hospital and became a pathologist in Bath. His syndrome was described in 1911.

32. CARL FRIDERICHSEN (b. 1886)
Danish paediatrician.

33. ALBERT LUDWIG SIEGMUND NEISSER (1855–1916)
Neisser worked with Wassermann on the complement fixation test for syphilis and with Ehrlich on treatment of syphilis with arsenic. Neisser and Ehrlich were very close friends. He was also interested in leprosy and introduced the scientific world to the work of Gerhard Hansen (1841–1912), the Norwegian who discovered the leprosy bacillus (leprosy was then still endemic in Norway and Iceland). In 1903 the Pasteur Institute, then headed by Metchnikoff and Roux, succeeded in infecting apes with syphilis. Neisser immediately had a large monkey house built in the garden of his house and had as many as 200 monkeys on which to experiment; however they were expensive and disease-prone, so he and two friends financed a private expedition to Java to continue primate experiments with syphilis.

34. SIR WILLIAM BOOG LEISHMAN (1865–1926)
Leishman was born and qualified in Glasgow. He joined the RAMC and was involved in some of the investigations into Malta fever. At Netley, the military hospital, he worked with Sir Almroth Wright who was then Professor of Pathology in the army; he studied phagocytosis and discovered the stain by which he is known. The organism of Leishmaniasis (trypanosomiasis) was discovered in a soldier dying of "dum dum fever". With Wright, Leishman worked on typhoid vaccination, which was tried out first during the Boer War and was remarkably successful when used in British and American troops in the First World War. Oddly, despite Germany's unrivalled knowledge of immunisation, her troops were not at first vaccinated, and consequently she lost many men from typhoid.

35. SIR DAVID BRUCE (1855–1931)
Born in Melbourne, his parents having gone to Australia from Scotland for the Australian gold rush, Bruce qualified in Edinburgh. He joined the army and was posted to Malta. Using Koch's techniques, he investigated Malta fever in the British troops, finding a "micrococcus" in the spleen of a patient with Malta fever (undulant fever). It was not until 1905 that goats were implicated in the causation of undulant fever (brucellosis). Bruce also investigated trypanosomiasis in Zululand, and nagana fever in cattle; he concluded that both were carried by the tsetse fly and were the same disease as the "tsetse fly disease" described by Livingstone in 1858. Bruce and his wife were at Ladysmith during the Boer War. He eventually became commandant of the Royal Army Medical College. His wife accompanied him on almost all his many assignments and acted as his laboratory technician. When she died he was so distraught that he himself was unable to go to the funeral and died while her funeral was taking place.

36. Kálmán Pandy (1868–1945)
Budapest psychiatrist.

37. Carl Friedrich August Lange (b. 1883)
Berlin physician.

38. August Paul von Wassermann (1866–1925)
Berlin bacteriologist.

39. Reuben Leon Kahn (b. 1887)
Lansing, Michigan serologist.

40. Adolf Jarisch (1850–1902)
Jarisch qualified in Vienna and became Professor of Dermatology first in Innsbruck and then in Graz. He was one of the first to study the histology of skin disorders systematically.

41. Karl Herxheimer (1861–1944)
Frankfurt dermatologist, incarcerated and probably killed by the Nazis.

42. George Sumner Huntington (1850–1916)
Huntington was born in Long Island, New York. A family from Suffolk afflicted with Huntington's disease had settled there and had been studied by Huntington's grandfather and father. He documented the clinical and hereditary nature of the condition in 1909.

43. James Parkinson (1755–1824)
Parkinson first published (at the age of 62) his six cases. It was not until 1912 that an American (Rowntree) linked the name of Parkinson with the "paralysis agitans" in the English literature, although on the Continent it had long been known as "maladie de Parkinson". This was due to Parkinson's revolutionary fervour; when young he was in sympathy with the French Revolution. He was thought to have been involved in a rather farcical plot to assassinate George III, and gave evidence which was severely challenged by the Attorney General at the Privy Council. During his lifetime he was better known as a geologist; he lived and worked in the East End of London.

44. Ernest Charles Lasègue (1816–1883)
Lasègue studied under Trousseau and Bernard. He wrote principally about neurology and described the first occurrence of a cerebrovascular accident as "loss of cerebral virginity". He devised his sign when asked by an army Inspector General to expose a recruit who was feigning sciatica; while watching its son-in-law tuning his violin he saw an analogy between the stretched sciatic nerve root produced by disc protrusion and a string stretched over the bridge of a violin.

45. Friedrich Theodor Schwann (1810–1882)
Like Henle, Schwann's significance is much underestimated. By 1838 he had produced his two devastatingly revolutionary ideas; the first was that fermentation was due to micro-organisms, thus anticipating Pasteur, and the second was that the human body is composed of cells. It is difficult to conceive these days that these two ideas probably had as much impact as the publication of Darwin's *Origin of Species*. Schwann, who was a deeply religious man, was sufficiently aware of the significance of the cellular theory to obtain the permission of his archbishop before publishing. Although German he became Professor of Anatomy in Liege (Belgium).

46. GEORGES GUILLAIN (1876–1961)
Paris neurologist.

47. JEAN ALEXANDER BARRÉ (1880–1967)
Strasbourg neurologist.

48. GEORGES FROIN (b. 1874)
Vienna physician.

49. OCTAVE LANDRY (1826–1865)
Landry worked through one cholera epidemic (for which he had a medal struck for him); however, in the next epidemic he died (with Charcot at his bedside). Guillain (1876–1961) always felt that Landry should not have his name associated with the syndrome which he and Barré (1880–1967) later described (because the technique of lumbar puncture had not been developed during Landry's lifetime). Guillain called the linking of his and Barré's name with the syndrome described by Landry as "une confusion nosographique absolue". Landry described ascending paralysis in 1865; Guillain and Barré wrote their paper on the dissociation between the cells and albumin in the CSF in 1916.

50. KARL WERNICKE (1848–1905)
Wernicke qualified in Breslau, where he worked with Neumann and then with Westphal in Berlin. He returned to Breslau and later went to Halle as Professor of Psychiatry. He was killed while riding his bicycle. He described his encephalopathy in 1877. He was opposed to Kraepelin's classification of psychiatric disorders.

51. SERGEI SERGEYEVITCH KORSAKOFF (1853–1900)
Korsakoff qualified in Moscow and was interested in psychiatry, alcoholic dementia and polyneuropathy. He introduced into the psychiatric hospital the system of Pinel, in which psychiatric patients are not restrained, and he advocated the concept of psychiatric hospitals having "family" farms worked by groups of patients.

52. ALOIS ALZHEIMER (1864–1915)
Alzheimer was born in Bavaria, and trained at the medical schools of Berlin, Wurzburg and Tübingen. He worked as a clinician in Frankfurt, where he met Nissl and studied the cellular morphology of the brain. In 1895 Alzheimer followed Nissl to Heidelberg and in 1902 went with Kraepelin to Munich. At Heidelberg, Alzheimer was friendly with Wilhelm Erb. Erb was treating a syphilitic banker who subsequently died. Alzheimer married the widow. In 1912 he was appointed Professor of Psychiatry at Breslau.

53. GUILLAUME BENJAMIN AMAND DUCHENNE (1806–1875)
Duchenne practised in Boulogne, but when his wife died he settled in Paris where he was friendly with Trousseau and Charcot. His inability to have post-mortems performed led him to develop the practice of tissue biopsy, which was more colourfully known as the "histological harpoon", and it is difficult to appreciate to-day the polemics which resulted from this idea of removing living tissue. He also described the function of skeletal muscles by stimulating individual muscles with electric currents.

54. BRIAN MCARDLE (b. 1911)

In 1951 McArdle described the syndrome of apparent intermittent claudication in a 30-year-old man, "George", who could not read or write, who was at a school for backward children, whose father had died when he was a small boy and whose mother had remarried. The remarkable aspect of McArdle's discovery was that he persevered with such a patient, eventually proving that George could not break down glycogen to lactic acid because of an absence of muscle phosphorylase, and that he was not a hysteric.

55. AUGUSTUS VOLNEY WALLER (1816–1870)

Waller was born in Kent, qualified in Paris, then entered general practice in London from 1842–1851. During this time he described nerve degeneration, but then gave up general practice, went to Berlin and worked on the nerve supply of the eye. He then moved to Paris and eventually became Professor of Physiology in Birmingham. His son, Augustus D. Waller, qualified in Aberdeen and was the first to show that the heart produced electrical impulses which could be recorded.

56. ASMUS JULIUS THOMAS THOMSEN (1815–1896)

Danish physician.

7

ENDOCRINOLOGY

Introduction

Endocrinology as a formal discipline began with Claude Bernard's[1] concept of organs of internal secretion and Brown-Séquard's[2] demonstration that death from adrenalectomy could be delayed by infusing blood from healthy animals. In 1902, Bayliss and Starling[3] demonstrated that squashed-up jejunal mucosa injected into a dog produced a rapid flow of pancreatic juice, and the presumed stimulatory substance they called "secretin". The resulting simple concept of a hormone produced by a gland acting at a distance on an end organ has had to be modified considerably with the discovery of the peripheral modulation of hormones and the role of hypothalamic stimulating and inhibitory substances. The simpler concepts have now to be amplified to accommodate new knowledge about the direct effects on other organs of some of the endocrine-gland-stimulating hormones of pituitary origin such as ACTH and TSH. For example, in hypothyroidism there is usually elevation of serum enzymes, particularly CPK and LDH. Increased TSH levels seen in myxoedema cause reduced ATP level in cell membranes, which predisposes to leakage of enzymes from cells.

The trophic hormone ACTH can be split into a number of components, which include alpha and beta MSH (melanocyte-stimulating hormone) and CLIP (corticotrophic-like intermediate peptide). These products have no physiological or pathological actions of their own. However, some tumours produce variants of ACTH, such as a polymer of ACTH ("big ACTH") or breakdown products useful as measures of tumour recurrence. ACTH is now known to be derived from "pro ACTH", which consists of normal ACTH plus lipotrophin (LPH). When ACTH is produced, lipotrophin is also released. Related to LPH are the enkephalins and endorphins which occur in the pituitary, binding to opiate receptors and having morphine-like activity. Thus, related to ACTH are several effects other than its control of adrenal function. It is involved with pain appreciation and response to opiate addiction.

Sometimes this new knowledge raises more questions than it answers; for example, thyrotrophin-releasing hormone (TRH), the hormone which releases TSH from the pituitary, is rapidly metabolised, but the degrading enzymes have to be controlled, in this case probably by circulating levels of thyroid hormones. Another method of influencing hormone action is modulation of hormone receptor sites; this can occur by altering their number or their affinity. In the case of TRH, the number of receptor sites is affected by circulating levels of T3. The prohormone concept, e.g. proinsulin, pro-ACTH and androstenedione (which part can be considered as a prohormone for testosterone), also includes thyroxine (T4), modulated in various peripheral tissues and cells to different breakdown products, and having different actions on different tissues, in a variety of physiological circumstances. For example, in febrile illness, malignancy, beta-blocker treatment and in the fetus, a greater proportion of circulating T4 may be converted to inactive reverse T3 (rT3) than to metabolically active T3. Excessive peripheral conversion of T4 to T3 is one of the factors responsible for T3 hyperthyroidism. One common variety of Graves' disease starts with elevated T3 levels and then progresses to raised levels of T4 as well. However, there are also reports of excess T4 production with normal T3 levels in response to acute illness. There have been reported a few cases of hyperthyroidism in which circulating thyroid-binding globulin is deficient, leading to excess free circulating T4 and T3 but with normal total T4 and T3 levels. The fact that T3 is found in the circulation emphasises the fact that peripheral conversion of T4 is not the only source of T3 (or rT3). It is known that both are secreted by the thyroid gland in response to TSH.

Antibodies to thyroid hormones have been reported; if present, the circulating levels of T4 and T3 may be very high, but they are metabolically ineffective and the patient has clinical features of myxoedema. There is also a situation in which normal circulating levels of hormones are ineffective at the periphery because of presumed alteration in thyroid hormone receptor sites.

THE ACTION OF HORMONES

Hormones act by two main mechanisms. Firstly, reaction with cell membrane hormone receptor sites; this leads to release within the cell of adenyl cyclase which produces cyclic AMP from ATP. The cyclic AMP acts on enzymes which cause cell proteins to be modified. Activated cyclic AMP is associated with increased cellular concentrations of calcium from the mitochondria. Calcium may inhibit the action of cyclic AMP. Calcium is often referred to as the "second messenger." Most peptide hormones act by this mechanism.

The other main groups of hormones, the steroids, act by a different mechanism. These enter the cell and bind with a cell protein, and then enter the cell nucleus and produce messenger RNA, which passes back into the cytoplasm, leading to increased protein synthesis and alteration of cell function.

ENKEPHALINS AND ENDORPHINS

It has been known for many years that some tissues contain opiate agonists and also that, using substances with a minor alteration of structure, antagonism could be produced, which implies that there are also opiate receptors. Opiate receptors in the brain were identified which bind naloxone, an opiate antagonist, as well as opiates themselves. The search was on for endogenous opiates in the brain which were deduced from the already discovered opiate receptors. In 1975 Kosterlitz of Aberdeen described the amino-acid sequence of two such peptides which he called enkephalins. It was established that the enkephalins were fragments of larger molecules (endorphins) which also have opiate activity. These in turn are fragments of a larger molecule from which ACTH is also detached. The release of beta

TABLE XV

THE HYPOTHALAMIC FACTORS IN PITUITARY HORMONE PRODUCTION

Hormone	Acting on	Diagnostic and Therapeutic Use
Thyrotrophin-releasing hormone (TRH)	TSH	Used in TRH test for thyroid function. Hyperthyroidism reduces TSH response to TRH
Gonadotrophin-releasing hormone (Gn-RH)	LH FSH GH	Used as test of pituitary function. Used to induce ovulation. Used to treat gonadotrophin deficiency in acromegaly and craniopharyngioma
Growth-hormone-releasing factor (GRF)	GH	
Prolactin-releasing factor (PRF)	Prolactin	
Growth-hormone-release inhibiting hormone (somatostatin)	GH TSH FSH Insulin Glucagon	
Prolactin release inhibitory factor	Prolactin	Stimulated by bromocriptine.

endorphin from the pituitary parallels that of ACTH and beta lipotrophin. It is now known that there are many different opiate receptors, some of which are specific for individual endorphins. The endogenous opiates are responsible for pain appreciation, the release of some pituitary hormones (GH, ACTH and vasopressin) and the inhibition of others (TSH and gonadotrophins).

Hypothalamic Factors

There are a variety of hypothalamic releasing and inhibitory hormones, some of which are used diagnostically and therapeutically.

THE THYROID

Iodine is absorbed mainly from fish and iodised salt; it is trapped by the thyroid gland so that the concentration of iodide in the thyroid is at least twenty times that in the serum. The trapping of iodide is inhibited by perchlorate and thiocyanate by competition for binding sites in the thyroid. Within the gland, iodide is oxidised to iodine, which is coupled on to mono- and diiodotyrosines, forming triiodo-thyronine (T3) and thyroxine (T4). This coupling takes place within the colloid of the gland. T4 and T3 are attached to the protein thyroglobulin and stored as such in the colloid. When required, T3 and T4 are split off the thyroglobulin by proteolytic enzymes, and then diffuse into the blood stream; the same proteolytic enzymes also split thyroglobulin into mono- and diiodotyrosines which are also freely diffusible. However, they do not normally appear in the blood as such because dehalogenase enzymes split off the iodine. This iodine is conserved in the thyroid; in the absence of dehalogenase, mono- and diiodotyrosines enter the blood stream and are excreted by the kidneys, resulting in loss of iodine from the body and severe iodine deficiency—this is a rare cause of congenital hypothyroidism.

In the serum a small amount of thyroxine exists free, but most of it is bound to an alpha globulin, thyroxine-binding globulin or TBG, which is normally about one-third saturated. If the amount of TBG increases (as in pregnancy) more thyroxine will be carried bound to it, although the quantity of free thyroxine in the serum remains the same. Thyroid-binding globulin is also increased in prolonged pheno-thiazine and clofibrate administration. It is lowered in hypo-proteinaemias, nephrotic syndrome, and in hydantoin and anabolic-steroid therapy. In pregnancy the T4 is raised but the metabolically active free thyroxine is normal. This also occurs in oestrogen therapy and is, therefore, of relevance when women are taking oral contraceptives, because their T4 may be higher than normal. Thyroid-stimulat-ing hormone (TSH) has an effect on all the aspects of thyroxine production from the uptake of iodides to the release of thyroxine from the thyroglobulin by the proteolytic enzymes. Antithyroid drugs such as thiouracil and carbimazole prevent the binding of iodine to the tyrosines, whilst thiocyanate and perchlorate prevent the uptake of iodide by the gland. Iodine can have a paradoxical action by blocking the further production of T4, and occasionally this can result in iodide myxoedema. Patients with Hashimoto's disease who have had thyroid surgery are abnormally sensitive to the blocking effect of iodine. Lithium inhibits release of T4 from its prohormone, thyroglobulin.

The Normal Thyroid Hormones

Thyrotrophin-releasing hormone (TRH).—TRH is rapidly destroyed in the blood by an enzyme which itself is influenced by the circulating level of thyroid hormones. There are also TRH receptors in the pituitary whose number is influenced by the thyroid hormones, the number being decreased by thyroid hormones and so limiting the influence of TRH on TSH secretion.

Thyroid-stimulating hormone (TSH).—TSH is a glycoprotein hormone which consists of alpha and beta chains. The alpha chain is the same as the alpha chain of LH and HCG; the specificity of action is conferred by the beta chain, although separate alpha and beta chains have no action on their own. The pituitary contains an excess of alpha chains. Some tumours produce an excess of circulating alpha or beta chains which have no biological activity but can be used as markers for the tumour. A fragment of TSH may be responsible for the exophthalmos of Graves' disease, although TSH itself, which is present in large amounts in myxoedema, has no exophthalmos-producing ability.

Thyroxine (T4) and triiodothyronine.—Thyroxine is metabolised to a variety of products by removal of a molecule of iodine. The clinically most important of the products are T3 and an isomer of T3 which is metabolically inactive called "reverse T3". It is clear that the peripheral metabolism (mainly in the liver) of the thyroid hormones is extremely complex. T4, T3 and reverse T3 bind to TSH-receptor sites in the thyroid and can block the action of the TSH on the thyroid. The peripheral modulation of hormones is affected by the speed with which receptor sites degrade the occupying molecule; this accounts for variation in stimulating ability which may not relate to circulating hormone levels.

Both T4 and T3 are bound in the plasma to thyroid-binding globulin (TBG). They are also bound to a pre-albumin (T4-binding pre-albumin or TBPA). T3 is not bound to TBPA and less firmly than T4 to TBG. A greater proportion of T3 therefore is free in the plasma.

The mechanisms for maintaining the level of circulating T4 and T3 probably only respond to the level of free hormone. T3 is the active hormone and 80 per cent of it is derived from peripheral conversion of T4; about 20 per cent is secreted by the thyroid. T4 and T3 are metabolised, T4 producing reverse T3 and acetate derivative tetrac. Reverse T3 is inactive, hence the proportion of active T3 and reverse T3 produced from peripheral T4 represents another mechanism for modulating the amount of peripheral thyroid activity. There are some disorders which affect the peripheral conversion of T4 to active T3. If this conversion is reduced the amount of reverse T3 and tetrac is increased. Reduced conversion of T4 to T3 occurs in old age, severe illness, trauma and beta-blocker administration.

Tests of Thyroid Function

Serum thyroxine (T4) and triiodothyronine (T3) levels.—These are now routinely and accurately measured by radioimmunoassay. The protein bound iodine (PBI) test has been largely superseded. The serum levels reflect the bound and unbound hormones; the free hormone levels can be measured, but only with difficulty.

T3 resin uptake and free thyroxine index.—This test is concerned with the amount of thyroid binding globulin which is binding T4. This gives an indirect measure of the amount of free T4. Normally only about a third of binding sites on TBG are occupied by T4. If more sites are occupied the more radioactive-labelled T3 is available for uptake by the resin. Hence the higher the saturation of TBG the higher the resin uptake. It follows that if the binding sites are largely saturated and the total T4 is normal, the quantity of free T4 in the serum is reduced.

The free thyroxine index is the product of total serum T4 and resin T3 uptake. Normally as one goes up the other goes down, so the product stays the same. If however there are more binding sites than normal (for example, if there is more TBG) then the T3 resin uptake is reduced, but the total serum T4 is normal; hence the T3 resin uptake is reduced but the total serum T4 is normal; hence the FTI will fall. If there is a fall in TBG or it is abnormal, the T3 resin uptake is increased, whereas the total serum T4 may still remain normal causing a raised FTI.

Serum TSH.—Serum TSH is raised in hypothyroidism (unless this is due to hypopituitarism). The TSH is low in hyperthyroidism (unless a rare TSH-producing tumour is present in the pituitary).

Thyrotrophin releasing hormone (TRH) test.—When TRH is injected into normal people the TSH level begins to rise after 10 minutes and reaches a peak between 20 and 40 minutes. If the pituitary TSH is being suppressed by increased amounts of thyroid hormone, as in hyperthyroidism, the TSH response to TRH will be less than normal. If hypothyroidism is present the TSH response will be greater than normal.

Radioactive iodine uptake tests and triiodothyronine suppression tests.—These have been largely superseded. The TRH test gives the same information as the T3 suppression test. The iodine or technetium uptake tests are used in the investigation of iodine trapping defects and dehalogenase defects.

Thyroid Autoimmune Antibodies

These are:

> Thyroglobulin antibodies
> Thyroid microsome antibodies
> Thyroid cell membrane antibodies
>> These antibodies may all be elevated in autoimmune thyroiditis (Hashimoto's disease)
> TSH receptor antibodies (TSH R-Ab)
>> Stimulating LATS
>> Non-stimulating LATS protector

Raised thyroglobulin antibodies usually occur in Hashimoto's disease but not in Graves' disease. Thyroglobulin antibodies may occasionally bind in the serum circulating T4 and T3, which are not then effective although apparently present. Microsomal antibodies to thyroid cells also occur frequently in Hashimoto's disease.

HLA status.—HLA – B8 is associated with a higher relapse rate in Graves' disease treated with antithyroid drugs.

HYPERTHYROIDISM

A simple feature of thyrotoxicosis, often overlooked, is that it may be due to two conditions. The first is a diffuse hyperplasia of the gland known as Graves' disease[4] and the second is a toxic nodule (adenoma) which may occur alone or in a gland in which there are multiple nodules. There are a number of working rules with regard to this classification which are useful for clinical purposes.

1. Eye signs only occur in Graves' disease, as do certain other manifestations, such as acropachy and pretibial myxoedema.

2. Patients who have Graves' disease may develop nodules in the gland as a result of repeated hyperplasia and regression.

3. In the absence of hyperthyroidism at the time, patients with some of the extrathyroid manifestations of Graves' disease eventually develop true hyperthyroidism.

4. Graves' disease when accompanied by high levels of antithyroid antibodies usually burns itself out and is best treated with antithyroid

drugs rather than partial thyroidectomy, as the latter will be accompanied by a high incidence of postoperative myxoedema.

GRAVES' DISEASE

Pathogenesis.—1. *Overaction of the autonomic nervous system.*— There is some evidence that psychological stress can cause hyperthyroidism; there is evidence of a sympathetic nerve supply to the thyroid, and that stimulation of the cervical sympathetic supply on one side can result in unilateral increase in thyroid hormone output. Furthermore, the impressive effect of beta blockers on the reduction of thyrotoxic features without affecting raised T4 levels and in the absence of raised catecholamine levels suggests involvement of the sympathetic nervous system.

2. *Disorder of hypothalamic/pituitary axis.* It was found in 1916 that hypophysectomy in amphibians led to failure to metamorphose and to atrophy of the thyroid. In 1931 it was shown that extracts of the pituitary could cause thyroid overactivity. For some years during the 1930s Graves' disease was treated in some centres by pituitary irradiation. However, there were occasional examples of hypopituitarism occurring with Graves' disease and exophthalmos. The hypothesis of altered regulation of TSH became less tenable with the discovery of LATS which is an IgG protein and is dissimilar from the peptides of pituitary origin. However the pituitary is certainly partially involved in the pathogenesis of Graves' disease. TRH tests have demonstrated that TSH secretion is unresponsive to TRH in Graves' disease. Furthermore it has been shown that fragments of TSH are capable of producing exophthalmos.

3. *Autoimmune hypothesis.* In 1956 LATS was discovered, and it was soon identified as an IgG produced by the lymphocytes in Graves' disease. LATS is thought to react with the membrane binding sites of the thyroid which normally responds to TSH. However, LATS is not found in all cases of Graves' disease, and sometimes occurs in normals who do not have Graves' disease. Another IgG, known as LATS protector, which is human specific, also acts as a thyroid stimulator and it is more closely correlated with the presence and severity of Graves' disease than is LATS. Both LATS and LATS protector are antibodies to thyroid plasma membrane antigen. LATS protector is an antibody to TSH receptors in the thyroid; it minimises the action of TSH on the TSH receptors. These thyroid stimulating antibodies therefore increase the secretion of thyroid hormones, inhibit the binding of TSH to receptor, and protect LATS from neutralisation by competing with LATS for LATS neutralising sites in the thyroid; hence the name LATS protector.

Exophthalmos (Havard, 1979)

Mild exophthalmos occurs with virtually all cases of Graves' disease when the thyroid is overactive; however, it can occur in the absence of any disorder of the thyroid, when it is referred to as ophthalmic Graves' disease. Thyroid stimulating antibodies bind to TSH sites in the retro-orbital tissue. TSH can be fragmented to produce EPS (exophthalmos producing substance). In addition a further IgG enhances the action of TSH and EPS on retro-orbital tissue. Thyroglobulin may be the protein which sensitises the retro-orbital tissue to TSH and EPS.

One of the cardinal symptoms of thyrotoxicosis is weight loss. Other features common to hyperthyroidism due to Graves' disease or a toxic nodule are diarrhoea, pigmentation, osteoporosis, myopathy and myasthenia. Features which are associated only with Graves' disease are an increased incidence of Addison's disease, eye signs and thyroid acropachy. The acropachy consists of clubbing and periosteal new bone formation; it is almost invariably associated with pretibial myxoedema and eye signs and is much commoner in males.

The eye signs of Graves' disease may occur in the absence of hyperthyroidism although hyperthyroidism is usually present at some stage of the disease, either before or after the eye signs. The commonest eye sign is lid retraction. This may be present all the time and account for the staring appearance and wide separation of the upper and lower lids or it may be present only when the patient attempts to look upwards (lid lag); in this case the superior rectus muscle is always weak and the levator palpebrae superioris is over-stimulated; both muscles are supplied by the oculomotor nerve and it has been postulated that an abnormal number of impulses pass down the nerve in an attempt to overcome the weakness of the superior rectus; the increased number of stimuli causes the levator palpebrae superioris to over-react.

Malignant exophthalmos is a rare condition and the definitive treatment is open to dispute; however, two procedures which may save the eyes are tarsorrhaphy and surgical decompression of the orbit, in which as much orbital tissue as possible is removed from behind the eye. Local treatment should include Predsol eye-drops (occasionally Predsol eye-drops *increase* the intra-ocular pressure), or guanethidine eye-drops (a "medical Horner's syndrome" is produced). The patient should sleep sitting upright. Other more controversial treatments are:

Thyroxine, on the grounds that TSH or other exophthalmos-producing substances may be inhibited.
Irradiation of the orbit.

High doses of corticosteroids as soon as the malignant exophthalmos begins to get worse.

Total ablation of the thyroid on the grounds that an antigen from the thyroid acting in the orbit causes an inflammatory reaction and exophthalmos.

Hypophysectomy.

Resection of Muller's muscle, which is the smooth-muscle component of the levator palpebrae.

Decompression of the orbit into the ethmoid sinuses.

Treatment of Hyperthyroidism

Graves' disease is usually intermittent and sometimes self-limiting; it can always be controlled with antithyroid drugs. However, these are accompanied by disadvantages which sometimes preclude their use.

The advantages of antithyroid drugs are:

Hypothyroidism is readily reversed.

Convenience and avoidance of a major operation.

In pregnancy, they control symptoms and are not harmful to the fetus in therapeutic doses, although in large doses they may produce goitre in the fetus.

The disadvantages are:

Treatment is long term, and close supervision is essential.

The gland is not reduced in size, hence pressure effects on the trachea will not be relieved and may be made worse. Antithyroid drugs should not be used if a retrosternal goitre is present.

Recurrent thyrotoxicosis is more resistant to drug treatment than the first attack of thyrotoxicosis.

The risk of side-effects from the drugs is always present.

Partial thyroidectomy is more suitable if there is a large goitre, a single nodule, tracheal distortion or relapse following drug treatment. The disadvantages are: damage to parathyroids, recurrent laryngeal nerve palsy, and possible hypothyroidism which is severe and will require life-long substitution therapy. Hypothyroidism developing many years after partial thyroidectomy is much more common than is generally appreciated. Its incidence is much the same as that following radioactive iodine treatment for hyperthyroidism.

In the immediate postoperative period after partial thyroidectomy the main problems are:

Laryngeal oedema
Haemorrhage
Stridor due to recurrent laryngeal nerve palsy

Tetany due to hypocalcaemia as a result of damage to the parathyroid, although this is usually transient.

Thyrotoxic crisis. This is now very rare, but when it does occur it is treated with hydrocortisone, fluid replacement, Lugol's[5] iodine and large doses of chlorpromazine.

Radioactive iodine is selectively concentrated in the hyperplastic gland and is a convenient way of irradiating it. It is conventional to give radioactive iodine only to patients over the age of 45 or if the patient suffers from some other disease which limits life expectancy to less than 20 years, although there is no evidence of an increased incidence of carcinoma or leukaemia following radioiodine. Radio-iodine is usually the treatment of choice for restrosternal goitre or for a recurrence of thyrotoxicosis following a partial thyroidectomy. The risk of myxoedema is more than with drugs or partial thyroidectomy, and about a third of patients develop transient myxoedema. The incidence of hypothyroidism increases each year following the treatment, hence patients need long-term follow up.

Radioactive iodine may be used for treating a single toxic nodule without any danger of myxoedema, because only the "hot" nodule will take up the radioiodine; the remainder of the thyroid being quiescent, it will not take up the radioiodine and will receive little or no irradiation. The disadvantage of treating "hot" nodules in this way is that it takes up to a year for the nodule to disappear.

In the treatment of thyrotoxicosis by antithyroid drugs the most suitable drug is carbimazole, which inhibits the organic binding of iodine to iodotyrosines in the formation of thyroxine. Other drugs such as thiouracil are used only if the patient develops side-effects to carbimazole. Potassium perchlorate is a drug which prevents the uptake of iodide by the gland; very occasionally a combination of perchlorate and carbimazole is used to treat a recalcitrant case. The starting dose of carbimazole is usually about 40 mg and this is continued for one month; thereafter the dose is reduced when the patient is euthyroid as judged by weight gain, normal pulse rate and improvement in thyrotoxic symptoms; 5 mg a day are given for 2–3 months. The symptoms do not usually begin to improve for two weeks after the drug has been started. It is obviously of great importance to tell the patient this.

In order to reduce the incidence of myxoedema, thyroxine is sometimes given with carbimazole; this has the disadvantage that much larger doses of carbimazole have to be used, with a consequent increase in side-effects which, on the standard dose, are minimal. The most important side-effects are agranulocytosis and aplastic anaemia. When the patient has remained euthyroid on the minimum dose for two months the drug can be stopped and a T4 estimation performed after a further two months. Thereafter, the patient should return if there is a recurrence of symptoms.

Carbimazole is used to make patients euthyroid before partial thyroidectomy, and it is given four weeks before the operation is due; iodide is given two weeks before the operation to reduce the vascularity of the gland which carbimazole causes as well as for its antithyroid effect. It is important to note that if iodine is given for a longer period, the vascularity of the gland increases again.

Biochemical evidence of thyroid activity following antithyroid drugs can be obtained by estimating the T4 and T3 two months after the drugs have been stopped. Radioactive iodine uptake by the thyroid is increased after antithyroid drugs and may remain so for some time even if the patient is euthyroid. However, evidence of suppression of I^{131} uptake with triodothyronine indicates that the thyroid is under the influence of TSH and that the patient is probably euthyroid.

Some Special Problems

Diagnosis and treatment during pregnancy.—The free thyroxine index is the best guide to the presence of thyrotoxicosis. Treatment with antithyroid drugs in the correct dose is generally better than thyroidectomy. Hypothyroidism during pregnancy should be treated with triiodothyronine (T3) rather than thyroxine (T4) because it crosses the placenta better.

Monitoring treatment (rarely necessary).—The radioactive iodine uptake tests after 2½ hours are affected by the antithyroid treatment; however the 20-minute radioactive uptake tests are *not* affected by treatment. Thyrotoxic patients who have gone or will go into remission will have a normal triiodothyronine suppression test. Non-suppressibility of the gland after six months' anthithyroid treatment indicates that sustained remission is unlikely and this is an indication for ablative thyroid therapy, either partial thyroidectomy or radioactive iodine therapy.

Thyroid function after thyroidectomy.—Free thyroxine index is the most reliable guide.

HYPOTHYROIDISM

The causes of hypothyroidism are:

> Primary failure of the thyroid (primary myxoedema)
> Autoimmune thyroiditis (Hashimoto's disease)
> Secondary failure of the thyroid due to pituitary failure (secondary myxoedema)
> Prolonged iodine deficiency

Antithyroid substances in the diet or given therapeutically
Inherited enzyme defects
Thyroidectomy or radioactive iodine therapy.

Primary Myxoedema and Hashimoto's Disease

The histology of the gland in these two conditions is very similar and the incidence of antithyroid antibodies in Hashimoto's disease is nearly 100 per cent, while in primary myxoedema it is about 60 per cent. The antithyroid antibodies are antibodies against thyroglobulin and an antigen within the thyroid cells. In Hashimoto's disease the patient may be euthyroid or hypothyroid; there is a high output of TSH and if the gland is not too badly damaged it can be stimulated to produce enough thyroxine to keep the patient euthyroid at the expense of developing a goitre—the alternative is a goitre with some hypothyroidism. However, in the end the patient always develops myxoedema. Occasionally, the patients with thyrotoxicosis have antithyroid antibodies and histological changes in the thyroid similar to those of Hashimoto's disease—these patients always end up eventually with myxoedema, and are usually treated with antithyroid drugs rather than partial thyroidectomy, because the drugs can be stopped as soon as the patient is euthyroid or hypothyroid. The diagnosis of Hashimoto's disease can be confirmed by the high levels of antithyroid antibodies and biopsy of the thyroid gland. The treatment of Hashimoto's disease is replacement therapy with thyroxine, which will inhibit TSH and reduce the size of the gland. If the gland remains large after thyroxine treatment, partial thyroidectomy is performed. Corticosteroids are not normally used.

The cause of Riedel's thyroiditis is not known. The gland is usually very fibrotic and the fibrosis may involve other structures in the neck.

Myxoedema Secondary to Pituitary Failure and Iodine Deficiency

Myxoedema due to pituitary failure is usually accompanied by a deficiency of ACTH and consequent adrenal hypofunction, as well as a failure of TSH secretion. Unlike other forms of myxoedema, the serum cholesterol is usually normal. The condition can be separated from myxoedema due to thyroid damage by the TSH stimulation test. If the thyroid itself is damaged, TSH will not affect radioiodine uptake or T4 levels, whereas if the thyroid itself is normal, exogenous TSH will stimulate it to take up radioiodine normally. In pituitary failure there is usually absence of body hair, and the skin is of fine texture despite the myxoedema. Occasionally when pituitary failure has been present for a long time, the thyroid itself may atrophy and will sometimes not respond to TSH.

Treatment of secondary myxoedema is by replacement with thyroxine. It is of the utmost importance to treat any coincidental adrenal hypofunction first, as treatment of myxoedema in the presence of adrenal hypofunction will precipitate an Addisonian crisis.

Prolonged iodine deficiency results in compensatory thyroid enlargement in an attempt to utilise all available iodine in the blood—the thyroid is extremely avid for iodine. Following this compensated state, frank hypothyroidism may ensue. The Medical Research Council have suggested that all table salt in this country should have iodide added to it.

Antithyroid substances.—Thyroid enlargement and hypothyroidism can occur with PAS, phenylbutazone, resorcinol and antithyroid drugs. Occasionally, excess iodides can cause hypothyroidism—the reason for this is not known. Certain foods and contaminants are goitrogenic, particularly the Brassica group of vegetables (cabbage and kale), swedes and turnips.

Inherited enzyme defects.—These are uncommon causes of myxoedema and goitre, but interesting from the point of view of inborn errors of metabolism. They are all inherited as autosomal recessives—the homozygote has goitre and hypothyroidism, whereas the heterozygotes usually have a goitre with normal thyroid function.

The enzyme defects are:

Iodide trapping defect

Defect in binding iodine with tyrosine: this is associated with congenital deafness (Pendred's syndrome)

Defect of coupling iodotyrosines to form thyroxine and triiodothyronine

Dehalogenase deficiency (tinker's disease) in which excess loss of iodine occurs in the urine.

Abnormal thyroxine-binding globulin, which is metabolically inactive and is unable to bind thyroxine.

Clinical Features of Myxoedema

The "myxoedema" is an accumulation of mucoprotein and water; an increase in body fat is not a cardinal clinical feature of myxoedema and the apparent obesity is due to the mucoprotein accumulation. Because of the lowered metabolic rate the patients are intolerant of cold, and their temperature is often subnormal. The slight yellow colour of the skin is due to deposition of carotene; normally carotene is converted to vitamin A, but in hypothyroidism the reduced metabolism slows this conversion so that carotene tends to accumulate. In the gastro-intestinal tract, motility is slowed so that constipation occurs and absorption across the intestinal mucosa is slower than normal resulting in a flat glucose tolerance curve.

The heart is involved in several ways: atheroma and coronary artery disease are more common, a pericardial effusion may occur, the myocardium itself may be damaged resulting in a diffuse fibrosis and a cardiomyopathy, and finally, adequate thyroxine is necessary for the proper metabolism of myocardial cells. The electrocardiogram may show a generalised reduction in voltage which is sometimes, but not invariably, due to a pericardial effusion, or there may be non-specific wave inversion and bradycardia. Most of the ECG changes are rapidly reversed when thyroxine is administered.

Anaemia is common in myxoedema and is due to several factors:

> Diminished peripheral oxygen requirements result in a physiological reduction in the red cell mass causing a normochromic, normocytic anaemia.
> Accompanying achlorhydria may contribute to an iron deficiency, microcytic, hypochromic anaemia.
> Pernicious anaemia occurs more commonly in myxoedema than in normals.

One of the most useful and constant signs of myxoedema is delayed relaxation of the tendon jerks. Occasionally the carpal-tunnel syndrome is a feature due to pressure from mucoprotein on the median nerve where it passes under the flexor retinaculum in the wrist. One presentation of myxoedema of great practical importance is a non-specific psychosis—"myxoedematous madness".

Hypothermia

Myxoedema coma is accompanied by hypothermia (defined as a rectal temperature below 90°F. or 32°C.)—the ordinary clinical thermometer does not read below 95°F. so that a special low-temperature thermometer should be used in a suspected case.

Any case of hypothermia should be suspected of suffering from myxoedema; hypothermia may also be precipitated by infection, chlorpromazine, Tofranil and other antidepressant drugs. The important physiological disturbances of hypothermia are:

1. Intense muscular rigidity which impairs ventilation of the lungs leading to an accumulation of carbon dioxide and respiratory acidosis. The respiratory centre is driven by the anoxic stimulus, hence oxygen therapy alone may be harmful.

2. Metabolic acidosis due to accumulation of metabolites in muscles. This may be more severe during rewarming, when muscular activity may be greatest due to the onset of shivering.

3. The cardiac output is reduced, but the blood pressure is often normal due to intense vasoconstriction; the viscosity of the blood is

also markedly increased. The characteristic J-wave may be seen in the ECG.

4. Renal and hepatic function are impaired.

5. There is an inability to utilise glucose, despite high blood levels of both glucose and insulin.

It is important to note that the normal methods of measuring blood gases and acid-base balance may be misleading. These estimations are normally performed at 37°C. Table XVI (Hockaday and Fell, 1969) shows that in hypothermia the true value is different from the apparent laboratory level.

TABLE XVI

	27°	37°
pH	7·19	7·32
Pco_2	80	52
Po_2	85	43
O_2 saturation	95·6	92
(HCO_3)	29·5	32·5

In the treatment of hypothermia it is recommended that rewarming should take place gradually in old people—the patient is put in a warm room and covered with blankets. In the case of young patients who have suffered from immersion in cold water, it is suggested that rewarming should be faster, and the patient should be placed in a warm bath. If respiratory acidosis is present, mechanical ventilation either via a tracheostomy or endotracheal tube will be required; respiratory stimulants such as nikethamide are justified in milder cases. Hydrocortisone and glucose are given intravenously, even though the blood glucose is sometimes high; there is probably always some adrenal insufficiency in the presence of hypothermia. Adrenal failure and hypoglycaemia will certainly be present if hypothermia is due to pituitary failure. The metabolic acidosis is corrected with parenteral bicarbonate. Hypothermia due to myxoedema is treated with a small dose of triiodothyronine, in addition to the other supportive measures. Arterial blood only should be used for the determination of electrolytes and blood gases, as venous blood is virtually completely stagnant in severe cases.

Confirmation of myxoedema.—The laboratory diagnosis of myxoedema is much less precise than that of hyperthyroidism. No one test is entirely suitable, and in practice reliance is usually placed on the clinical features, PBI, serum cholesterol and CPK. The presence of antithyroid antibodies is suggestive of thyroid damage, although the titre of antibodies is no guide to the severity of the thyroid lesion.

Radioiodine tests alone are of limited value; however, used in conjunction with TSH stimulation, they are probably about the best laboratory tests.

Treatment of Hypothyroidism

L-thyroxine is given in a dose of 0·1 mg daily for 2–4 weeks and then is gradually increased until the patient is euthyroid. The usual maintenance dose is 0·2–0·4 mg daily. Elderly people, and those with coronary artery disease, should be started on a lower dose and the dose increased more gradually, with frequent monitoring of the patient's symptoms and ECG; there is great danger of precipitating angina and cardiac failure if the condition is corrected too rapidly. The patient is judged to be euthyroid on clinical grounds and by the sense of well-being. PBI estimations are higher than the clinical state of the patient would suggest, due to binding of the administered thyroxine by TBG.

Carcinoma of the Thyroid

Most thyroid cancers are well-differentiated into papillary (with long columns of cells) and follicular in which almost normal thyroid follicles are seen. The minority of carcinomas are undifferentiated or anaplastic; these are commoner in the elderly and are treated with external irradiation and surgery if they are compressing the trachea or other structures in the neck.

Papillary carcinomas are unlike all other carcinomas in that they are equally common in all age groups and furthermore they are not more malignant in the younger age groups. Some thyroid carcinomas are dependent on TSH; hence the administration of thyroxine, which will reduce endogenous TSH, leads to regression, and this is particularly true of the papillary type. Papillary carcinomas tend to metastasise to local lymph glands and to be very slow growing—the primary may be exceedingly small. Follicular carcinomas are commoner in the older age groups and metastasise via the blood vessels, the contralateral lobe of the thyroid is involved in over half the cases. They commonly develop in a previous long-standing goitre.

Well-differentiated (papillary and follicular) carcinomas and their metastases do take up a small amount of radioiodine, but very much less than normal thyroid tissue. For this reason, any "cold" nodule, i.e. one which does not take up much radioiodine, should be assumed malignant until proved otherwise—a benign cyst will also appear as a "cold" nodule on a thyroid scan.

As a general rule, well-differentiated thyroid carcinoma is treated with total removal of the thyroid and the local lymph glands if they are involved with growth. Following thyroidectomy, radioiodine scanning and excretion tests are performed. The scan will reveal any radioiodine accumulation in carcinoma remnant or metastases and the excretion test will measure the amount of radioiodine retained in the remnants.

One of the greatest problems is that both primary and metastatic thyroid carcinomas only concentrate a small amount of radioactive iodine; however, they can be made to take up more radioactive iodine by: removing all normal thyroid tissue, stimulation with TSH, and administration of carbimazole, which increases the vascularity of the tumours.

Normal thyroid tissue is removed either by thyroidectomy or a dose of radioiodine. Opinions differ as to which is the best way of promoting the tumours and their metastases to take up iodine; whichever method is employed large doses of radioiodine are given once the tumours have been made as iodine-avid as possible. Further doses of radio-iodine may be necessary if excretion and uptake tests indicate that tumour deposits are still present.

THE ADRENAL CORTEX

One of the problems which has bedevilled adrenal physiology for the non-expert is the varied terminology used for the adrenal steroids.There are three groups of adrenal hormones all ultimately derived through intermediaries from pregnenolone and cholesterol:

Cortisol
Aldosterone
Adrenal androgens.

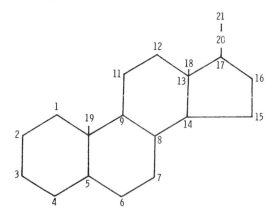

Fig. 35.—This shows the numbering of the carbon atoms on the basic 4-ring structure of all steroids.

TABLE XVII

THE VARIATIONS IN ATTACHMENT TO THE BASIC 4-RING STEROID STRUCTURE OF DIFFERENT GROUPS
OF THE MAIN ADRENAL STEROIDS

Steroid carbon atom to which each group is attached	Pregnanelone	Progesterone	Cortisol	Aldosterone	Adrenal Androgens	Testosterone	Oestrogen
C3	OH	=O	=O	=O	=O Androstenedione –OH (DHEA)	=O	OH
C11	–	–	OH	–	–	–	–
C18	CH_3	CH_3	CH_3	CH0	CH_3	CH_3	CH_3
C17	–R=O	–R=O	<ROH	–R=O	=O	–OH	–OH

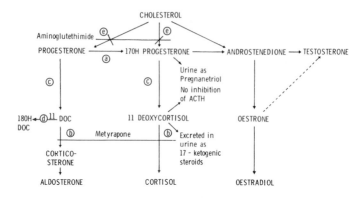

FIG. 36.—This shows the production of the steroid hormones together with their precursors and the site of action of various enzyme deficiencies and blocking drugs.

Site of Defect	Result of Defect
a	17α hydroxylase deficiency leads to cortisol deficiency and increased ACTH which increases corticosterone, causing salt retention and hypertension. There is also reduced sex-hormone production.
b	11β hydroxylase deficiency (or metyrapone administration) leads to reduced cortisol and therefore increased ACTH and raised deoxycorticosterone and other intermediaries, which leads to hypertension. It also causes raised progesterone and androgens (and therefore virilism). Metyrapone causes low cortisol levels and raised ACTH, leading to increased deoxycortisol, which is excreted in the urine as 17-ketogenic steroids.
c	21 hydroxylase deficiency. This is the commonest enzyme defect and results in reduced aldosterone and cortisol and therefore salt loss. 17 OH progesterone accumulates and leads to increased androgens and virilisation, and increased pregnanetriol in the urine.
d	Isolated increase in 18 DOC hydroxylase will lead to 18 OH DOC excess and hypertension.
e	Aminoglutethimide inhibits steroidogenesis and has been used to treat Cushing's disease and secreting adrenal carcinomas.

Aldosterone and its metabolites in the urine cannot be measured in routine clinical practice.

All adrenal androgens have a ketone ($=O$) group at C17. Ovarian and testicular androgens have an OH group at C17 but are metabolised to 17-ketosteroids.

The adrenal androgens are excreted in the *urine* as 17-ketosteroids and so are testicular and ovarian androgens. Normally two-thirds of the urinary ketosteroids are derived from adrenal androgens.
Cortisol has an OH group and a side-chain at C17
Cortisol is metabolised by three reactions:

1. C11 OH group becomes ketone group
2. C3 ketone group becomes an OH group. When there is a side-chain on C17 (as in cortisol) these substances can be measured by the Porter-Silber chromogens (used more in the USA than in the UK)
3. Changes in the side-chain at C17.

All three of the metabolites in 1, 2, and 3 can be treated to remove the side-chain from C17 and to add a ketone group at C17 instead, converting them to 17-ketosteroids. The amount of urinary 17-ketosteroids derived from C17 side-chain plus OH group substances (all from cortisol) can be calculated if the amount of 17-ketosteroids derived from adrenal androgens has already been estimated. These derivatives of cortisol which yield ketosteroids when treated are called ketogenic steroids. The 17-ketogenic steroids are therefore measures of cortisol production. 17-hydroxycorticosteroids (17-OHCS) are urinary derivative which contain a 17-OH group and side-chain on C17 (all derived from cortisol). They are measured by a different method from that used to produce the derived value for 17-ketogenic steroids mentioned above. Cortisol is usually measured in the blood indirectly by measuring either the plasma 17-OHCS or the plasma 11-OHCS, both of which positions of the OH group are reasonably specific for cortisol, although the 11-OHCS will include some 11-OH androstenedione.

CUSHING'S[6] SYNDROME

Like malabsorption this is a condition in which a high clinical index of suspicion is important if mild cases are not going to be missed. The incidence of the well-known manifestations varies in different series but most agree that in over 75 per cent of the cases obesity, hypertension, glycosuria and hirsutism will be present. Other impressive initial features are muscular weakness, depression and osteoporosis. One point worth emphasising is that the disease often fluctuates and spontaneous improvement may occur. Suggestive simple laboratory investigations are a diminished lymphocyte and eosinophil count, elevated blood sugar and a hypokalaemic alkalosis.
The diagnosis of Cushing's syndrome falls into three parts: 1. suspicion; 2. confirmation; 3. finding the cause. Cushing himself

described the clinical features of excess cortisol excretion which he attributed to a pituitary basophil adenoma causing excess ACTH production. The exact role of the pituitary in the pathogenesis of bilateral adrenal cortical hyperplasia is not certain. Histological changes in the basophil cells of the pituitary can occur following corticosteroid therapy and small pituitary tumours can be demonstrated in up to one-half of the patients with Cushing's syndrome.

The syndrome is caused by:

> Bilateral adrenal hyperplasia usually due to excess pituitary ACTH: 80 per cent
> Benign adenoma: 5 per cent
> Adrenal carcinoma: 1 per cent
> Carcinoma elsewhere: 15 per cent
> Rarely, adrenal hyperplasia occurs in the absence of excess pituitary ACTH

In approximately 10 per cent of cases of adrenal hyperplasia due to excess ACTH the adrenals develop nodular hyperplasia. This type represents the adrenal equivalent of tertiary hyperparathyroidism, in the sense that the hyperplastic adrenal becomes more or less autonomous and that suppression of pituitary ACTH with dexamethasone may not result in suppression of steroid output from the adrenals. It is important to appreciate that the adrenals frequently also develop multiple adenomata which are not pituitary induced, and the increased steroid output causes low levels of ACTH. *But* dexamethasone response is the same in both types, for in the latter type the multiple adenomata are already autonomous, so that suppression of ACTH with dexamethasone is irrelevant.

Confirmation of the Clinical Diagnosis of Cushing's Disease

The fundamental abnormality is increased secretion of cortisol (hydrocortisone) from the adrenal cortex. Cortisol secretion rates can be estimated using radioactive labelled steroids but this is still a research tool and is not available for general use. Other measurements are used as circumstantial evidence of increased cortisol production. The most important of these are:

> Serum level of cortisol at any one time
> Urinary free cortisol excretion
> 24-hour urinary excretion of 17-hydroxycorticoids (17-OHCS)
> 24-hour urine excretion of 17-ketogenic steroids (17-KGS).

There is a diurnal variation in the rate of cortisol secretion by the adrenals; at night, during sleep, the need for adrenal steroids is low; at the beginning of the day the secretion and, therefore, the blood level is high. In Cushing's syndrome this diurnal variation is lost and output of cortisol is more or less constant throughout the day and night.

Many laboratories estimate the 24-hour urinary excretion of 17-hydroxycorticoids and 17-ketogenic steroids to confirm the diagnosis of Cushing's syndrome; however, it is worth pointing out that these estimations may miss many patients who have Cushing's syndrome. The most conclusive evidence of Cushing's syndrome is the demonstration of failure of the diurnal rhythm of cortisol secretion. This can be demonstrated simply by finding a high level of serum cortisol or hydroxycorticoids in the late evening or at midnight. Obesity can cause a real increase in the urinary ketogenic steroids, which fall to normal when the patient regains a normal weight; one point of practical importance is that ketone bodies in the urine (which may occur during strict weight reduction) may interfere with the estimation of the urinary ketogenic steroids.

Confirmation of the Cause

Metyrapone test.—This is really a test of the ability of the pituitary to respond by producing more ACTH to a negative feedback stimulus. *Metyrapone* inhibits the adrenal 11-beta-hydroxylase enzyme and therefore blocks cortisol production at the level of 11-deoxycortisol, which, unlike cortisol, does not inhibit ACTH production. In normals there is a rise in ACTH levels in the blood and an increase in 17-ketogenic steroids in the urine. In Cushing's disease caused by increase in ACTH there is no rise in urinary ketogenic steroids since ACTH output is already maximal. There are unfortunately some false positives with adrenal adenomas and ectopic ACTH production.

The dexamethasone suppression test.—This is used much less often now than previously because patients with obesity and severe depression may not suppress normally, and adrenal adenomatas may suppress. A shortened form of suppression test has been advocated in which a dose of dexamethasone is given at midnight and serum cortisol estimations performed the following morning.

Patients with Cushing's syndrome from any of the causes mentioned produce excess cortisol which is not controlled by ACTH; reduction of the plasma ACTH level will not reduce the output of cortisol from the adrenals. In the normal, cortisol production is controlled by ACTH and any reduction of ACTH causes a lowered cortisol output. ACTH output from the pituitary can be diminished by administering a powerful steroid such as dexamethasone, which has the great advantage of not being broken down to hydroxycorticoids, and hence urine and blood estimation of hydroxycorticoids are not altered by the dexamethasone itself. The diagnosis of Cushing's syndrome may be confirmed if there is failure to suppress the level of plasma cortisol or hydroxycorticoids, or the 24-hour urine excretion of 17-hydroxycorticoids with dexamethasone (2 mg daily for two days).

In obesity and hyperthyroidism there is an increase in the rate of metabolism of cortisol, and therefore the urinary metabolites of cortisol (17-ketogenic steroids and 17-hydroxycorticoids) are increased. The circulating levels of cortisol are, however, normal.

Treatment of Cushing's Syndrome

Bilateral hyperplasia.—There are two orthodox approaches, one is bilateral adrenalectomy and the other is partial ablation. Pituitary ablation is the treatment of choice if there is evidence of high ACTH output or if the pituitary fossa is enlarged. The disadvantage of total adrenalectomy is that the pituitary continues to pour out ACTH and may develop a chromophobe adenoma (Nelson syndrome). This may be a serious complication and the pituitary tumours may become locally malignant. For this reason the pituitary approach is most frequently recommended. Later the adrenals can be removed if there is evidence that they have become partly autonomous.

Adenoma or carcinoma.—These are treated by surgical removal; the opposite adrenal will be atrophic and is not removed.

Ectopic ACTH production.—The commonest primaries to produce ACTH are bronchus and thymus. The patient is usually thin, severely pigmented and has profound uncontrollable hypokalaemia. Death usually occurs from the adrenal hyperfunction; if the prognosis of the primary tumour warrants it total bilateral adrenalectomy is indicated.

Addison's[7] Disease

The main causes of Addison's disease are:

Idiopathic adrenal cortical atrophy
Tuberculosis
Pituitary-hypothalamic disorders such as suppression of ACTH production by therapeutic corticosteroids
Other replacements of the adrenals such as amyloidosis and sarcoidosis
Haemorrhage or infarction of the adrenals.

It is worth emphasising at the outset that nine-tenths of both adrenals have to be destroyed before the clinical features of Addison's disease are seen, and even people with only a small amount of functioning adrenal tissue left are able to survive without stress; but in a stress situation which demands increased steroid output they will develop features of adrenal insufficiency. It is not known how many patients develop undiagnosed adrenal insufficiency following stress situations such as an emergency operation or myocardial infarction, but it is probably more common than is generally appreciated. American workers lay emphasis on the value of an eosinophil count— in a stress situation the increased output of cortisol in a normal person will lower the eosinophils below $50/mm^3$ but in a patient with adrenal insufficiency the eosinophil count is above $50/mm^3$.

Idiopathic adrenal cortical atrophy accounts for at least half the cases of Addison's disease in this country. In this group there is a high incidence of anti-adrenal and antithyroid antibodies, there is also a higher-than-normal incidence of thyrotoxicosis, myxoedema, diabetes, hypoparathyroidism, atrophic gastritis and pernicious anaemia.

Clinical features of importance (which are so common in a gastro-enterological clinic that Addison's disease may not be suspected) are weight loss, vomiting, abdominal pain and diarrhoea.

Some of the metabolic effects of cortisol are not well understood; this is partly due to the fact that cortisol has some mineralocorticoid activity like aldosterone, but it is not known to what extent aldosterone is also deficient in many cases of Addison's disease. What *is* known is that aldosterone is not controlled by ACTH. Cortisol seems to be essential for the proper functioning of a large number of structures, for example:

Renal tubules.—Without cortisol the renal tubules are unable to dilute the urine, so they cannot excrete a sudden water load. It is possible that cortisol normally acts in competition with ADH, and so in cortisol deficiency ADH can act unopposed. Cortisol appears necessary for aldosterone to be able to exert its action on the renal tubules. One of the features of prolonged Addison's disease is dehydration, possibly because in the absence of cortisol aldosterone is unable to retain sodium and water. Note that Addison's disease has two effects on water excretion: on the one hand there is dehydration, possibly because of end-organ unresponsiveness to aldosterone, and on the other there is inability to excrete an increased water load at normal rate, presumably as a result of tubular dysfunction in the absence of cortisol.

Blood vessels.—Cortisol is necessary for the blood vessels to respond to circulating catecholamines; hence, the appearance of hypotension in Addison's disease and the improvement in clinical shock that may occur when hydrocortisone is given. In Addison's disease there is failure of the normal arteriolar reflexws; despite hypotension there may be peripheral vasodilatation.

Gastro-intestinal tract.—In Addison's disease there may be increased excretion of faecal fats, suggesting that cortisol is necessary for the functional integrity of the small-intestinal mucosa. The hypoglycaemia and weight loss of Addison's disease are also due to this mechanism.

Glomerular filtration.—This is generally reduced in Addison's disease and is probably the cause of the rise in blood urea which occurs.

Diagnosis

A chest x-ray, abdominal plain x-ray and Mantoux test are necessary to pick up those cases due to tuberculosis; idiopathic atrophy of the adrenals does not cause adrenal calcification. It is important to pick up those cases due to tuberculosis because replacement therapy with corticosteroids may light up the dormant tuberculosis. Most patients with Addison's disease do not have tuberculosis as the cause; they have an autoimmune cause and the adrenal antibodies are usually raised as are other organ-specific antibodies such as antithyroid, intrinsic factor and antiparietal-cell antibodies. As with Cushing's disease the laboratory diagnosis involves first of all confirming the clinical diagnosis and then discovering the cause.

The diagnosis of Addison's disease is confirmed by administering exogenous ACTH and estimating the steroid output before and afterwards; either the serum cortisol or hydroxycorticoids or the urinary 17-hydroxycorticoids are measured. The ACTH is usually given intramuscularly as this diminishes the incidence of allergic reactions compared with giving it intravenously. Synacthen is a synthetic preparation of ACTH which does not produce allergic effects, however, its duration of action is short.

Besides primary failure of the adrenals due to atrophy or replacement there may be adrenal insufficiency for two other reasons: first the pituitary-adrenal axis may be impaired, and secondly the pituitary or hypothalamus may not be able to respond normally to stress. In pituitary-adrenal axis dysfunction the normal feed-back mechanism of cortisol is impaired, so that the pituitary does not put out more ACTH in response to a lower level of cortisol. Cortisol itself is the only substance which will inhibit ACTH secretion from the pituitary. The precursors of cortisol do not inhibit ACTH but are excreted in the urine as 17-hydroxycorticoids.Metopirone (metyrapone) is a substance which blocks the synthesis of cortisol at a late stage so that the feed-back mechanism is destroyed, but the early precursors of cortisol are still produced and excreted as 17-hydroxycorticoids. Thus, if Metopirone is given to a normal person cortisol will be diminished, ACTH will be secreted stimulating the adrenal to produce more cortisol (via its precursors), but cortisol production is blocked so that the increased precursors are excreted in the urine as excess 17-hydroxycorticoids. In a patient with pituitary-adrenal axis dysfunction the fall in cortisol after Metopirone is given does not stimulate the production of more ACTH, so that the urinary level of 17-hydroxy-corticoids from cortisol precursors does not rise. It is essential to note that before the Metopirone test is performed the adrenals must be shown to function normally in response to an injection of ACTH. It should also be noted that impairment of the feed-back mechanism does not mean that the adrenals cannot respond normally to stress. The response to stress involves stimulation of the pituitary or hypothalamus which then stimulate the adrenals. The hypothalamus stimulates the pituitary to produce ACTH by a corticotrophin release factor. Lysine vasopressin (lypressin) is a substance which acts like the corticotrophin release factor and can be used to assess the ability of the pituitary and adrenal to respond to potentially stressful situations. Insulin-induced hypoglycaemia also stimulates the secretion of corticotrophin release factor but the hypoglycaemia has to be quite profound.

Treatment of Addison's Disease

In an Addisonian crisis the patient will require cortisol, water, saline and glucose quickly. Replacement therapy is with cortisone and fludrocortisone 0·1 mg b.d.

WITHDRAWAL OF LONG-TERM STEROIDS

The four problems are:

1. Relapse of the disease for which they were prescribed.
2. Reduction of adrenal mass and therefore reduced cortisol output (aldosterone is not affected because it is not under ACTH control).
3. The fact that with steroid withdrawal symptoms may occur which are unpleasant but do not necessarily indicate danger. Nausea, malaise, and aches and pains occur on steroid withdrawal.
4. Impairment of pituitary ACTH-releasing mechanism
   (a) under normal circumstances
   (b) under stress circumstances.

The fourth problem, in practice, is the greatest. Usually the adrenals take several months to recover if the dose of prednisolone has been over 20 mg/day and has been given for a year or more; occasionally however the adrenals recover quickly even after prolonged therapy. Fortunately the estimation of plasma cortisol is not affected by simultaneous administration of prednisolone, neither is the measurement of urinary 17-ketogenic steroids or 11-hydroxycorticosteroids. In general, urinary measurements are preferable to plasma measurements, since the binding globulins may be avid for even small amounts of cortisol, giving falsely high plasma levels. The regime for reducing steroids is:

1. Cut prednisolone to physiological levels, i.e. 5·0–7·5 mg per day.
2. Perform short, and if necessary long, ACTH or Synacthen stimulation tests to establish if the adrenals can produce endogenous cortisol.
3. If they do not, ACTH injections will be needed to restore the adrenal cell mass to normal; this should take 3–4 weeks of daily ACTH.
4. If the adrenals do respond to ACTH stimulation, the level of circulating ACTH should be measured and if there is detectable ACTH and the adrenals can produce cortisol, the prednisolone can be cut from 5·0 mg per day to 5·0 mg on alternate days for 4 weeks, then stopped.
   On the day on which the prednisolone is not given, many patients will get non-specific symptoms of malaise and odd joint pains.
5. Low or absent levels of circulating ACTH mean that the alternate-day regime of prednisolone must be continued for much longer. After 6 months the ACTH level should again be measured and an ACTH stimulation test performed. ACTH may need to be given for 4–5 days before a maximum adrenal response is observed. ACTH may need to be given to restore the adrenal mass.
6. Once the patient is off steroids, a prolonged Metopirone (metyrapone) test will establish the ability of the pituitary to produce ACTH. Patients should be warned that under periods of stress the adrenal reserve may not be enough and there may be continued impairment of the ACTH-releasing mechanism. Patients should receive physiological doses of prednisolone if they develop a severe infection or require an operation.
7. The ability to respond to stress can be tested by insulin-induced hypoglycaemia after which ACTH and cortisol are measured, although it is not often necessary to perform this test. It is safer to assume reduced adrenal and pituitary reserve for 2 years after steroids have been stopped.

   Fortunately there is evidence that if the adrenals and pituitary ACTH-releasing mechanism are suppressed, the ACTH-releasing mechanism usually recovers before the adrenals. In practice this means that if the adrenals have recovered (as shown by producing cortisol in response to ACTH), it can usually be assumed that the pituitary has also recovered.

DIABETES

Definition of Diabetes (British Diabetic Association)

Potential diabetes.—A normal glucose tolerance test with:
(1) Both parents diabetic
(2) Identical twin a diabetic
(3) One parent diabetic and the other parent having a near relative a diabetic
(4) A woman who has given birth to a baby weighing 10 lb or more.

Latent diabetes.—A normal glucose tolerance curve which is known to have been diabetic in type during pregnancy, stress or obesity.

Asymptomatic diabetes.—No symptoms of diabetes but where the glucose tolerance test is diabetic in type.

Clinical diabetes.—A diabetic glucose tolerance test with symptoms and/or complications of diabetes.

Pre-diabetic.—This refers to the period in the life of a diabetic before the diagnosis is made.

Diagnosis

The incidence of diabetes is increasing in the developed countries, which is probably due to the prevalence of obesity and the longer average survival of the individual, because there is a deterioration in glucose tolerance with age, even in non-diabetics.

A number of factors are known to be associated with the development of diabetes and there are large numbers of undiagnosed patients who either have diabetes or who are destined to develop it. It is not yet established whether the complications of diabetes can be prevented by prompt and careful treatment.

Patients who have a high risk of developing diabetes are said to have pre- or latent diabetes; the three factors which are known to increase the risk are a family history, giving birth to overweight babies and an abnormal stress glucose tolerance curve. Corticosteroids delay the uptake of glucose by the peripheral tissues and any tendency to develop diabetes will be reflected in an abnormally high glucose blood level after corticosteroids have been given (stress glucose tolerance test). A person who has a normal glucose tolerance test but who has had an abnormal one in a period of stress (e.g. pregnancy, infection or obesity) is also a pre-diabetic.

The oral glucose tolerance test is still the method of choice to confirm the diagnosis of diabetes. It is influenced by a number of factors other than the presence of diabetes: a previous low carbohydrate intake will produce a diabetic type curve, there is also a small increase in blood sugar in women, and with ageing. The level of blood sugar attained will also be affected by disorders of absorption. The intravenous glucose tolerance test has not circumvented these difficulties, and in practice is no more suitable than the oral test in distinguishing diabetics from non-diabetics.

Aetiology and Pathogenesis

There are often genetic as well as acquired factors responsible for the development of glucose intolerance. There are a few patients in whom one group of factors is predominant. About a third of diabetics give a history of diabetes in a close member of the family. There is a rare diabetic syndrome which is purely inherited and is often referred to as DIDMOAD which is an acronym for the main features: diabetes insipidus, diabetes mellitus, optic atrophy and deafness.

Diabetes may be classified in management terms into those who require insulin and those who do not. These two types are referred to as Type I juvenile onset or IDD (insulin dependent diabetes) and Type II maturity onset or NIDD (non-insulin dependent diabetes). There is some evidence of a genetic aetiology in both types.

Type I is associated with the presence of certain histocompatibility antigens (HLA), whereas most Type II cases are not related to HLA status. However, there is a form of Type II diabetes which is inherited as an autosomal dominant; in this form there is evidence of glucose intolerance, but it occurs in relative youth and does not require insulin; it is referred to as MODY, an acronym for maturity onset diabetes of youth. There are also ethnic differences in the diabetic syndrome which are not readily explicable in terms of diet and different environmental factors. Diabetes in one of its various forms often accompanies a wide variety of inherited disorders. The incidence of diabetes in the offspring of diabetic parents is not usually more than 10 per cent, suggesting that "idiopathic" diabetes may be due to a large number of different inheritable factors.

The incidence of diabetes in monozygotic (identical) twins varies in different series but it is certainly not 100 per cent. Concordance refers to the presence of a disorder in both members of a twin pair, and discordance refers to the disorder in only one member of a pair. In identical twins diabetes is usually concordant if there is also evidence of diabetes in a close member of the family, and when the diabetes develops after age 40 (Pyke and Nelson, 1976).

There are significant correlations between Type I diabetes and HLA status, particularly HLA−BY and BW 15. There is also a *negative* correlation with HLA−B7. The situation is complicated by the fact that defective insulin production, transport, uptake and utilisation may play a part in the pathogenesis of diabetes (see Table XVIII).

Table XVIII

Possible Causes of Hyperglycaemia Related to Defect of Insulin in Different Sites

Site	Abnormality of insulin
Beta cell	Defective synthesis of pro-insulin
	Defective conversion of pro-insulin to insulin
	Defective release of insulin
	Abnormal structure of insulin
Circulation	Abnormal insulin binding
	Abnormal permeability of vessel walls to insulin
Liver	Excessive degradation
	Excessive binding of insulin
Target cells	Defective membrane receptor
	Defect in adenyl cyclase system
	Defect in rate-limiting enzymes

In both the main types of diabetes there is usually a deficiency in insulin production although in Type II the circulating insulin levels are only slightly below normal. It is *not* now believed that insulin output is actually increased in this type of diabetes, if the appropriate correction factors are used in interpreting insulin levels when obesity is present. In Type I diabetes there is lymphocyte infiltration and hyalisation of the pancreatic islet cells (islets of Langerhans[8]). There are also antibodies against islet cells (PICA—pancreatic islet cell antibodies) early in the disease but these usually disappear later, although there is a sub-type in which the islet-cell antibodies persist much longer (Type 1B).

Insulin is synthesised in the beta cells from pro-insulin, a large, single-chain polypeptide which splits into two by removal of a connecting strand of 35 amino acids known as C-peptide. The resulting two peptide chains form the double-chain insulin molecule. Insulin and the C-peptide are stored together in granules and are discharged together by the appropriate hyperglycaemic stimulus. Insulin release is biphasic and is ultimately dependent on calcium mediated contraction of the storage granules. In order to stimulate insulin release the perfusing glucose itself must react with glucose receptors on the beta cells. Insulin secretion is stimulated by other factors such as amino acids and the gastro-intestinal hormones, which explains why insulin release is greater when glucose is given orally than when given parenterally. The C-peptide, always being secreted with insulin, can be used as an indicator of endogenous insulin production. It can be used to document a phenomenon sometimes observed soon after the onset of Type I diabetes, in which there is often temporary reduction in exogenous insulin requirement (the honeymoon or Brush effect) and evidence of an increase in endogenous insulin production. The temporary reduction in insulin requirements may be due to reduced glucagon synthesis, reduced requirement due to removal of hyperglycaemia and temporary recovery from islet viral change before the development of secondary autoimmune viral damage. Diabetics who are difficult to control usually have no evidence of any endogenous insulin production.

The relatively high levels of insulin in Type II diabetes are due to a reduction in the number of insulin receptors on the surface of cells. The failure of insulin to promote the uptake of glucose by the cells results in a persisting high level of glucose and further stimulation of insulin production. For unknown reasons reduction of obesity causes the number of peripheral insulin receptors to increase.

There is now some evidence that Type I diabetes may be caused by the interaction of three aetiological factors. The first is related to inherited HLA status, the second to virus infection and the third to an immunological reaction. In children, diabetes may follow a serious viral infection and the establishment of diabetic registers has shown new cases of diabetes with remarkable clustering in the winter months. The part immunological aetiology is postulated on the basis of increased antibodies to islet cells early in the onset of diabetes. (Bloom, 1978).

The binding of protein and polypeptide hormones to surface receptors must occur before the hormones can influence the target organ. However, circulating hormone can be bound by receptor sites without initiating a response. In Type II diabetes there is known to be a deficiency of insulin receptor sites; receptor sites may also develop an enhanced ability to degrade insulin and antibodies to receptor sites may develop, all of which may lead to insulin resistance. In Type I diabetes there may be an autoimmune basis. Type I diabetes occurs more frequently in other autoimmune diseases such as idiopathic Addison's disease, there are sometimes thyroid and gastric antibodies present in diabetes, and there may be islet-cell antibodies detectable in a majority of newly diagnosed diabetics.

Management of Diabetes

Hyperglycaemia, glycosuria and ketonuria are still the main parameters by which control of diabetes can be judged. Longer-term control can be assessed by the level of HbA_{1c} (glycolysated haemoglobin). The level in normal adults is about 5 per cent of normal haemoglobin; in poorly controlled diabetics the level rises to over 15 per cent. The level of HbA_{1c} reflects the control of diabetes over the preceding 3–4 weeks.

The level of blood sugar at which glycosuria occurs varies in different individuals. Before relying on levels of glycosuria to adjust insulin dosage it is essential to determine the renal threshold for glucose; this is usually done during the glucose tolerance test. The objectives in treating diabetes will depend on the type of diabetes, the age of the patient and the complications present. Type I diabetes requires insulin treatment to avoid ketoacidosis, weight loss and other complications.

Insulin

Insulin consists of two amino-acid chains; the smaller A chain contains the antigen sites. Pro-insulin consists of the two insulin chains linked by another peptide chain (the C-peptide) which is removed when the insulin is secreted. The C-peptide, which is biologically inactive, is secreted in the same proportion as insulin itself. In high concentrations or in the presence of divalent cations (such as zinc) insulin forms hexamers. Pork insulin differs from human insulin in only one amino acid, whereas beef insulin differs in four and is therefore more antigenic.

The number of commercial insulins available in the UK are now so many that some confusion from proprietary names which are rather similar is inevitable. In Canada, Australia, New Zealand and the United States all insulin is now supplied as 100 units per ml (called U100). In the UK also from 1983 all insulin is available as U100.

There are no commercial sources of human insulin; all insulin comes either from beef cattle or pigs. Porcine insulin differs from human insulin by only one amino acid, bovine insulin differs by four amino acids; of the two, therefore, there are marginal advantages in porcine insulin. When insulin was first manufactured in 1922, the University of Toronto, in which it was discovered by Banting and Best, established an institute to standardise insulin strength, and licensed certain manufacturers to produce it commercially. Among these was the Novo company of Copenhagen. Workers in this same company discovered the value of certain divalent cations, such as zinc, in prolonging the action of insulin. The Novo company have continued to produce insulin and were the first to produce highly purified insulins (monocomponent insulins). When extracted from animal sources insulin contains contaminants and breakdown products as well as pro-insulin, all of which may be antigenic. The production of highly purified insulins leads to lower levels of antibody formation, although the practical value of this is still debatable. There is no real evidence that the complications of diabetes are related to circulating insulin antibody levels, nor that insulin resistance is directly related to antibody production. However, there are some advantages in using monocomponent insulins, such as the undoubted lower incidence of insulin-induced lipoatrophy.

Table XIX
Examples of Commercial Insulins

			Duration of Action	Source
Actrapid MC	Novo		0–6 hours	Pork
Velosulin (HP)	Nordisk		0–6 hours	Pork
Semitard MC	Novo	Amorphous	4–10 hours	Pork
Ultratard MC	Novo	Crystalline	8–30 hours	Beef
Insulatard (HP)	Nordisk	Crystalline	4–20 hours	Pork (Isophane)
Monotard MC	Novo	Mixed amorphous & crystalline	6–20 hours	Pork suspension
Rapitard MC	Novo	25% Actrapid 75% Ultratard	2–20 hours	Beef/Pork
Mixtard (HP)	Nordisk	30% Velosulin 70% Insulatard	0–20 hours	Pork
Initard (HP)	Nordisk	50% Velosulin 50% Insulatard	0–20 hours	Pork

The easiest regime to get used to is: Twice-daily injections of a mixture of Velosulin and Insulatard, or twice-daily Mixtard or Initard. Whenever possible patients should be persuaded to have twice-daily injections of insulin as this ensures much smoother control of blood sugar. The regime of a mixture of Velosulin and Insulatard is the best because the dose of the short-acting and intermediate-acting insulin can be altered independently depending on the individual patient's meal-times and physical activities.

In older patients who require insulin, the need for the best possible control is less because there is less time for the development of the complications of diabetes. The main aim in these patients is to avoid ketoacidosis. A suitable once-daily regime is a mixture of Monotard and a variable amount of Actrapid to combat the early-morning and after-breakfast hyperglycaemia.

Insulin Resistance

Occasionally patients on insulin require very high doses. Only rarely is this due to insulin antibodies; these antibodies are present, sometimes at high levels, in all diabetes treated with conventional insulins. The most usual cause of insulin resistance is a disturbance of insulin receptors due to excessive surges in blood sugar and insulin levels. The insulin resistance in these patients can usually be abolished if they are treated with continuous low-dose insulin infusion for several days.

The Somogyi Effect

Excess of long-acting insulins given in the morning may lead to nocturnal hypoglycaemia which is, of course, asymptomatic because it occurs during sleep. The hypoglycaemia results in a rebound hyperglycaemia and glycosuria in the morning specimen of urine; as a result the patient gives himself *more* insulin, and so the cycle is repeated.

Type II—Maturity Onset Diabetes

In the majority of maturity-onset diabetic patients dietary control alone should be sufficient. It is unwise to give sulphonylurea drugs if the patient is overweight as they may induce mild hypoglycaemia, which merely increases his appetite. The three main sulphonylureas are chlorpropamide, tolbutamide and glibenclamide. Tolbutamide has to be given at least twice a day, but in the elderly this is a positive advantage because chlorpropamide is liable to cause nocturnal hypoglycaemia. The drugs are excreted by the kidneys so that minor degrees of renal impairment will further delay the excretion of chlorpropamide and its metabolites, which also have hypoglycaemic properties. The sulphonylureas often take two weeks or more to exert their maximum hypoglycaemic action. Generally tolbutamide is the safest drug, particularly if there is renal or hepatic impairment. There are a number of other sulphonylureas, and whereas none is clearly superior to the older drugs, individual patients may respond to one better than another. The sulphonylureas probably act by increasing endogenous insulin secretion and by reducing the production of glucose by the liver. All the sulphonylureas produce hypoglycaemia and with chlorpropamide this effect of the drug may last for several days. They are protein bound and therefore may be displaced by certain drugs such as salicylates, probenecid, phenylbutazone and oral anticoagulants. Chlorpromazine may inhibit the action of sulphonylureas.

With chlorpropamide facial flushing may occur with alcohol in genetically susceptible individuals. The sulphonylureas also have effects not related to their effect on blood sugar. For example, chlorpropamide has an antidiuretic action in patients with diabetes insipidus; this is believed to be due to potentiation of very small amounts of ADH. Tolbutamide has the opposite effect and increases water excretion.

The UGDP Controversy

In 1970 the University Group Diabetes Program in the USA, which was trying to establish whether diabetic complications could be influenced by the quality of diabetic control, published evidence that there was an increased incidence of cardiovascular complications in overweight, middle-aged, asymptomatic diabetics. There may be doubts about the long-term benefits of using sulphonylureas and the UGDP controversy has underlined the importance of treating overweight diabetics with strict dietary treatment before starting sulphonylureas.

Biguanides

These compounds promote the uptake of glucose by the cells in the presence of small amounts of insulin and they reduce gluconeogenesis in the liver. They cause an increase in blood lactate and pyruvate; because of this they are prone to result in lactic acidosis. Phenformin is not used in the USA. Metformin is less likely to cause lactic acidosis. Metformin is indicated in maturity-onset diabetes if weight reduction has not been achieved or has not resulted in normoglycaemia. They are sometimes used with a sulphonylurea if the sulphonylurea alone has not been successful. The biguanides may cause weight loss largely as a result of gastric irritation. Metformin should be given with meals—a daily dose of 500–1000 mg may be necessary.

Quality of Control and Incidence of Complications

Table XVIII (p. 431) shows the possible causes of hyperglycaemia related to insulin; if one adds to these the other factors known to influence the blood glucose, such as glucagon secretion, cortisol secretion, catecholamine secretion and vasoactive intestinal polypeptide, it is not surprising that there is continuing debate on whether good control of diabetes prevents its complications. Even good control is difficult to define; in the non-diabetic the blood sugar varies very little even after a meal or starvation. Constant monitoring of the blood sugar even in well controlled diabetics shows surprising fluctuations of blood sugar levels over quite short periods. It is well documented that complications are frequently absent many years after the onset of insulin-requiring diabetes.

The complications of diabetes are almost always attributable to changes in the microvasculature of the eyes, kidneys and arteries, due to thickening of the capillary basement membranes. The neuropathies and cataracts may be related to deposition of fructose and sorbital, because the insulin lack results in failure to metabolise glucose through the normal glycolytic pathway. The damage to the capillary basement membranes may be due to slight tissue hypoxia resulting from changes in the oxygen dissociation curve of haemoglobin: a slight shift of the curve to the left increases the affinity of haemoglobin for oxygen and therefore reduces the release of oxygen at tissue level. The uptake of oxygen by haemoglobin is influenced by 2-3-diphosphoglycerate (DPG) and uptake is increased by low levels of DPG. The often persistent mild acidosis of diabetes influences haemoglobin synthesis, leading to the formation of increased amounts of variants of normal haemoglobin which have a *high* oxygen affinity. These haemoglobins are known as HbA_1 and normally comprise about 5 per cent of normal haemoglobin A. The main HbA_1 which are sometimes called "fast" haemoglobins because on chromatography they move faster than normal HbA, is HbA_1C, which differs from normal haemoglobin in that the amino group of the beta chain is occupied by glucose and is unable to react with 2,3,DPG, which results in a haemoglobin with high oxygen affinity but which is more stable than normal HbA and therefore is less willing to give up oxygen in the tissues. These haemoglobins, which are attached to glucose, are also called glycolysated haemoglobins. Increased levels of these glycolysated haemoglobins remain elevated for 3–4 weeks, even although diabetes is brought under control, following an episode of ketoacidosis. Measurement of HbA_1C therefore gives a measure of the quality of control in diabetes over the preceding 3–4 weeks.

There are in addition other important abnormalities in diabetes which contribute to the damaging complications.

These are:

Increased platelet aggregation
Increased blood viscosity
Decreased spontaneous fibrinolytic activity in the blood
Hypertriglyceridaemia
Decreased lipolytic activity of plasma

Probably a fair generalisation of current policy is to advise manipulation of diet and insulin so as to avoid large changes in the blood sugar throughout the 24 hours. Most studies agree that those patients who seem to have been well controlled have less vascular disease than those who have been poorly controlled. However, this controversy is still unresolved; experienced diabetologists can cite good evidence to support either viewpoint.

Diabetic Ketoacidosis

It is now believed that ketoacidosis in diabetics is not simply due to insulin deficiency. It has long been known that hypophysectomised and pancreatectomised patients do not usually develop severe ketoacidosis, and there is now evidence that increased amounts of glucagon and cortisol are present early in the development of ketoacidosis. Furthermore, those factors known to precipitate ketoacidosis such as infection, trauma and myocardial infarction are all associated with increases in cortisol, glucagon and catecholamine output. The precise cause of coma in ketoacidosis is still obscure; there is, for example, no obvious correlation between levels of consciousness and levels of ketones and pH, although there is a relationship to increased plasma osmolality.

Hyperglycaemia occurs because of reduced peripheral uptake of glucose and increased hepatic gluconeogenesis because of failure to suppress adenyl cyclase in the liver cells through insulin deficiency. Increased lipolysis is necessary to produce the substrates for increased gluconeogenesis. There is an excess of acetyl coenzyme A produced from fatty-acid breakdown, and this is not sucked into the Krebs cycle because of a simultaneous inhibition of citrate synthetase activity. (Normally acetyl coenzyme A combines with oxaloacetic acid to form citrate and so enters the Krebs cycle.) The acetyl coenzyme A is metabolised instead of acetoacetate and ketones.

Treatment of Ketoacidosis

The mortality from ketoacidosis is still 10–15 per cent and most cases have lost at least 5·0 litres of fluid as well as 500 mmol of sodium and potassium. Most cases are precipitated by infection and it is usual to give a broad-spectrum antibiotic whether or not there is definite evidence of infection. This is particularly so if it is decided to catheterise the patient; most physicians feel that catheterisation is necessary and that the dangers of introducing infection have been overemphasised. In the elderly an accurate measure of central venous pressure is necessary to prevent fluid overload.

Fluids

The high blood glucose causes an osmotic diuresis and the patient is severely dehydrated; the excess loss of water in the urine causes secondary salt depletion. Thus, patients in diabetic coma are short of both salt and water but the shortage of water is the greater. It is usually safe enough to give 3 litres of normal (isotonic) saline; if there is evidence of severe haemoconcentration then the saline can be given with an equal volume of water. One disadvantage of giving solutions which are more dilute than plasma is that they may cause haemolysis. Half normal saline should be used if the serum sodium is raised. There is a danger of rapid decrease in extracellular osmolality, particularly if there is also a rapid fall in glucose and urea levels. This fall in extracellular osmolality can precipitate cerebral oedema.

The most suitable replacement fluid is 0·5 normal saline. Often 3–4 litres will be required in the first 6 hours. When the blood glucose level has fallen the saline can be replaced by 5 per cent dextrose. The risks of circulatory overload and intravascular haemolysis should be always considered.

Insulin

Treatment of diabetic ketoacidosis has been simplified and improved by the introduction of constant insulin infusion in doses lower than those which were previously thought necessary. Soluble or Actrapid insulin are infused intravenously in a dose of 5–10 units per hour. These low doses of insulin have been shown to reduce liver production of glucose (reduced gluconeogenesis) and to promote the uptake of glucose by peripheral cells. Insulin given intravenously has a half-life of only about 5 minutes; it is therefore not surprising that continuous infusion of smaller doses of insulin are as effective as boluses of much larger doses. It is known that diabetics with ketosis are relatively insulin resistant and this resistance may be increased by hypothermia, acidosis, infection and insulin antibodies.

The general policy is to infuse insulin in a dose of 5 units per hour increasing to 12 units per hour if the blood sugar continues to rise after the first hour.

Potassium

In ketosis the total potassium deficit is often 500 mmol. The usual regime to give 20 mmol per hour of potassium increasing this to 40 mmol per hour if the potassium level falls below 4·0 mmol per litre.

Bicarbonate

There is still debate about the importance of correcting the metabolic acidosis with bicarbonate. Insulin may be less effective in the presence of acidosis, and severe acidosis may cause vasodilatation, hypotension and reduced cardiac output. Nonetheless, bicarbonate may precipitate hypokalaemia because bicarbonate causes a reduction in hydrogen ion concentration both outside and inside the cells, and potassium enters the cells in exchange for hydrogen. Rapid reversal of acidosis may have a deleterious effect on the oxygen dissociation curve and can cause a paradoxical lowering of pH in the CSF. If bicarbonate is used, these counter arguments should be considered.

The number of milliequivalents of bicarbonate which the patient may require is calculated by considering the level of the serum bicarbonate and hence the number of milliequivalents per litre that he is depleted, remembering that the normal serum bicarbonate is 25 mEq per litre. The bicarbonate ion is both an intracellular and an extracellular ion and it has been found empirically that bicarbonate is distributed through a volume (in litres) equivalent to one-quarter of the body weight in kilograms, i.e. in a 60 kg man this will be 15 litres. For example, if the serum bicarbonate is 15 mEq/1 then each litre is (25 − 15) mEq short of bicarbonate; there are 15 litres to be considered so that the patient requires $15 \times (25-15) = 150$ mEq. This is given as isotonic sodium bicarbonate (which contains 167 mEq of sodium and bicarbonate per litre).

It is essential to monitor the electrolytes, acid-base status and blood sugar at frequent intervals (at least hourly for 3–4 hours). One hour after the first dose of insulin has been given the blood sugar is repeated. If the blood sugar has risen the dose of insulin is doubled, if the blood sugar remains the same the same dose of insulin is infused, and if the blood sugar is falling the insulin infusion rate is reduced. After 3–4 hours most patients develop hypokalaemia, so that potassium has to be given; this is best administered as potassium chloride into the infusion bottle (1 g of potassium chloride contains 13·4 mEq potassium).

Phosphate

In diabetic ketoacidosis there is phosphate depletion which may be made worse by fluid replacement and insulin treatment. Phosphate depletion causes depletion of diphosphoglycerate (DPG) in the red cells. Low levels of DPG shift the oxygen dissociation curve to the left and decrease the oxygen which can be delivered to the tissues. It is thought that high doses of phosphate may prevent the depletion of DPG.

The other facets of treatment of diabetic coma are:

Antibiotics to counteract probable precipitating infection
Gastric tube to prevent gastric atony and vomiting
Catheterisation of the bladder
Treatment of hypotension.

Hyperosmolar coma.—Sometimes a mild diabetic has some impairment of glucose metabolism but not enough to cause the body to turn to fat as a source of energy, and in these patients there may be a rise in blood sugar but no ketosis. The rise in blood sugar promotes an osmotic diuresis and the patient becomes severely dehydrated and eventually comatose. The hall-marks of this condition are, therefore, severe haemoconcentration (with a high serum sodium and packed-cell volume), hyperglycaemia and glycosuria, but little or no ketosis. These patients require large amounts of fluids and only small amounts of insulin. Occasionally mild diabetes presents as hyperosmolar coma and when the patients recover they usually give a history of a sudden onset of a craving for sweet foods (and liquids) some weeks before.

Hypoglycaemia

At a serum level of 2·0 mmol/1 of glucose there will usually be symptoms of hypoglycaemia, although it is important to note that some normal people tolerate a blood level of 1·7 mmol/1 without developing symptoms and others develop symptoms of hypoglycaemia at a higher level if there has been a rapid fall from a previously high level.

The precise clinical manifestations of hypoglycaemia depend on the speed of onset, the level to which the blood sugar falls and the degree of cerebral atherosclerosis. The early symptoms are hunger, nausea, tremor palpitations and sweating, which may progress to personality change and automatism with subsequent amnesia (subacute neuroglycopenia). Chronic neuroglycopenia refers to the state in which persistent low blood sugars result in organic cerebral damage which eventually leads to dementia. The important causes of hypoglycaemia are:

1. Functional hypoglycaemia. This occurs two hours after a meal and is due to excessive outpouring of insulin in response to the meal. It tends to occur in the psychiatrically ill.
2. Excessive insulin or sulphonylureas.
3. Liver disease.
4. Post-gastrectomy and malabsorption states.
5. Early diabetes. In the early stages there may be attacks of spontaneous hypoglycaemia after meals. In early diabetes there seems to be a delayed response to a meal but when the response does occur excess insulin is produced causing hypoglycaemia.
6. Sensitivity to alcohol.
7. Addison's disease and pituitary failure.
8. Insulinoma.
9. Non-pancreatic neoplasms, such as mediastinal or retroperitoneal sarcoma, hepatic carcinoma and adrenal tumours.
10. Pregnancy. In diabetics who become pregnant the dose of insulin required usually increases. However, following delivery there is a sudden fall in insulin requirement and failure to appreciate this may lead to profound hypoglycaemia.
11. Liver and renal disease. These can both contribute to hypoglycaemia in diabetics, probably because of reduced breakdown or excretion of insulin. In renal failure there is often retention of guanidine, which is known to cause hypoglycaemia.
12. Autonomic neuropathy. In long-standing diabetics the development of autonomic neuropathy affecting the sympathetic system may lead to loss of warning symptoms that hypoglycaemia is developing.

Diagnosis

1. Plasma insulin levels. The insulin is inappropriately high for the level of hypoglycaemia if an insulinoma is present. Also the C-peptide level is raised.
2. Prolonged fast. Normal subjects have a normal blood sugar even after a fast of 72 hours. If an insulinoma is present patients will develop symptoms usually after 24–48 hours' fast.
3. Tolbutamide test and glucagon test. These tests are not usually necessary if an insulinoma is present, because the fasting test will be positive. They are highly specialised tests and should not be performed casually.
4. The clinical relevance of C-peptide measurements firstly are in the estimation of beta cell reserve, when the presence of insulin antibodies prevents the measurement of insulin, and secondly as a test for insulinomas, in which the pro-insulin level does not fall in the presence of hypoglycaemia. Pro-insulin measurements are useful in the detection of islet-cell tumours in which pro-insulin levels may be much higher than insulin levels.

Acromegaly

There is still doubt as to whether acromegaly is primarily a disorder of the pituitary or of the hypothalamus. Certainly growth-hormone production can be reduced by infusion of the growth-hormone-release-inhibiting hormone (somatostatin), but this hormone also reduces the output of other hormones such as insulin, glucagon and vasoactive intestinal polypeptide (VIP).

The mortality of acromegalics is approximately twice that of normals. The diagnosis of acromegaly is confirmed by finding high levels of growth hormone during a glucose tolerance test in which insulin secretion is stimulated. There is a poor correlation between the levels of growth hormone and the severity and progression of acromegaly. Acromegaly which is causing pressure symptoms from enlargement of the pituitary fossa should be treated by direct pituitary surgery. Bromocriptine, a dopamine agonist which increases growth hormone in normals, has an unexplained paradoxical action in acromegaly in that it reduces growth hormone secretion in most patients. Prolactin levels are also raised in some cases of acromegaly; bromocriptine may lead to a reduction in the raised prolactin levels which may be the cause of the impotence and loss of libido often occurring in acromegaly. Bromocriptine causes nausea and constipation; it should always be given with meals, and started in small doses which are gradually increased to the optimum dose.

Hirsutism

Idiopathic hirsutism is caused by a disturbance of the adrenals *and* ovaries. In some women in whom all the known virilising hormones and their precursors are normal it is necessary to postulate an increased sensitivity of hair follicles to normal amounts of circulating hormones. Testosterone and small amounts of oestrogen are transported in the blood bound to a specific globulin, sex hormone binding globulin (SHBG); only about 1–2 per cent of total testosterone is unbound, but this is the form in which it is active. Alteration in the binding properties of the protein or displacement of testosterone may result in virilism. Androgens decrease the amount of SHBG while oestrogens increase it: this may be one of the mechanisms by which oestrogens sometimes improve hirsutes, that is, by increased SHBG binding more testosterone. Reduced levels of SHBG may result in increased circulating levels of unbound hormone. The difficulties are compounded by the fact that some non-virilising hormones may be converted at cellular level into virilising hormones. In women, up to 50 per cent of circulating testosterone is of adrenal origin, derived from androstenedione, although only a small minority of patients with Cushing's disease have hirsutism. If a small increase in the circulating testosterone is derived from androstenedione it can be suppressed with dexamethasone. When confronted with a patient who complains of hirsutism it is necessary to obtain a detailed history of menstruation, drug taking, date of onset, weight gain and familial propensity to hirsutism. Physical examination would aim to demonstrate signs of Cushing's disease, hair distribution and amount and other evidence of virilisation such as voice change, acne and clitoral enlargement.

The main causes of hirsutism are:

Idiopathic
Polycystic ovaries (Stein[9]-Leventhal[10] syndrome)
Adrenal hyperplasia
Ovarian tumours
Adrenal tumours.

In idiopathic hirsutism both ovarian and adrenal androstenedione (which is derived from progesterone) and testosterone levels may be slightly raised. Androstenedione may be converted in the liver and the skin into testosterone. There is no clear differentiation between idiopathic hirsutism and the polycystic ovary syndrome, although the periods are usually regular in the former and very irregular in the latter. In the polycystic ovary syndrome the testosterone and androstenedione levels may be raised in addition to the serum gonadotrophin (LH) level being elevated, while the specific sex hormone binding level may be reduced. In idiopathic hirsutism and the polycystic ovary syndrome, serum prolactin levels may also be raised as one of the causes of the hirsutism. Insofar as any of the causes of hirsutism may result in increased quantity of C19 steroids with a ketone group in the 17 position, there will be elevation in the 24-hour urinary 17-ketosteroids. The 17-ketosteroids may contain a contribution from C21 steroids, and so an increase in the virilising hormones in the plasma may not be reflected in raised urinary 17-ketosteroids (which are derived from metabolites and precursors of cortisol and progesterone). When virilism is due to adrenal or ovarian tumours, the urinary 17-ketosteroids cannot be suppressed with dexamethasone 2 mg/day; if they do suppress, an ovarian or adrenal tumour is unlikely.

There are several varieties of congenital adrenal hyperplasia syndrome, but the commonest is partial absence of the 21-hydroxylase enzyme which is normally involved in the synthesis of cortisol and aldosterone (see Fig. 36). If cortisol production is reduced, ACTH is produced in excess, leading to overproduction of those adrenal hormones not dependent on the 21-hydroxylase enzymes; these are mainly virilising hormones. Occasionally the raised ACTH levels bring the cortisol levels back to normal if the 21-hydroxylase deficiency is only partial. Congenital adrenal hyperplasia usually causes virilisation and salt loss in childhood, but some cases present after the menarche in which case menstruation may be normal. Cases of suspected congenital adrenal hyperplasia should not be given ACTH. The cases of congenital adrenal hyperplasia presenting as hirsutism in adult life nearly all have raised levels of urinary pregnanetriol, derived from progesterone which is increased by the failure of ACTH inhibition from normal levels of glucocorticoids.

Treatment of Idiopathic Hirsutes

Apart from the usual cosmetic treatments if no cause is detected, the usual treatment is to try to suppress the presumed slightly excessive ACTH drive by giving a small dose of prednisolone (7·5 mg per day). 5·0 mg of this should be given at night to suppress the normal morning surge of ACTH. This treatment is usually required for at least 6 months before any beneficial effect is to be seen. If prednisolone suppression fails, cyclical oestrogens should be given a 6-month trial (these may act by increasing SHBG or decreasing the sensitivity of hair follicles to circulating androgens). Cyproterone inhibits the effects of androgens on hair follicles; it should not be used in women who could become pregnant. Cyproterone also suppresses ACTH slightly; this effect may be masked by the fact that metabolites of cyproterone in the urine may colorimetrically resemble those of cortisol.

Investigation of Hirsutism

Full clinical assessment
Exclude Cushing's disease by

> diurnal cortisol
> urinary 17-ketogenic steroids (17-hydroxycorticoids)
> urine free cortisol test
> ACTH levels

Plasma testosterone
Serum luteinising hormone (LH)
Urinary 17-ketosteroids (as a measure of adrenal and ovarian androgens)
Sex hormone binding globulin level
Plasma androstenedione (an androgenic metabolite of progesterone)
Prolactin
Dexamethasone suppression test if either testosterone or urinary 17-ketosteroids raised. If there is no suppression, an ovarian or adrenal tumour should be suspected. If the testosterone suppresses, polycystic ovaries are likely. If the 17-ketosteroids suppress, congenital adrenal hyperplasia (or Cushing's disease) is likely. Congenital adrenal hyperplasia is confirmed by finding raised urinary pregnanetriol or raised plasma dehydroepiandrosterone.

Delayed Puberty

Delay in puberty is commoner in boys than girls; by the age of 15 the majority of children will have some evidence of pubertal development or pubertal growth spurt, which occurs 1–2 years later in boys than girls. There is good evidence that delayed puberty with subsequent normal development is an inherited predisposition which is not sex linked, so that a family history of delayed puberty in the mother or father is important. Before embarking on investigation for an endocrine cause it is important to exclude a generalised systemic disease and chromosome disorders such as Klinefelter's syndrome (boys) and Turner's syndrome (girls). Important early investigations are chromosome karyotyping, skull x-ray to see if there is any enlargement of the pituitary fossa indicative of a chromophobic adenoma, and x-rays to assess bone age. The ability of the pituitary to produce growth hormone. TSH and gonadotrophins should be established. A growth-hormone level (during insulin-induced hypoglycaemia) and TSH and gonadotrophin levels (FSH and LH in boys and girls) in response to injected gonadotrophin and thyrotrophin-releasing hormones should be measured. If these results are within the normal range or the levels of gonadotrophins are elevated, then the diagnosis is primary gonadal failure.

The causes of delayed puberty are:

Physiological

Chronic unrelated diseases (the easiest to miss are mild steatorrhoea and renal tubular disorder)

Low gonadotrophin hormone production (LH and FSH). Reduced production may be associated with other pituitary hormone deficiencies if the pituitary has been damaged by tumour, meningitis or histiocytosis. The deficiency of gonadotrophin may by isolated. LH alone may be affected. Both LH and FSH are affected in Kallmann's syndrome, which also includes anosmia.

Hypergonadotrophic. Gonadal agenesis and dysgenesis (Klinefelter's syndrome in boys and Turner's syndrome in girls) and disorders of testosterone synthesis.

THE MENOPAUSE

At the menopause ovarian follicles fail to develop normally in response to pituitary FSH and LH. The failure of follicles to develop results in depleted oestradiol levels and persistent high levels of LH and FSH because of lack of negative feedback. Oestrogen levels are generally lower in the menopause than in premenopausal women, but the levels are variable and oestrogens are seldom completely absent. It is known that there is considerable interconversion of oestrogens and androgens and that at the menopause there are alterations in interconversion; there are also alterations in hormone peripheral receptor-site binding ability by which circulating levels of a hormone do not always match its ability to act at the target organ. This may be the case with the vagina and account for the fact that dyspareunia does not always correlate with physiological levels of circulating oestrogens. Oestrogens in postmenopausal women are produced by the adrenal and other tissues; there is evidence that after the menopause the adrenal produces increased amounts of androstenedione, which is converted in the liver and adipose tissue into oestrone, a much less active oestrogen than oestradiol, the main oestrogen in premenopausal women.

The main reasons for considering treatment of the menopause are:

Vasomotor symptoms (hot flushes)

Dyspareunia

Prevention of secondary disorders related to decline in oestrogen levels, such as osteoporosis and cardiovascular disease.

Circulating oestradiol levels are the same in the presence or absence of flushing attacks, but levels are lower in women who have both flushing attacks *and* dyspareunia (Hutton *et al.*, 1979). Nevertheless pharmacological doses of oestrogens usually reduce both symptoms, presumably because of interconversion to a metabolite which *is* related to pathogenesis of symptoms, or because of a change in receptor-binding sites.

The improvement in symptoms with oestrogens usually takes at least 4 weeks to become evident and increasing improvement can be expected for as long as 6 months.

The FSH level may be a guide to oestrogen responsiveness (Chakravarti *et al.*, 1979). The incidence of myocardial infarction in women increases rapidly after the menopause in that 3 years after the menopause the incidence is the same as in men at the same age. The implication therefore is that the atherogenic tendency in postmenopausal women is much greater than in men, who have a gradual increase in coronary artery disease from their twenties. After the menopause there is a rise in all the major lipid fractions, and with oestrogen treatment the cholesterol and phospholipids fall but not usually the triglycerides. On the basis of the increased tendency to thrombosis in premenopausal women on the contraceptive pill, it is arguable whether the benefit of oestrogens on the lipids is more advantageous than their presumed effect on the tendency to thrombosis. The evidence is not yet convincing enough to recommend oestrogen therapy solely on the basis of possible prophylaxis against cardiovascular disease.

There is now good evidence that osteoporosis is related to a decline in oestrogen levels and that the development of osteoporosis is most rapid within the first few years of the menopause, and thereafter there is a more gradual but still increased tendency to loss of bone matrix. There is also evidence that osteoporosis can be delayed by treatment with oestrogens. The absence of oestrogens may increase the resorption of bone mineral induced by normal amounts of parathyroid hormone.

Assessment of Menopausal Patients

There is considerable overlap in the levels of individual oestrogens between pre- and postmenopausal women. However, in general, FSH and LH levels are higher after the menopause, and the ratio of FSH to LH is altered even if absolute levels are not raised. Circulating oestradiol and oestrone levels and their main urinary excretory metabolite, oestriol, are lower after the menopause; testosterone levels are not usually altered. Measurement of oestradiol and oestrone are not widely available and it is usually sufficient to measure FSH, LH and 24-hour total oestrogens (oestriol). These measurements are helpful in determining whether the symptoms are due to the menopause or to some other reason. Additional gynaecological assessment of menopausal patients who have vaginal bleeding is essential.

The causes of postmenopausal bleeding in patients receiving oestrogens are:

> Genital carcinoma
> Breakthrough bleeding from continued oestrogen stimulation
> Withdrawal bleeding when oestrogens are stopped
> Vaginal-wall bleeding from excess oestrogen.

Treatment

There are three types of oral oestrogen treatment:

1. "Normal" oestrogen tablets which contain oestrone (Harmogen) and oestradiol (Progynova)
2. Synthetic oestrogens
3. "Natural" oestrogens, such as Premarin.

The advantage of "normal" oestrogen tablets is that the oestrone and oestradiol levels which result from their administration can be measured, whereas the oestrogens from synthetic and natural oestrogens cannot easily be measured. Patients being treated with "normal" oestrogens should have oestrone and oestradiol measured occasionally to ensure that the levels are around the physiological, i.e. $10\,\mu g/l$. High levels of oestrogens result in endometrial hyperplasia and bleeding, but this can be avoided if oestrogen levels are kept around $100\,\mu g/l$ by dosage control. If the oestrogen treatment is withheld every fourth week, withdrawal bleeding occurs but at a predictable time; it usually ceases when oestrogens are restarted; if it does not, the dose of oestrogen should be temporarily increased or progestogen given for one week; this produces a withdrawal bleed which should then be followed with a regime of low-dose continuous oestrogen. After a progestogen-induced bleed, further breakthrough bleeding on a small dose of continuous oestrogen does not usually occur for several months, if at all. An alternative and probably preferable regime is the administration of continuous oestrogens with the addition of a progestogen every fourth week, which produces a small amount of bleeding soon after the progestogen is given (sequential mestranol/norethisterone (Menophase)). This regime can be timed so that the progestogen is given for the first few days of each calendar month. Monthly shedding of the endometrium is likely to reduce the largely theoretical risk of increased liability to endometrial carcinoma with oestrogen therapy. There was a fear that oestrogens used to treat symptomatic menopausal women will increase the risk of developing breast carcinoma or endometrial carcinoma. It is now believed that there is little or no increased risk.

REFERENCES

BLOOM, A. (1978) *J. roy. soc. Med.*, **71**, 170.

CHAKRAVARTI, S., COLLINS, W. P., THOM, M. H. and STUDD, J. W. (1979) *Brit. med. J.*, **1**, 983.

HAVARD, C. W. H. (1979) *Brit. med. J.*, **1**, 1001.

HOCKADAY, T. D. and FELL, R. H. (1969) *Brit. J. hosp. Med.*, **2**, 1083.

HUTTON, J. D., JACOBS, H. S. and JAMES, V. H. T. (1979) *J. roy. Soc. Med.*, **72**, 835.

PYKE, D. A. and NELSON, P. G. (1976) *The Genetics of Diabetes Mellitus* (Ed. Creutzfield, W., Kobberlung, J. and Neel, J. V.). New York: Springer-Verlag.

GENERAL REFERENCES

BONDY, P. K. and ROSENBERG, L. E. (1980) *Metabolic Control and Disease*, 8th edit. New York: Saunders.

HALL, R., ANDERSON, J. R., SMART, G. A. and BESSER, M. (1980) *Fundamentals of Clinical Endocrinology*, 3rd edit. Tunbridge Wells: Pitman Medical.

STANBURY, J. B., WYAGAARDEN, J. B. and FREDERIKSON, D. S. (1978) *The Metabolic Basis of Disease*, 4th edit. New York: McGraw-Hill.

EPONYMS

1. CLAUDE BERNARD (1813–1878)

Bernard at first worked with Magendie. His fundamental contributions included the elucidation of the functions of the anterior and posterior nerve roots, that of the pancreas in fat digestion, the autonomic nervous system, and the demonstration of continued gluconeogenesis after death and of glucose in the blood of starved animals. The fact that the urine of herbivores could be made acid by starvation suggested to him that the body attempted to maintain the constancy of its composition even if it meant the breakdown of its own tissues. In physiological terms Bernard conceived of the body as a whole unit, but was not opposed to the cellular concept, believing that the body was a chemical protoplasm while being anatomically cellular. Never having been a clinician, he thought of all diseases as disordered physiology; he could not accept the existence of disease in a parasitic sense, and opposed some of Pasteur's ideas.

2. CHARLES EDOUARD BROWN-SÉQUARD (1817–1894)

Brown-Séquard succeeded Bernard as Professor of Physiology at the College of France. Bell's methods of galvanic stimulation to study nerve function were being widely applied, and Brown-Séquard, using the techniques, made some significant observations. He became involved in revolutionary activities in Paris and had to depart for the United States but, speaking little English, almost immediately returned to France. On Pierre Broca's recommendation he was offered a post in the Medical College of Virginia, but his imperfect English and his anti-slavery views again saw him back in Paris, where he built up a neurological practice which culminated in a three-year appointment at the National Hospital for Nervous Diseases in London. He demonstrated that adrenalectomised animals die, but could be kept alive by blood transfusions from healthy animals.

3. ERNEST HENRY STARLING (1866–1927)

Starling qualified at Guys Hospital and after studying in Europe he joined Schafer's laboratory at University College Hospital, London. His contributions to physiology were enormous and included fundamental work on secretin and the concept of hormones, renal function, capillary pressure and cardiac function. He was dubbed "the clinician's physiologist."

4. ROBERT JAMES GRAVES (1796–1853)

Dublin physician.

5. JEAN GUILLAUME AUGUSTE LUGOL (1786–1851)

French physician whose daughter married Pierre Paul Broca.

6. HARVEY WILLIAMS CUSHING (1869–1939)

Cushing qualified at Harvard and worked in Baltimore where he knew Osler well (he later wrote the definitive biography of Osler, for which he received the Pullitzer Prize in 1926). He also worked with William Halsted (who performed the first mastectomy, and introduced rubber gloves into surgery). Cushing eventually became Professor of Surgery at Harvard. In 1919 he removed a large meningioma from the Chief of Staff of the US Army, who returned to official duties within a month of the operation. During the First World war Cushing joined the Harvard Unit which served with the British Expeditionary Force before the United States entered the war.

7. THOMAS ADDISON (1793–1860)

Addison received his medical education in Edinburgh, and described adrenal insufficiency in 1855. Armand Trousseau in Paris first called the disease "maladie d'Addison". Addison married at the age of 52, was a severe depressive, and attempted suicide on several occasions. That he was eventually successful was the reason that no obituary notices appeared in the *British Medical Journal* or *Lancet*.

8. PAUL WILHELM HEINRICH LANGERHANS (1847–1888)

Langerhans qualified in Berlin and studied under Virchow. Like many of his countrymen he became involved in the Franco-Prussian war. He developed pulmonary tuberculosis, and for this reason settled in Madeira until his death. He discovered the pancreatic islet cells in 1869.

9. IRVING FREILER STEIN (b. 1887)

Stein qualified in the University of Michigan and worked as a gynaecologist in Chicago.

10. MICHAEL LEO LEVENTHAL (b. 1901)

Leventhal was born, qualified and worked as a gynaecologist in Chicago.

8

RENAL DISEASES

Clinical Features

Pain from the kidney is referred to the skin in the distribution of the 10th, 11th and 12th thoracic nerves. The pain of ureteric colic is felt in the same distribution but often extends to the cutaneous distribution of L.1 and to the testicle or labia. Tenderness from renal disease may be elicited by firm palpation posteriorly in the angle between the 12th rib and erector spinae ("renal angle").

The right kidney is 1½ cm below the left and the lower pole of the right kidney is generally higher than anticipated; it is level with a point 2½ cm above the umbilicus.

There is considerable movement of the kidneys during respiration, but for practical purposes, the hilum is considered to be at the level of L.2. Clinical examination of the kidneys should include auscultation to exclude a bruit from stenosis of the renal artery. The best sites for auscultation are in the lumbar region opposite L.2 and on the anterior wall of the abdomen, 1 in. lateral to the umbilicus; at this site, the stethoscope can be pressed firmly into the abdomen.

The course of the ureters is variable but usually lies over the tips of the transverse processes of the lumbar vertebrae and across the front of the sacro-iliac joints. The ureters are narrowed in three places: at their origin from the renal pelvis, where they pass over the pelvic brim, and at their entrance to the bladder. These sites are the most common for impaction of renal stone.

Examination of the Urine

Proteinuria is usually due to disease of the glomeruli despite the fact that glomerular filtrate normally contains 10–20 mg/dl of protein which is reabsorbed by the tubules. "Tubular proteinuria" occurs in conditions affecting tubular function, such as the Fanconi syndrome, and heavy-metal poisoning. Lysozyme and beta 2 microglobulin and other low-molecular-weight proteins are reabsorbed by normal tubules but appear in the urine if the tubules are diseased. Urinary protein may also be present as a result of disease in the lower urinary tract; however, heavy proteinuria (5 g/l) will usually be due to a functional disorder of the glomeruli. Smaller amounts of urinary protein arise from inflammation of the lower urinary tract or blood loss. The rate of protein loss by the kidney in renal disease is fairly constant throughout the day, it is therefore important to know the specific gravity of a specimen of urine in which protein is found. A trace of protein in a dilute urine will be more serious than a trace of protein in a more concentrated urine. With the stick tests for urine testing it is important to note that a false positive result for proteinuria will occur if the urine is alkaline or the test strip on the stick is already wet. The presence or absence of urinary casts is helpful in deciding the site of the protein loss. Hyaline casts are complexes of albumin and other proteins secreted by the tubules and cast in the shape of the renal tubules, and if present in excess in a fresh specimen of urine, they indicate that the proteinuria is of renal origin. Epithelial casts consist of freshly shed epithelial cells from the renal tubule, and they indicate that the disease process is affecting the tubules. Granular casts are probably degenerate epithelial casts. Electrophoresis of the urinary protein may give some indication as to the site of origin: disease of the glomeruli causes loss of albumin, while disease of the tubules causes mainly loss of alpha and beta globulins.

Normal urine contains red cells, white cells and hyaline casts. Addis (1949) defined the normal excretion of them in 24 hours. Subsequently, alternative methods of expressing the rate of excretion have been devised. The average normal excretion is 0–200,000 red and white cells per hour.

RADIOLOGY OF THE KIDNEYS

A straight x-ray of the abdomen may show the shape, size and position of the kidneys, as well as renal stones or calcification within the kidneys. A lateral x-ray will help to locate the site of a radio-opaque stone; most renal stones are radio-opaque, whereas the majority of gall-stones are radiotranslucent.

Intravenous Pyelogram (Excretion Nephrogram) or Intravenous Urogram

Some compounds containing iodine are radio-opaque and are both filtered through the glomeruli and actively excreted by the proximal tubules. To diminish the urine flow and increase the concentration in the urine, the patient is dehydrated. Excretion from the kidneys and emptying of the ureters are delayed if external pressure is applied to the lower abdomen, which compresses the lower part of the ureters.

In the presence of renal failure and raised blood urea, a nephrogram can be performed by infusing the contrast medium intravenously over a long period and taking the x-rays at a longer time interval than usual. The conventional IVP will usually not give meaningful results if performed when the blood urea is above 150 mmol/l.

There is some variation of size of normal kidneys between the two sides and at different times. General anaesthesia and hypotension may cause a diminution in size of the kidneys. As a practical rule, the length of the long axes of the kidneys is 12–14 cm; there should not be more than 1·5 cm difference between the two kidneys. An imaginary line should always be drawn joining the tips of all the renal pyramids, and the distance between this line and the renal outline should be constant. This is known as the "renal substance". Any localised depression or bulging of the renal outline should be noted; depression of the renal outline is due to scarring and fibrosis due to infarction or infection. Occasionally in normals the outline may have a lobulated appearance, particularly at the upper poles. The renal substance may be diminished in old age, renal-artery stenosis, fibrosis and back-pressure on the kidney. The renal substance and length of the kidney may be increased in hypertrophy due to disease of the opposite kidney. Hypertrophy of one kidney is suggestive of severe damage to the opposite kidney even if the radiological appearances are normal or near-normal.

The calyces drain into the renal pelvis; projecting into each calyx is a pyramid of renal tissue into which the collecting ducts drain. Any increased pressure or infection in the calyces will tend to destroy the delicate renal pyramid, leading to the appearance of a rounded, enlarged end to the calyces—"clubbing of the calyces". In ureteric obstruction the rate of urine formation is diminished, the ureter and pelvis may be dilated, the calyces are clubbed and the renal substances is diminished. In its extreme form, this is the appearance of hydro-nephrosis. Space-occupying lesions within the kidney, such as tumours, cysts or abscesses, may cause bulging of the renal outline and displacement or distortion of the calyces. Renal arteriography should always be performed in the presence of a space-occupying lesion; carcinomas usually have an abnormal vascular pattern, whereas cysts are usually avascular. However, it is important to note that cysts may undergo malignant change, and that a carcinoma may be avascular if it is necrotic or if its nutrient artery is thrombosed. Renal cysts do not cause hypertension, although hypernephromas may do so.

Pyelonephritis causes localised narrowing of the renal substance, due to focal scarring, and clubbing of the calyces which is at first restricted to one or two calyces. If all the calyces are involved it suggests that there is obstruction in the ureters or lower urinary tract. The pyelonephritic kidney is usually smaller than normal.

Scarring of the surface of the kidney may be due to infection or ischaemia; in general, scars due to infection will be associated with abnormal calyces whereas the calyceal pattern is usually normal in ischaemia. Rarely, scarring may be due to tuberculosis, in which case the scar is likely to be calcified and possibly associated with evidence of a tuberculous infection elsewhere in the urinary system—such as a contracted bladder.

The course of the ureters should be noted; peristalsis in the ureters may cause great variation in their apparent size. Particular attention should be paid to anatomical sites where narrowing normally occurs. In the standard IVP external abdominal compression is applied to compress the lower ureters, in order to delay the contrast leaving the renal pelvis. The abdominal pressure may distort the position of the ureters; in addition, the pressure may not affect both ureters equally so that excretion of the dye may appear to be delayed on one side, giving an appearance suggestive of renal-artery stenosis. For this reason it is important not to base the diagnosis of renal-artery stenosis on an IVP taken with abdominal compression. The sites of narrowing of the ureters are the most likely ones for impaction of a small calculus which may be very difficult to see. In the IVP a small calculus will be seen as a filling defect. At the pelvi-ureteric junction there may be a small filling defect, due to an aberrant renal artery, such as may occur in unilateral renal-artery stenosis. Rarely, such an artery may be the cause of ureteric obstruction. Reduplication of the ureters is a common cause of continuing urinary infection; the diagnosis is usually easy if the ureter drains functioning kidney, which will excrete the dye normally; however, sometimes the second ureter drains non-functioning kidney and will not fill with contrast. A second ureter draining non-functioning kidney should be suspected if there are fewer calyces on one side, if part of the kidney does not appear to have calyces or if the long axis of the kidney is altered by displacement of the organ by an inflammatory swelling.

Retroperitoneal fibrosis causes narrowing of the ureters over a distance of several centimetres. The ureters gradually widen out again to attain the normal size. As well as being narrowed, the ureters are pulled towards the midline. The condition is almost invariably bilateral, but both sides are not always affected equally.

At the end of the IVP, contrast material should be seen in the bladder, and the amount remaining in the bladder after micturition should be noted. Normally there should not be more than a small amount. Incomplete bladder emptying suggests infection or obstruction at the bladder neck or in the urethra. Prostatic enlargement will cause increased trabeculation of the bladder wall and a filling defect at the lower end of the bladder. Hypertrophy of the bladder wall with lower urinary obstruction may result in diverticulae of the bladder; if large, they may give rise to the symptom of "double micturition"—a desire to pass urine twice within a short space of time. This symptom may also occur if there is reflux of urine up dilated ureters during micturition (vesico-ureteric reflux). Such reflux will be seen in the majority of patients suffering from chronic pyelonephritis if a micturating cystogram is performed. The investigation is somewhat tedious, and is usually only performed if the IVP shows a definite abnormality in the kidney.

Renal Isotope Scanning

Isotopically labelled iodohippurate is used for assessing uptake, transit through the kidney and removal from the kidney. The value of renograms is in the detection of renal-artery stenosis and in establishing whether or not there is obstruction to outflow either within the kidney or lower in the renal tract. The value of the renogram may be improved using frusemide to try to speed the transfer of isotope through the kidney. Frusemide is of value in the presence of dilated calyces to help establish whether there is an obstruction to urine flow. Hippuran is excreted solely by tubular excretion and therefore it tends to be affected by obstructive lesions. DTPA (labelled with technetium) is filtered by glomeruli and therefore gives better anatomical localisation of a cyst, Grawitz[1] tumour or scarring.

The characteristic findings with hippuran are shown in Table XX.

TABLE XX

RENAL ISOTOPE SCANNING: FINDINGS WITH HIPPURAN

	Uptake	Parenchymal transit time	Pelvic transit time
Normal with dilated pelvis—no obstruction	N	N	Prolonged
Anxiety, pain and polycystic disease	N	Prolonged	N
Obstruction in normal kidney	N	Prolonged	Prolonged
Parenchymal renal damage but no obstruction	Reduced	N	N
Dilated pelvis, some renal damage but no obstruction	Reduced	N	Prolonged
Renal ischaemia	Reduced	Prolonged	N
Obstruction, reduced plasma flow and parenchymal renal damage	Reduced	Prolonged	Prolonged

THE MECHANISM OF CONCENTRATION AND DILUTION OF THE URINE

In the proximal convoluted tubule, the concentration of the fluid remains exactly the same; nevertheless, large amounts of water and solutes are reabsorbed but in the same proportions. With water, some sodium and chloride, and all the glucose are reabsorbed. Chlorothiazide acts on the proximal tubules, preventing reabsorption of sodium and chloride, and hence water. Fluid isotonic with plasma is delivered to the descending limb of loop of Henle[2]; the wall of the descending limb is permeable to water but not to sodium; the distal limb of the loop of Henle actively pumps out sodium into the interstitial fluid. The resulting increased concentration of sodium in the interstitial fluid draws out water from the proximal (descending) limb of the loop. This process continues down the proximal limb—water being removed by concentrated interstitial fluid—so that urine flowing down the proximal limb becomes more and more concentrated, as does the interstitial fluid; the concentration reaches a maximum at the tip of the loop of Henle. As fluid ascends the distal limb, sodium is pumped out, causing it to become more dilute again. Near the tip of the loop the urine leaving the proximal limb is highly concentrated so that a great deal of sodium is available for pumping out into the interstitial fluid near the tip of the loop. This is the principle of the counter-current multiplier system. The points that are usually not made clear are that the system has two purposes:

1. To produce a high concentration of solutes near the tip of the loop of Henle.
2. To *dilute* the urine ascending the distal limb. It is important to note that the primary purpose of the system is to concentrate the interstitial fluid near the tip of the loop of Henle.

The microscopic anatomy of the kidney is such that the tips of the loop of Henle of all the nephrons lie close to the collecting ducts into which the distal tubules drain. Dilute urine from the distal limb of the loop of Henle enters the distal convoluted tubule and collecting ducts. This dilute urine in the collecting duct comes into contact with the areas of high concentration of solutes in the interstitial tissue. Water is withdrawn from the collecting ducts and the urine becomes more concentrated. The amount of water which crosses the collecting tubules is controlled by altering the permeability of their walls. This is done with antidiuretic hormone (ADH)—when the hormone is secreted the wall becomes highly permeable to water which is withdrawn into the interstitial fluid leading to a concentrated urine (antidiuresis). The confusion about the counter-current system arises because the loop of Henle *taken with* the collecting duct is a mechanism for concentrating the urine, *but* the urine leaving the loop of Henle is dilute.

Functions of the Tubules

The ability to concentrate and dilute the urine is the single most important function of the tubules and the one most useful in assessing tubular function. The tubules also actively excrete potassium, hydrogen ion and ammonium salts, independently of glomerular filtration. Phosphate excretion depends on glomerular filtration, it is not actively excreted by the tubules, hence renal (glomerular) failure is accompanied by a rise in serum phosphate. Conditions which cause phosphaturia (i.e. excessive loss of phosphate) are due to a defect in the tubules preventing reabsorption of phosphates from the glomerular filtrate. Similar defects are responsible for inability to reabsorb amino acids; thus, there are two ways in which tubular defects may be manifest:

1. Inability to excrete actively
2. Inability to reabsorb.

Inability to excrete actively.—Loss of excretory function of the tubules causes an elevation of the serum potassium and an inability to excrete hydrogen ion and ammonium salts. Inability to excrete hydrogen ion may also be due to an inherited tubular defect (renal tubular acidosis). Retention of hydrogen ion leads to acidosis and a fall in plasma bicarbonate; the fall in bicarbonate is accompanied by an increase in chloride (hyperchloraemic acidosis) in order to keep the anion content of the blood constant. Often the blood urea is not much raised, and the clue to the condition is the very low plasma bicarbonate with only slight elevation of the blood urea.

Inability to reabsorb.—Sodium is largely reabsorbed in the proximal tubules; chronic renal failure may be associated with excessive loss of sodium and patients will need a high salt intake.

Sodium deficiency is a cause of renal failure and is one of the causes of uraemia in Addison's disease. Other conditions associated with loss of sodium can also cause renal failure, e.g. diabetic coma, vomiting, diarrhoea, although these are associated with dehydration as well. Normally the tubules reabsorb glucose, phosphate and essential amino acids; congenital or acquired loss of ability to reabsorb all of these is the Fanconi[3] syndrome. In addition to the collective disorder which constitutes Fanconi's syndrome, isolated tubular defects of reabsorption may occur. The most important of these are:

Renal glycosuria (inability to reabsorb glucose)
Renal diabetes insipidus (inability to reabsorb water due to unresponsiveness of collecting tubule to ADH)
Vitamin D-resistant rickets (inability to reabsorb phosphate)
Cystinuria (inability to reabsorb cystine).
(Cystinuria should not be confused with cystinosis which is part of the Fanconi syndrome. As well as an inherited defect of tubular reabsorption in cystinosis, there is an inherited defect

of protein and amino-acid metabolism, leading to accumulation of cystine in the tissues.)

Acquired disorders which may cause isolated tubular defects of reabsorption without causing more severe renal damage are:

Potassium deficiency
Sickle-cell anaemia
Chronic pyelonephritis
Heavy-metal poisoning (gold, lead and copper)
Myelomatosis.

Tests of the Ability of the Tubules to Reabsorb and Excrete

Ability to reabsorb.—The ability to reabsorb water to produce a concentrated urine is the simplest test of tubular reabsorptive capacity. The test can be performed by inducing fluid deprivation or injecting ADH. The ability to reabsorb sodium can be tested by sodium deprivation or giving a salt-retaining hormone.

Glucose is normally completely reabsorbed in the proximal tubule. If glucose appears in the urine it is either because the blood (and hence glomerular filtrate) level is abnormally high, or because there is a congenital defect in the ability of the tubule to reabsorb glucose (renal glycosuria). There is a point at which glucose will appear in the urine if the blood level is gradually raised, i.e. despite reabsorption from the tubule, some glucose is getting through to the urine. This is the point at which the tubule is reabsorbing maximally.

The maximum amount of glucose reabsorbed (maximum tubular reabsorption of glucose, or Tm_g) will be the amount presented to the tubules less the amount in the urine in one minute, or

(glomerular filtration rate × plasma glucose) −
(urine glucose × urine volume)

The normal value is 320 mg/min (52 mmol).

Ability to excrete.—A substance actively excreted by the tubules which is easy to measure in blood and urine is para-aminohippuric acid (PAH). The maximum amount actively excreted (Tm_{pah}) is PAH excreted in the urine less the amount filtered by the glomeruli, or

(urine PAH × urine volume) −
(glomerular filtration rate × plasma PAH)

The normal Tm_{pah} is 70 mg/min (11 mmol).

Other tests of tubular function of importance are:

Ability to produce an acid urine (tested by loading with ammonium chloride).
Ability to conserve sodium on a low-sodium diet or with salt-retaining hormone (fludrocortisone).
Ability to excrete potassium (level of serum potassium).

Ability to conserve amino acids (chromatogram of urine for abnormal urinary amino acids).

Renal Tubular Disorders

The tubules have homeostatic functions which involve either absorption or excretion. Congenital disturbances of tubular function are usually due to an enzyme deficiency leading to increased excretion of precursors or accumulation of precursors which are toxic. As a rule toxic damage to the tubules causes failure of all tubular functions. This means that there is:

Proteinuria	Aminoaciduria
Glycosuria	Disturbed acid-base
Phosphaturia	balance.

Toxic damage to the tubules can be either *congenital* as in the case of Wilson's disease, galactosaemia or cystinosis, or *acquired*, e.g. heavy-metal poisoning, multiple myeloma, drugs (expired tetracycline, streptomycin, salicylates) or hypokalaemia. Many other tubular disorders are due to a deficiency in one enzyme only and hence other tubular functions are not affected. The most important disorders of *single* tubular functions are:

Renal glycosuria
Specific aminoaciduria, e.g. cystinuria (cystine stones)
Vitamin D-resistant rickets (inability to reabsorb phosphates)
Renal tubular acidosis (defective reabsorption of bicarbonate)
Resistance to antidiuretic hormone (nephrogenic diabetes insipidus).

Glomerular Function

Bowman's[4] capsule acts as a simple filter. The properties of filters which are of importance are the amount of fluid they let through, whether they stop substances which should be allowed through, or allow through substances which should be retained. Glomerular filters can fail in all three functions:

1. By a reduction in the amount of fluid which passes them— reduced glomerular filtration rate
2. By retaining substances which should be filtered, e.g. urea and creatinine
3. By allowing substances through which should be retained, e.g. plasma proteins.

Glomerular filtration rate.—A substance which is not absorbed or excreted by the renal tubules will appear in the urine at the same rate that it is filtered through the glomeruli. Such a substance is inulin. The fluid in the proximal tubule is isotonic with plasma, hence the concentration of a substance in the glomerular filtrate is the same as in the plasma. The glomerular filtration volume in one minute is:

$$\frac{\text{Conc. inulin in urine} \times \text{volume of urine}}{\text{Conc. inulin in plasma}}$$

In practice, creatinine clearance is used to estimate glomerular filtration rate. Creatinine is an endogenously produced substance, whose plasma concentration remains uniform throughout the day, and which is not absorbed or excreted by the renal tubules to an extent which interferes with its usefulness. Because the level of creatinine in the serum remains constant only one blood estimation is necessary. The urine is collected for 24 hours, thus minimising errors due to incomplete bladder emptying and inaccuracies of timing.

"Clearance" is an entirely theoretical concept. It may be defined as the volume of plasma which contains the amount of the substance which appears in the urine in one minute, assuming the plasma to be completely "cleared" of the substance.

If u = urinary concentration of the substance
v = urine flow per minute
p = plasma concentration of the substance

Clearance = $\dfrac{uv}{p}$

i.e. $\dfrac{\text{amount in urine (per minute)}}{\text{amount in plasma (mg per cent)}}$

The normal creatinine clearance is 100–120 ml/minute (in effect this is the volume of the glomerular filtrate). The value normally falls with age, so that at 80 the normal creatinine clearance is 65 ml/minute. The retention of substances in the blood which should be filtered does not occur until there is a marked fall in glomerular filtration rate. The blood urea and blood creatinine on a normal diet do not start to rise until the creatinine clearance is below 50 ml/min (i.e. 50 per cent of normal). The glomeruli allow through protein if they are damaged; however in very severe renal failure protein may disappear from the urine because of widespread loss of functioning glomeruli (i.e. the filter is completely "clogged up").

The individual components of renal function and their tests are:

Glomerular function:
Glomerular filtration rate (creatinine clearance)
Blood urea and creatinine
Proteinuria
Serum phosphate.

Tubular excretory function:
Serum potassium

Tubular reabsorptive function:
Concentration and dilution of urine
Serum sodium (and urine sodium)
Glycosuria
Urinary amino acids.

Urinary Acidification

The body produces an excess of hydrogen ions which are excreted into the urine as carbonic acid and ammonium compounds; as a result the tubules have to:

1. Reabsorb bicarbonate
2. Produce ammonia from ammonium bicarbonate and thus produce (or regenerate) bicarbonate.

If there is a reduced ability to reabsorb bicarbonate there may be compensatory increased ammonia production, i.e. a reduced ability to reabsorb bicarbonate will lead to increased regeneration of bicarbonate, large amounts of bicarbonate in the urine (and therefore an alkaline urine), which can be neutralised by adding acid. Thus the amount of acid needed to neutralise the bicarbonate is a measure of increased bicarbonate production which in turn is a measure of increased ammonia production. Thus *excess excretion* of bicarbonate is a measure of inability to *reabsorb* bicarbonate. *Reduced ammonia* in the urine is a measure of the *inability to regenerate* bicarbonate from ammonium bicarbonate, hence a reduced urinary ammonia is a measure of failure to regenerate bicarbonate.

GLOMERULONEPHRITIS

"General Physicians yearn for a classification of nephritis that will make this complicated subject simple; trying to provide one is an occupational disease of nephrologists." (Kerr, 1978.)

Clinical Presentation

Chronic progressive inflammation of the kidneys presents commonly in only five ways:

1. Symptomless proteinuria
2. Nephrotic syndrome
3. A nephritic illness
4. Chronic renal failure
5. Hypertension.

Three aspects of glomerulonephritis are accepted as uncontroversial:

1. There is an acute form of nephritis associated with haematuria and previous streptococcal infection
2. About 5 per cent of cases of acute nephritis develop a chronic, long-standing and eventually fatal disease
3. There is a chronic form of nephritis associated with albuminuria and eventual renal failure in which there is no history of preceding acute nephritis.

Immunological Classification

Most cases of glomerulonephritis fall into the following broad immunological groups:

1. Immune complex associated disease (commonest, although still rare)
2. Complement-mediated disease (mainly post-streptococcal)
3. Anti-basement membrane antibody associated disease (mainly Goodpasture's syndrome)
4. Cell-mediated immune disease.

Pathological Classification

Minimal change lesion
Focal nephritis
Membranous
Membranoproliferative (now called mesangiocapillary)
(a) dense deposit types
(b) subendothelial type
Rarer types

Immune Mechanisms in Renal Disease

Immune complex disease
(a) endogenous antigen
(b) exogenous antigen
Complement alternative pathway mediated disease
Anti-basement membrane antibody
Cell-mediated immune disease.

Immune-complex-mediated renal disease.—This is the commonest form of immune damage to the kidneys. Circulating antibody-antigen complexes localise in certain sites preferentially, such as heart valves, choroid plexus and even large blood vessels at sites of turbulent-flow. The complexes will release inflammatory mediators and activate Cl_q and the classical complement cascade; some antibodies can, however, activate the complement alternative pathway. The offending antigen is eventually used up but antibody production may continue, leading to the formation of very large immune complexes from circulating immunoglobulins. The smaller immunoglobulins can pass into the extracellular fluid, so that immune complex formation need not always be intravascular. The antigens which give rise to immune complexes are either exogenous, such as micro-organisms, or endogenous.

Complement-associated injury (often post-streptococcal).—Tissue injury may occur because of activation of both complement pathways. Some forms of nephritis are associated with low circulating levels of C3. Persisting low C3 levels may allow persistence of antigens and may be an adverse prognostic feature following acute glomerulonephritis.

Anti-basement membrane injury.—Circulating IgG antibody binds with antigen in the capillary wall of the glomeruli. The formation of immune complexes *in situ* leads to the formation and release of various potentially harmful mediators such as vasoactive peptides, complement and coagulation factors, leading to damage to the basement with resultant leakage into Bowman's capsule, and also proliferation and inflammation of the capillaries, leading to obstruction to flow and reduced glomerular filtration rate. The disease becomes self-perpetuating by virtue of persistent antibody production in response to the triggering circulating IgG antibody.

This type of immune damage is relatively uncommon but is important because of the relative ease with which it can be produced and studied in experimental animals. The archetypal disease in humans produced by anti-basement membrane immune injury is Goodpasture's syndrome, in which the nephritis is usually associated with haemoptysis due to lung purpura.

In Goodpasture's syndrome there are circulating antibodies to glomerular basement membranes, the characteristic immunofluorescent-demonstrable linear deposition of IgG is found, and there is circulating antibody which can cause the disease in transplanted kidneys, and also in other primates.

Cell-mediated glomerular and tubular damage.—Sensitised lymphocytes are responsible for transplant rejection, but may also be involved in spontaneously occurring disease.

The three main presentations of glomerulonephritis are the syndrome of acute nephritis, the nephrotic syndrome (which may lead to chronic renal failure) and persistent urinary abnormalities without associated clinical features. There are also a number of broad histological features which do not always correlate closely with the clinical manifestations. The principal groups of disordered histology are:

1. Minimal-change disease.—This is primarily a disease of children. The main histological feature is patchy glomerulosclerosis and mesangial hypertrophy. The glomerulosclerosis is focal within each affected glomerulus, and also global in that it may affect all glomeruli. One problem is the fact that these same changes occur with increasing age. In adults the response to steroids is partly related to the degree of mesangial hypertrophy. Most adult patients have at least one relapse. Relapse is least likely if initial response to steroids has been rapid and complete. Steroids are the first choice of treatment, with cyclophosphamide as a reserve if steroids do not produce a remission or if relapse occurs despite steroids.

2. *Membranous glomerulonephritis.*—The cardinal feature is thickening of the capillary loops within the glomeruli due to deposition of IgG and C3. Clinically these patients have non-selective proteinuria and nephrotic syndrome. This type of glomerulonephritis seldom starts with an acute nephritic presentation. The prognosis is dependent on age of presentation; in childhood the condition has a good prognosis. In adulthood the outcome is unpredictable: some patients survive for many years with symptomless proteinuria, some recover spontaneously usually within 5 years of onset. About half the adult patients progress slowly to renal failure. There is still debate as to whether patients with this disease respond to treatment.

3. *Focal segmental glomerulosclerosis.*—This subgroup is more difficult to define. The disease is patchy, not all glomeruli within an affected area are involved, and within the affected glomeruli the lesions may be segmental. There is usually associated patchy tubular atrophy, adhesions to Bowman's capsule, inflammatory cell infiltration and capillary thrombi.

4. *Proliferative glomerulonephritis.*—Unlike the three main types of membranous nephritis, which present as proteinuria or nephrotic syndrome, proliferative nephritis tends to present as an acute nephritis or with recurrent haematuria. Generally recovery is more likely the younger the patient. There are several histological varieties of proliferative nephritis including mesangial, crescentic and focal proliferative nephritis. Goodpasture's syndrome consists of crescentic glomerulonephritis with lung purpura, in which there is a deposition of antiglomerular basement membrane antibody between the basement membrane of the glomerular capillaries and Bowman's capsule. The crescentic type of glomerular nephritis follows acute nephritis in about 5 per cent of cases, and when it does it has a better prognosis than a similar disease arising without an antecedent nephritic illness. Focal proliferative nephritis occurs with Henoch-Schönlein purpura, systemic lupus erythematosus and subacute bacterial endocarditis.

Treatment of Glomerulonephritis

It was established in an MRC trial that minimal-change nephritis almost always responds to steroids, but that they were not indicated for membranous or proliferative nephritis. However, it is now believed that slight histological features suggesting the more serious forms of nephritis are not a contra-indication for a therapeutic trial with steroids.

Acute Nephritis

Acute nephritis almost invariably follows previous infection with a nephritogenic strain of beta-haemolytic streptococcus. The most usual site of infection is the throat, although, rarely, infection in other sites may be responsible, for example streptococcal endocarditis or infected burns. The interval between infection and the onset of nephritis is usually 2–3 weeks but the limits are probably 48 hours to 4 weeks.

The disease usually starts suddenly with oliguria, oedema, haematuria, proteinuria and hypertension. The oedema is caused by hypoproteinaemia, and by water retention due to excessive tubular reabsorption of salt. The reasons for the diminished protein production and excessive salt absorption are not known. The hypertension may cause hypertensive encephalopathy and left ventricular failure, which will be exaggerated by the fluid retention. The urine contains albumin, red blood cells, granular and cellular casts.

Treatment.—Prophylactic penicillin is given to the contacts of a patient who has developed acute nephritis. Penicillin is also given in established cases, usually for the duration of the haematuria. The main disorder of function is fluid retention and oliguria which is accompanied by a rise in blood urea. The aim of treatment is to promote a diuresis and limit the harmful effects of oliguria, hence salt, water and protein intake should be limited if oliguria and uraemia are present. Bed rest alone usually promotes a diuresis. Protein and casts may continue in the urine for several years after the acute attack. The patient should be allowed out of bed when the red-cell excretion in the urine becomes constant. Conditions which may simulate acute nephritis are Henoch-Schönlein purpura, subacute bacterial endocarditis and acute polyarteritis nodosa.

Nephrotic Syndrome

The syndrome consists of proteinuria, hypoproteinaemia and oedema. There is often, but not invariably, a rise in serum lipids and a fall in serum calcium which may lead to tetany. The calcium is normally carried bound to the plasma albumin, but if the amount of circulating albumin is reduced, less calcium can be transported. The hypoproteinaemia and fluid retention cause oedema which results in secondary hyperaldosteronism which occasionally causes hypokalaemia. The nephrotic syndrome does *not* include a rise in blood urea or hypertension.

Causes of Nephrotic Syndrome

Glomerulonephritis
Pyelonephritis
Diabetes
Amyloid disease
Systemic lupus erythematosus and polyarteritis nodosa
Renal-vein thrombosis
Drugs, such as gold and mercury
Rare causes such as malaria, renal carcinoma and hypersensitivity states.

The nephrotic syndrome is treated with a high protein intake (to compensate for renal loss of protein) and a no-added-salt diet (to diminish fluid retention due to hypoalbuminaemia and salt retention). Thiazide diuretics, frusemide and spironolactone are used to reduce fluid retention. Potassium supplements may not be necessary if potassium retention accompanies the glomerular failure. Gross oedema may result in hypovolaemia. Occasionally a diuresis can be induced with a plasma expander such as dextran, but the benefit is usually short-lived.

The use of steroids and immunosuppressives in the nephrotic syndrome.—The indication and effectiveness of these drugs in the nephrotic syndrome are not clear. They may be valuable in some cases of chronic glomerulonephritis. They are almost certainly of less value when the nephrotic syndrome is secondary to pyelonenephritis, diabetes, amyloidosis and renal vein thrombosis. There are two main ways of judging the prognosis and assessing the functional abnormality in chronic glomerulonephritis, viz:

1. The severity of changes in the renal biopsy
2. Whether the loss of protein is selective or unselective.

With regard to assessing the effect of treatment there are three main considerations:

1. Immediate improvement in renal function
2. Effect of the treatment on the structural damage
3. Whether the duration or rate of progress of the disease is affected.

Selectivity of proteinuria.—The renal clearance of normal proteins with different molecular weights is compared with the clearance of one protein (transferrin). If smaller amounts of high-molecular-weight proteins than low-molecular-weight proteins appear in the urine the proteinuria is said to be "selective". If large amounts of high- and low-molecular-weight proteins appear in the the urine the proteinuria is said to be "unselective".

The quantity of protein in the urine does not correlate with selectivity of proteinuria, nor does the quantity of proteinuria give any indication as to the outcome of the attack; alteration in the daily output of protein either spontaneously or as a result of treatment does not alter the selectivity of proteinuria. There is a correlation between severity of biopsy appearances with selectivity of proteinuria—the less damage to the glomeruli the more selective the proteinuria; however there are many exceptions; occasional cases of severe proliferative glomerulonephritis have a highly selective proteinuria. If the biopsy shows epithelial crescent formation, this is always associated with unselective proteinuria. There is usually a good correlation between a response to steroids and a selective proteinuria.

The MRC trial of corticosteroids in the nephrotic syndrome indicated that only patients with minimal change glomerular lesions are *likely* to respond to steroids; also, steroids can be harmful in other forms of glomerulonephritis. However individual patients with more severe glomerular changes can be improved. Patients with membranous changes and unselective proteinuria given steroids may have improved renal function and develop remission in the nephrotic syndrome, although without improving the histological appearances of the glomeruli. The steroids may have to be given for as long as six months before deciding that they are not going to help.

Use of immunosuppressive drugs.—For proliferative glomerulonephritis it is worth trying either azathioprine or cyclophosphamide; these patients hardly ever respond to steroids alone, although steroids given with immunosuppressives may permit a higher dose of the latter to be given without producing serious side-effects.

For patients with minimal-change or membranous glomerulonephritis who fail to respond or who become resistant to steroids, a trial of azathioprine or cyclophosphamide should be considered. There is general agreement that nephrotic syndrome secondary to other conditions such as diabetes, renal-vein thrombosis, pyelonephritis and amyloidosis is unlikely to respond to either steroids or immunosuppressives. These cases almost invariably have an unselective proteinuria; in the rare instance of proteinuria being selective these drugs should probably be considered.

URINARY TRACT INFECTION

The essential feature which is often overlooked is that the infection is not only in the urine but also in the interstitial tissue of the kidneys and walls of the renal pelvis and ureters. All cases of pyelonephritis have minute abscesses within the renal substance. These abscesses heal by fibrosis and are most frequently found in the medulla near the collecting tubes which drain into the renal pelvis. The tubules are much more susceptible to damage than the remainder of the kidney. Two other aspects of the pathology of pyelonephritis are important: the first is a usually marked fibrosis surrounding the glomeruli in concentric layers (periglomerular fibrosis) and the second is the frequency of vascular involvement by the inflammation, leading to secondary ischaemic changes. Involvement of the kidneys is usually bilateral except when the infection arises as a result of unilateral obstruction; the involvement is also patchy so that a normal renal biopsy does not exclude the diagnosis. Progressive fibrosis leads to shrinking of the kidneys, inflammation leads to scarring and depression of the surface and involvement of the arteries leads to wedge-shaped areas of infarction, which also cause depression of the renal surfaces. Infection may destroy renal pyramids within the calyces, leading to clubbed calyces.

Hypertension may cause narrowing of the renal arterioles, exaggerating the areas of infarction which may occur as a result of inflammation. Pyelonephritis is common in hypertension and in other causes of renal damage, e.g. glomerulonephritis and diabetes. The main point of distinction between the IVP appearances of renal damage due to ischaemia alone and that due to infection is that the calyceal pattern will be normal in ischaemia but abnormal if the renal scarring is due to long-standing pyelonephritis. In renal damage due to chronic back-pressure the calyces are dilated uniformly throughout both kidneys, whereas pyelonephritis causes patchy involvement. In essence, therefore, the structural changes in the kidneys in chronic pyelonephritis which are reflected in the IVP are:

Decrease in size of the affected kidney
Focal scarring and decrease in renal substance
Abnormal calyces.

With regard to these changes, two other factors should be considered. It is now believed that clubbing of the calyces and focal scarring almost always occur as a result of renal infection during childhood. The renal changes due to pyelonephritis acquired in adulthood are diffuse interstitial fibrosis which leads to contraction of the kidneys. Coarse scars may be present if there is associated infarction due to hypertensive changes. The structural changes in the kidneys and the histological appearances of the interstitial tissue are not specific for pyelonephritis—a large number of other conditions can cause an identical histological picture. Any pre-existing renal damage predisposes to infection; the clinical significance of this is that the x-ray appearances of a small kidney with a biopsy appearance of interstitial fibrosis and evidence of infection in the urine does not mean that the structural changes in the kidneys are due to the infection. Among conditions which may cause interstitial fibrosis of the kidneys are:

Potassium depletion
Sulphonamide excess
Phenacetin excess
Hypertension
Radiation
Ureteric obstruction
Ageing.

Recommended Terminology of Urinary-Tract Infection (*British Medical Journal*, 1979)

Urinary-Tract Infection (UTI)
The presence of micro-organisms in the urinary tract.

Bacteriuria
The presence of bacteria in bladder urine. For epidemiological purposes this may be detected by quantitative urine culture; its presence is usually indicated by finding of > 100,000 colony forming units (cfu) per ml of freshly voided urine, and any growth from urine obtained by suprapubic aspiration.

Bladder bacteriuria
The presence of bacteria in urine obtained from the bladder by catheter or by suprapubic aspiration.

Covert bacteriuria (CB)
Significant bacteriuria detected by the screening of apparently healthy populations.

Upper-tract bacteriuria
The presence of bacteria in urine collected from the renal pelvis or ureter(s), or both. This may indicate renal infection, but in the presence of vesico-ureteric reflux the organisms may derive from the bladder.

Bacterial cystitis
A syndrome consisting of dysuria and frequency of micturition by day and night. Bladder bacteriuria is present and is usually associated with pyuria and sometimes haematuria.

Acute bacterial pyelonephritis

A syndrome consisting of loin pain, tenderness, and pyrexia, accompanied by bacteriuria, bacteraemia, pyuria, and sometimes haematuria. The condition is associated with bacterial infection of the kidney.

Chronic pyelonephritis

The terms *chronic interstitial nephritis* or *chronic tubulo-interstitial disease* are preferred.

Chronic interstitial nephritis (syn: chronic tubulo-interstitial disease)

A chronic inflammatory disease affecting the renal interstitium and tubules. The condition may lead to progressive shrinkage of the kidney(s) due to interstitial fibrosis. Tubular dysfunction is more pronounced than the reduction of glomerular filtration suggests. The condition has many causes including bacterial infection, excessive analgesic consumption, x-irradiation, crystal-induced nephropathies, methicillin nephropathy and lead poisoning. These aetiological factors have been identified, but in many instances the cause is unknown. Bacterial infection may prove to be a rare cause of chronic interstitial nephritis and is characterised by the presence of inflammatory changes in the renal pelvis. Interstitial disease produced by analgesics is often associated with papillary damage.

Radiological Definitions

Focal reflux nephropathy (syn: *coarse renal scarring (chronic), atrophic pyelonephritis, chronic childhood pyelonephritis*)

Focal scarring of the kidney(s), often predominantly polar in localisation and usually with related calyceal clubbing or blunting. The scars vary from small fissures to large zones of parenchymal atrophy; in unaffected regions there may be compensatory hypertrophy. There is a strong association with past or present vesico-ureteric reflux and often also with symptomless or symptomatic infections. The affected kidneys are often smaller than normal, and they may cease to grow during periods of infection or severe vesico-ureteric reflux or both.

Generalised reflux nephropathy

A condition associated with past or present vesico-ureteric reflux (most often grade 3 (see below)). It is characterised by generalised dilatation of the calyces and reduction of the renal parenchyma.

Vesico-ureteric reflux (VUR)

Reflux of urine from the bladder into the ureter due to incompetence of the vesico-ureteric valve mechanism. The severity of the condition has been graded in several ways; the use of three grades is recommended:

Grade I (mild) Contrast medium flows into the ureter but does not reach the kidney

Grade II (moderate) Contrast medium flows into the ureter and reaches the kidney without distension of calyces or ureter

Grade III (severe) Contrast medium flows into the ureter, reaches the kidney, and distends the calyces, ureter, or pelvis, or all three. (This grade may be subdivided depending on the degree of dilatation.)

The severity of VUR is influenced by several factors which include:

The severity of the anatomical and functional derangement at the vesico-ureteric region: this tends to lessen with age, and reflux may therefore disappear

The presence of bladder outlet obstruction or unstable bladder contractions or both

The vigour and efficacy of ureteric contractions, and

Technical factors such as the rate of contrast infusion, the volume of contrast used, and whether the examination is performed under general anaesthesia (which is not recommended).

Intrarenal reflux
Backflow of contrast medium from the calyces into the collecting tubules, which is occasionally seen in association with severe VUR. It is commonest in the polar regions of the kidney and is seldom seen in children after the age of 4 years.

Response to Treatment
Response
Disappearance of bacteriuria after treatment.

Relapse
Post-treatment recurrence of bacteriuria due to the same organism as that originally isolated. Relapse of infection usually occurs within six weeks of cessation of treatment.

Persistent infection
Bacteriuria persisting during and after treatment.

Reinfection
Recurrence of bacteriuria after treatment due to an organism different from that originally isolated. Reinfection with the same organism cannot be distinguished from relapse.

Criteria for cure

In all treatment, trials should be carefully defined. Urine specimens should be collected at specified times after completion of treatment, over a defined period (not usually less than six weeks). If the follow-up specimens show no evidence of infection, or if reinfection is found, the subject is considered to have been cured of the original infection. If the post-treatment specimens show a relapse, or the bacteriuria persists, treatment may be deemed to have failed.

Mechanisms of Renal Infection

It is now established that bacteriuria occurs commonly in asymptomatic women and may persist or disappear frequently and spontaneously often without causing symptoms or apparent renal damage. The high prevalence of chronic pyelonephritis found at routine postmortems is probably not related to recurrent asymptomatic bacteriuria.

There is good experimental evidence that bacteria will survive in a surface film of urine after a vessel has been emptied; also, flow mechanics have shown that when fluid flows down a tube there is an upward movement of a thin layer of fluid adjacent to the wall of the tube. In the ureters this would explain infection of the kidneys in the absence of ureteric reflux.

The renal medulla is peculiarly susceptible to infection, and the main reasons for this are:

> High concentration of ammonia in the medulla interferes with the antimicrobial action of complement.
>
> Hypertonicity of the interstitial fluid interferes with the action of phagocytes and allows the survival of protoplasts. Protoplasts are organisms which have lost their pathogenicity because of loss of a vital component of the cell membrane. They can only survive in hypertonic solutions, and they may become pathogenic again under suitable circumstances.
>
> The blood supply of the medulla is meagre compared with that of the cortex. This leads to a reduced supply of phagocytes; the blood supply to the medulla can be increased by promoting a diuresis, and this has been shown to prevent and eliminate infection.
>
> The medulla is susceptible to damage from other causes which may predispose to stasis.

Factors Predisposing to Infection

Catheterisation of the bladder
Urinary obstruction
Disorder of micturition due to neurological reasons
Diabetes mellitus

Coitus and pregnancy
Gout
Potassium deficiency
Nephrocalcinosis and nephrolithiasis
Hypertension and other causes of renal damage (e.g. collagen disorders)
Phenacetin ingestion
Sickle-cell trait.

Evidence of Infection

Infection may be present without symptoms or signs; there may be non-specific evidence (fever, leucocytosis and increased sedimentation rate). Although in pyelonephritis the essential infection is in the interstitial tissue of the kidney, the urine will provide a sample of the fluid within the interstitial tissue. Examination of the urine may demonstrate the infecting organism or evidence of renal damage. It is now well-established that careful collection of a normally voided specimen of urine will usually give evidence of infection when present. Direct bladder puncture or catheterisation is not usually necessary for the collection of samples. One of the problems is that even with very careful cleaning, there is always some contamination. However, this problem has been overcome by the demonstration that in asymptomatic people, bacterial counts in the urine below 10 000/ml do not indicate infection, but suggest contamination of the specimen with organisms at the introitus. Counts above 100 000/ml indicate infection in 85 per cent of cases (Kass, 1957). Bacterial counts between 10 000 and 100 000/ml are equivocal and a further specimen should be examined. Further evidence of infection is the growth of a single organism; the presence of several organisms suggests contamination. Evidence of inflammation may be given by an abnormally high excretion of leucocytes and casts. It is essential to appreciate that pyelonephritis may be present in the absence of white cells or pus cells in the urine. The presence of white cells in the urine indicates inflammation but this is not necessarily due to infection. White cells in a sterile urine may indicate pyelonephritis, renal tuberculosis, typhoid fever, acute glomerular nephritis, nephrolithiasis or phenacetin nephropathy.

Normal urine contains some white cells, and the number of these in normal urine has been defined and is up to 200 000/hour. There is an overlap between normals and patients with pylonephritis; however, the excretion of white cells in a patient with pyelonephritis can be increased by an intravenous injection of 40 mg of prednisone although it is rarely necessary these days to resort to this test. Further evidence of structural renal damage is the presence of proteinuria and an inability to concentrate and dilute the urine, due to involvement of the distal tubule, which is more susceptible to damage than the glomeruli; the patient may develop nocturia and an inability to concentrate the urine before there is any rise in blood urea or impairment of creatinine clearance. Rarely, a salt-losing syndrome due to tubular damage in the presence of a normal blood urea is the presenting feature.

Urine is an almost ideal culture medium for the most common organism responsible for urinary infection—*Escherichia*[5] *coli*. Urinary infections are due to only a very few serotypes of *E. coli*. Its pH, glucose content, osmolality and lack of humoral and cellular antibacterial substances make urine a good reservoir for bacteria. This is analogous to the situation in chronic bronchitis in which the sputum is an ever-present home for potentially pathogenic bacteria. *Symptomatic* renal and lower urinary-tract infections are undoubtedly associated with infection and micro-abscess formation within the tissues of the urinary tract. It follows from the above that the successful treatment of symptomatic urinary infections, or infections in which there is other evidence of tissue infection, demands a high tissue level of antibiotic to which the organism is sensitive, *and* steps to render the urine a less comfortable home for the offending organisms. However, another issue follows—if the urine is such a suitable place for the organisms to grow perhaps they grow there doing *no* harm; it is certainly true that bacteriuria is very common in the absence of any symptoms or other evidence of infection.

Evidence of *tissue* infection would be leucocytosis, raised sedimentation rate, pus cells, increased urinary enzymes (lactic dehydrogenase and glutamic oxaloacetic transaminase) and an increased titre of circulating antibodies to organisms grown from the urine. It has already been indicated that there are nearly always some pathogenic organisms in all urine—less than 10 000 organisms per ml is regarded as normal, more than 100 000/ml indicates urinary infection in 85 per cent of cases—this is regarded as "significant" bacteriuria. It is accepted that *transient* "significant" bacteriuria is common in normal women and girls; an "abnormality" is only likely in an asymptomatic patient with no renal damage when "significant" bacteriuria is *persistent*, i.e. has occurred in *three* successive speciments of urine. In the presence of urinary symptoms or other evidence of urinary infection, of course, one urine specimen containing 100 000 organisms per ml is highly significant and should be treated (v.i.). Pyuria (i.e. 5+ white cells per high-power field) when present usually indicates *tissue* infection; however, *tissue infection can be present in the absence of pyuria*.

In the absence of symptoms bacteriuria should not be considered significant unless there are more than 100 000/ml in at least *three* specimens; furthermore, pus cells may be absent from the urine even though infection is significant, because:

Pyuria is often intermittent

The concentration of pus cells is very dependent on rate of urine flow

Pus cells may be lysed in the urine

Pus cells are often absent from the urine even in clinically obvious pyelitis.

If there is doubt about the significance of pus cells a prednisone provocation test may be indicated. *Absence* of pus cells from the urine in the presence of bacteriuria should *not* lead to complacency.

In order to try to resolve some of the difficulty about the significance of persisting bacteriuria, attempts have been made to establish whether infection is involving renal parenchyma. The ways of doing this are:

Serum antibodies to the O antigen of *E. coli* found in the urine only occur when infection is involving the renal parenchyma.

Urine concentration. Ascending renal infection affects the efficiency of the collecting ducts and distal tubules leading to impairment of concentrating ability.

Excretion of enzymes in the urine known to result from inflammation of renal medulla, e.g. SGOT and LDH.

The presence of inflammatory cells.

Ureteric catheterisation.

Renal biopsy culture.

Urine obtained by Fairley techniques. This is a method of obtaining urine direct from the kidneys. The bladder is catheterised and sterilised with neomycin and well irrigated with sterile water. Samples are taken via the catheter every 10 minutes after inducing a diuresis.

The clinical importance of these techniques is to help assess whether recurrent asymptomatic bacteriuria is really due to infection within the kidneys or whether the organisms are harmless parasites or are contaminants.

The preliminary investigation of urinary infection should include an IVP and a micturating cystogram if there is a relapse or reinfection. It is usually not possible to eradicate organisms from the urine if there is anatomical abnormality in the urinary system.

One of the great enigmas about repeated urinary infections is the frequency with which they are followed by progressive renal damage and chronic pyelonephritis; and another whether persistent significant bacteriuria in the absence of other evidence of infection is to be regarded as a true urinary *tract* infection. Most authorities agree that *repeated* urinary *tract* infections during childhood often lead to chronic pyelonephritis. In adults, opinion is divided; some authorities regard *asymptomatic bacteriuria* in the absence of other evidence of infection as a benign condition.

Undiagnosed, asymptomatic pyelitis is widely regarded as a "missing link" between the frequent finding of chronic pyelonephritis at autopsy and the absence of any symptoms during life. However, the incidence of chronic pyelonephritis is equal in the two sexes, while bacteriuria and urinary infections are much commoner in women; many diseases other than repeated urinary infections can lead to histological appearances identical to pyelonephritis.

The incidence of chronic pyelonephritis is less common than was formerly believed and is of the order of 3 per cent, which corresponds with the incidence of undiagnosed structural disorders of the urinary tract which no one denies do lead to damaging infection and chronic pyelonephritis. Nevertheless, despite the conflicting evidence, ten working rules can be laid down for the clinician dealing with urinary tract infection:

1. Asymptomatic bacteriuria *alone* may indicate chronic pyelonephritis.
2. Repeated urinary infections *can* lead to progressive renal damage in the adult.
3. Repeated urinary infections *do* lead to progressive renal damage in children.
4. Patients who have *recurrent* urinary infections frequently have a structural abnormality of the urinary tract.
5. Suppression of recurrent asymptomatic bacteriuria *can* prevent progressive renal damage if given early, although successful suppression does not *always* prevent progressive damage.
6. Asymptomatic bacteriuria and urinary tract infections of pregnancy are associated with fetal prematurity and subsequent attacks of acute pyelonephritis in a quarter of women affected.
7. Persistent significant bacteriuria does not *always* mean infection in the kidney; infection may be localised to the bladder.
8. Asymptomatic bacteriuria with *any* evidence of tissue infection should be treated vigorously.
9. Hypertension complicates an unknown but probably small number of chronic renal infections.
10. Pyuria is *not* always present in urinary tract infections.

Following antibiotic treatment the incidence of further infection either with the same or different organism is very high. The rate of reinfection is not related to the length of the course of antibiotics; the rate of reinfection is 70–80 per cent regardless of whether the acute infection is treated for 14 days or 18 months. It is worth emphasising that the symptoms of pyelitis usually subside spontaneously even though bacteriuria and pyuria continue unchanged.

Numerous series have shown that recurrence rate following an acute urinary infection is around 80 per cent either with the original infecting organism or a different organism. For this reason it is *absolutely mandatory* that any patient with a urinary infection should be followed up for a minimum of 2 years with urine cultures every month for 6 months, then every 3 months for 18 months. *The available evidence does not in any way support the common practice of discharge of an asymptomatic patient after one or two token out-patient visits.*

Over 70 per cent of urinary infections are due to *E. coli* and 15 per cent to *Proteus vulgaris*. Sulphonamides are the drugs of choice for a first infection. In this country the evidence suggests that for the first symptomatic urinary infection, short, sharp courses of chemotherapy are as good (or bad!) as continuous treatment. In America, Kass believed that urinary infections in pregnancy should be treated with chemotherapy continuously until delivery; in this country there is a tendency not to use continuous chemotherapy *provided* there is *no* persistent bacteriuria. There is general agreement that pyelitis and continuing bacteriuria during pregnancy predispose to toxaemia and prematurity. It is also agreed that a high proportion (probably 20–30 per cent) of women who have symptomatic or asymptomatic bacteriuria of pregnancy will develop acute pyelonephritis and will have an abnormal IVP after pregnancy—it is not yet known what proportion of these women had bacteriuria (or urinary infection) before the pregnancy started.

The exact risk of developing renal damage with persistent bacteriuria is not known; however, it is known that *some* patients with persistent bacteriuria develop renal impairment and chronic pyelonephritis; furthermore this can happen when the bacteriuria is being actively treated. It should follow that an attempt should be made to eliminate persistent bacteriuria; however, there is genuine dispute as to whether the proportion (how small or large is not known) of patients who do develop progressive renal damage justifies routine treatment of asymptomatic bacteriuria in the remainder. It is suggested that those who develop renal damage will do so whether the bacteriuria is treated or not. There are several pieces of evidence that are difficult to interpret.

1. Bacteriuria occurs commonly in young girls without leading to renal damage.
2. Bacteriuria occurs very commonly (20–30 per cent) in elderly hospital patients.
3. Urinary infections are much commoner in women but the

incidence of pyelonephritis at post-mortem is equal in men and women.

4. The histological features of "pyelonephritis" can be caused by agents other than bacterial infection.

Recurrence of symptoms, significant bacteriuria or other evidence of infection is an indication for further *short* courses of chemotherapy.

In some centres facilities are available for measuring the circulating antibody titres to *E. coli* organisms which are grown from the urine. The antibody titre falls to zero within 6 weeks when the infection has been eliminated. Persistence of a raised titre indicates persisting infection or relapse of the original infection. Recurrence of infection due to a different organism is strong presumptive evidence of a structural abnormality of the urinary tract which should be fully investigated. One of the commonest causes of frequent relapses (due to the original infecting organism) or recurrence of an infection (i.e. due to a different organism) is reflux of urine from the bladder up the ureters—this may be demonstrated by a micturating cystogram. Evidence of dilatation of the calyces of the *upper* poles of the kidneys is particularly common with ureteric reflux.

Repeated recurrence of infection due to a different organism is an indication for long-term, continuous chemotherapy. This is best given continuously in the early stages; later it may be possible to give intermittent chemotherapy (e.g. for one week in three). The same antibiotics should be used continuously or for the intermittent courses. It is *not* recommended that alternating courses of different antibiotics be given as this is a sure way of producing antibiotic-resistant organisms. Nalidixic acid given with an acidifying agent such as mandelic acid is often suitable as a urinary antiseptic when recurrences are frequent. High concentrations are reached in the urine but not in the tissues; however, this may not matter if ascending infection of the urine is the route by which the organisms reach the kidneys.

Treatment of acute urinary infection.—Sulphonamides are the initial drug of choice for most urinary infections; a loading dose of 3·0 g is followed by 1·0 g 6-hourly for 10 days. A long-acting sulphonamide such as sulphadimethoxine (Madribon) 0·5 g can be given once daily instead. One disadvantage of a long-acting suphon-amide is that should the patient develop a hypersensitivity reaction, such as the Stevens-Johnson syndrome, the adverse reaction is usually more severe than with the shorter-acting drugs. All sulphonamides are bound to the plasma proteins but to a variable extent; the more free drug there is in the serum the higher is the effective tissue concentration of the drug. Sulphonamides are excreted by the kidneys after they have been acetylated; however, the acetyl derivative has no antibacterial properties. The drugs of choice in urinary infection are:

sulphadimidine, sulphamethizole (Urolucosil) and sulphafurazole (Gantrisin). Sulphamethizole and sulphafurazole are less bound to plasma proteins and are only about half acetylated, the remainder of the drug being excreted unchanged and hence in an active form in the urine.

Sulphonamides should be used with care if there is renal impairment. If one kidney is more damaged than the other, most of the drug will be excreted by the best kidney; hence almost no effective drug concentration will occur in the urine of the most damaged kidney.

Sulphadiazine is hardly bound at all to the plasma proteins and hence reaches a high tissue concentration; the concentration in the CSF may be 80 per cent of that in the blood, making it the drug of choice in the treatment of meningococcal meningitis. Unfortunately the solubility of the acetyl derivative is low, which makes the risk of crystalluria very high, particularly if there is oliguria. It should not be used in urinary infections.

The sulphonamides are most effective and the risk of crystalluria minimal if the urine is kept *alkaline* for *E. coli* infections. For *Str. faecalis* infections they work better in an acid urine.

If the sulphonamides fail to control infection or if there is symptomatic or bacterial evidence of a relapse they should be followed by 10-day courses of the following chemotherapeutic agents, provided the organisms cultured have been shown to be sensitive to them:

1. Septrin or Bactrim—a synergistic mixture of trimethoprim and a sulphonamide (urine pH should be alkaline).
2. Ampicillin 500 mg *q.d.s.* (unaffected by urinary pH).
3. Cephalexin.

The relapse rate following successful treatment of acute urinary infection is high; 60 per cent of patients relapse within 6 months and 80 per cent within 18 months. It therefore follows that all patients who have an acute urinary infection should be followed at *monthly intervals* for 6 months and 3-*monthly intervals* for a *further* 18 *months*.

Other antibiotics are sometimes necessary for the treatment of severe and persistent acute infections. The pH of the urine may be important because the effectiveness of the antibiotics is often pH-dependent. In all urinary infections the patient should be persuaded to have a high fluid intake—this creates the least hospitable invironment for the organisms; the dilution of the antibiotics in a dilute urine is less important than the production of other factors hostile to the infecting organisms.

Urinary pH for optimum antibacterial effect

Alkaline	*Acid*	*Unaffected by pH*
Sulphonamides	Tetracycline	Nitrofurantoin
(and trimethoprim)	Cycloserine	Ampicillin
Penicillin		
Streptomycin		
Erythromycin		
Gentamicin		

RENAL FAILURE

Renal failure implies failure of normal function of both glomeruli and tubules. By convention, isolated congenital or acquired tubular defects are not included. Chronic renal failure is not synonymous with irreversible renal failure, because chronic renal failure can sometimes be reversed by removing the cause, e.g. obstruction of the urinary tract or eradication of infection.

Functional Disturbances

One feature of renal failure which should be emphasised is that the glomeruli and tubules usually fail together. Any reduction in glomerular filtration due to disease affecting the glomeruli generally results in a diminution of blood supply to the tubules, resulting in a combination of glomerular and tubular failure ("total nephron failure").

Water excretion.—A reduction in glomerular filtration rate of solutes results in a rise in the serum concentration of urea, uric acid, urochromogen, phosphates and sulphates. These substances greatly increase the osmotic load and induce an osmotic diuresis, which results in polyuria and dehydration if water intake is not increased. Secondary tubular impairment (due to total nephron failure) results in inability to concentrate the urine, although the urine can often still be diluted if the kidney is presented with a water load. Inability to concentrate the urine results in nocturia, as the normal kidney concentrates urine at night. Later the kidney loses its ability to dilute, so that the urine has a fixed specific gravity—isosthenuria. Despite the ability to dilute the urine, the kidney is unable to excrete a water load as quickly as in a normal person because the total number of functioning nephrons is reduced. Patients with chronic renal failure are, therefore, vulnerable from the point of view of both overtransfusion and dehydration from vomiting and diarrhoea.

Acidosis.—Hydrogen ion is excreted in three forms:

1. Combined with ammonia (NH_3) to form ammonium (NH_4) salts

2. Combined with bicarbonate (NaHCO$_3$) to form carbonic acid (H$_2$CO$_3$)
3. Combined with disodium hydrogen phosphate (Na$_2$HPO$_4$) to form sodium dihydrogen phosphate (NaH$_2$PO$_4$).

The lowered glomerular filtration rate results in retention of phosphates which are then not available in the tubules for the formation of NaH$_2$PO$_4$. Tubular failure results in inability to produce ammonia and causes a leakage of bicarbonate, which is therefore not available for the formation of carbonic acid.

The increased hydrogen ion concentration in the blood is probably partly buffered by calcium buffers derived from the bones as well as the normal bicarbonate/carbonic acid buffers. Retention of hydrogen ion tends to cause a reduction in serum bicarbonate and hence a compensatory reduction in carbonic acid; CO$_2$ is blown off by hyperventilation (Kussmaul or acidotic breathing).

Sodium excretion.—Tubular impairment results in inability to reabsorb as much filtered sodium as normal. In the later stages of renal failure, overt sodium depletion may be present, which can be treated by increasing the dietary intake of sodium. However, this should be done carefully, because by this stage the kidney will have lost its ability to excrete increased amounts of solutes.

Potassium excretion.—Potassium is excreted by active tubular excretion as well as by glomerular filtration. Total nephron failure results in diminished filtration as well as impairment of active tubular excretion. Rarely, diseases which affect the renal tubules more than glomeruli (Fanconi syndrome and pyelonephritis) result in tubular damage and failure to reabsorb any filtered potassium, resulting in "potassium-losing nephritis". Hypokalaemia itself may cause tubular defects and increase the susceptibility to nephritis.

Calcium metabolism.—(See p. 523).

Anaemia.—There are many factors responsible for the anaemia of renal failure. The most important are:

1. Increased haemolysis
2. Bone-marrow depression due to reduced production or inhibition of erythropoietin.
3. Failure to incorporate iron bound to transferrin into red cells
4. Bleeding due to ulceration of the gastro-intestinal tract and purpura due to a platelet deficiency or increased capillary fragility.

The treatment of the anaemia of uraemia is unsatisfactory, as repeated blood transfusions have only a transient beneficial effect and sometimes they are positively harmful. When the haemoglobin level is raised by transfusion (and the PCV rises), the proportion of plasma in the blood falls; in chronic renal disease, the renal blood flow is usually fixed, so that less plasma will be flowing through the kidneys, and so the blood urea may rise.

Non-metabolic disturbances which may occur in uraemia are: pericarditis, "uraemic lung", peripheral neuropathy, coma, epilepsy, and hypertensive encephalopathy if there is associated hypertension.

ACUTE RENAL FAILURE

The main causes are:

> Sudden deterioration in pre-existing chronic renal failure
> Cardiogenic or septicaemic shock
> Ureteric obstruction
> Electrolyte imbalance (e.g. following severe vomiting and dehydration)
> Drugs (antibiotics and analgesics) and heavy metals
> Mismatched blood transfusion and haemolysis
> Malignant hypertension.

The main problem when confronted with a patient who is oliguric and uraemic is to decide whether dehydration and hypovolaemia are the cause, or whether there is damage to the kidney itself. This is an extremely important distinction, for in the one fluids will be required, and in the other they will be contra-indicated.

The clinical features may be vital in establishing the cause of the oliguria. It is essential to note:

> Any cause for dehydration (vomiting, diarrhoea, intestinal fistulae, excessive diuretics or diabetes)
> Duration of oliguria
> Previous history of renal disease (pyelonephritis, nephritis and polycystic kidneys) or urinary symptoms, particularly of prostatism or cystitis
> Presence of any cause of acute renal failure, for example shock, blood transfusion reaction, renal infarction or urinary infection.

If definite answers can be given to the above, it is usually easy to decide whether oliguria is due to dehydration or acute renal failure superimposed on normal or previously diseased kidneys. However, often reliable answers are not available and one has to rely on circumstantial evidence for obtaining the necessary information. The following information is necessary on all patients who are being treated for oliguria:

1. A definite decision as to whether dehydration is present or not.
2. Previous information with regard to renal function if available, for example a routine blood urea taken at an earlier admission.
3. A careful record of the exact volume of urine passed.
4. Examination of the urine will help decide whether oliguria is due to dehydration or damage to the kidneys, for example the presence of casts on microscopic examination.

   (a) *Concentration*—If the specific gravity is above 1015, severe renal damage can usually be ruled out. The colour of the urine is *no* indication as to its concentration. Urochrome pigments are excreted even in renal failure and may make the urine very dark in colour even though it is dilute.
   (b) *Urine urea.*—Over 150 mmol/l suggests normal kidneys and prerenal uraemia. Less than 150 mmol/l suggests established tubular necrosis. In prerenal uraemia the urinary/plasma urea ratio should be 10:1.
   (c) *Urine sodium.*—On a normal diet the normal urinary sodium is roughly 100 mmol/l. In oliguria due to dehydration or circulatory failure the urinary sodium is usually very low (less than 10 mmol/l.); this is because aldosterone secretion is stimulated and is causing sodium retention; the fact that the kidneys are able to respond to aldosterone and conserve sodium means that renal damage is not severe. In the presence of *oliguria* a urine sodium of more than 80 mmol/l suggest renal damage because the kidneys are not responding to aldosterone. It is possible to estimate chloride in the ward using a kit; the chloride levels correspond well with the sodium levels.
   (d) *Urine osmolality and specific gravity.*—The specific gravity of plasma without the plasma proteins is approximately 1010. In acute renal failure due to cortical necrosis, any urine passed has approximately this specific gravity. In prerenal oliguria the urine passed is much more concentrated due to the affect of ADH secretion. The specific gravity depends on the weight of dissolved substances regardless of their osmotic potential: osmolality measures the osmotic potential. Glucose, urea and other substances increase the specific gravity much more than the osmotic potential. It is more accurate to measure osmolality than specific gravity. The osmolality of plasma is 330 mOsm/l; in prerenal uraemia with maximal ADH secretion the osmolality of the urine should be at least 500 mOsm/l and may reach 1200 mOsm/l. In acute renal failure the osmolality of any urine passed is around 300 mOsm/l.

(e) *Urinary casts.*—A large number of casts suggest renal damage.

(f) *Culture of the urine.*—A heavy growth of a single organism suggests renal infection.

(g) *Urinary protein with electrophoresis.*—Large amounts of albumin (low molecular weight) suggest glomerular damage. Large amounts of globulin (high MW) suggest inflammation in the lower urinary tract.

5. Serum electrolytes and urea. It should be noted that an increase in all the electrolytes may indicate haemoconcentration and, therefore, dehydration.

6. Haemoglobulin and packed cell volume (PCV). Chronic renal damage often causes anaemia. Changes in the PCV are one of the ways of assessing the extracellular fluid state.

7. Plain x-ray of the abdomen to demonstrate kidney size and the presence or absence of the calculus which may be causing ureteric obstruction. The presence of one small kidney will indicate long-standing renal disease. If oliguria is due to unilateral ureteric obstruction the affected kidney may be slightly larger than normal.

8. Daily or twice-daily ECG.

9. Routine weighing of the patient if possible. An increase of weight is an indication of fluid retention.

Management of Acute Renal Failure

The management of acute renal failure is based on the premise that provided the cause is removed acute renal failure is potentially reversible. However, the accumulation of metabolites and waste products may cause death before the kidneys have a chance to recover. The most important substances which accumulate are:

Water
Urea
Electrolytes, particularly potassium
Acid metabolites such as sulphates.

Under normal circumstances, approximately 1000 ml water is lost daily in the sweat and faeces. However, many of the metabolic processes of the body produce water as a waste product—"water of metabolism"; usually this is about 500 ml but it may be considerably more in hypercatabolic renal failure (*v.i.*). This means that up to about 500 ml water can be given even if the patient has complete anuria.

The basal calorie requirement of the body at rest is about 1000—this is essential for voluntary and involuntary muscular movements, etc. If the patient is starved, body protein will be broken down to provide these basal calorie requirements, hence adequate carbohydrates must be given in order to prevent the harmful breakdown of body protein. There is evidence that by giving an excess of calories as carbohydrate or fat almost no body protein need be metabolised. The importance of sparing body protein is that patients who lose weight rapidly due to protein loss are prone to develop systemic infection and complicated electrolyte disturbances, and acidosis. Another important reason for preventing protein breakdown is that more urea and electrolytes are produced. The aim of treatment is, therefore, to conserve as much of the body's own protein as possible.

If a condition is present which is likely to cause acute renal failure (for example, shock, surgical operation, burns) there is now good evidence that administration of mannitol given prophylactically will prevent it. It increases extracellular fluid volume and renal blood flow; its osmotic action is probably not important.

Mannitol can also be used to determine whether renal failure is due to dehydration. Infusion of 100 ml 20 per cent mannitol over 15 minutes should result in a diuresis of 100 ml in the next 2 hours in the presence of dehydration but not if there is renal impairment.

Fluids.—500 ml plus the equivalent of the previous 24-hour urine volume.

Electrolyte requirements.—If the patient is passing no urine at all, no electrolytes are needed. The sodium and urea content of all urine passed should be measured if possible. Electrolytes should be replaced according to the amount lost in the urine.

Diet.—The diet should contain the basal quantity of calories plus an excess in order to spare endogenous protein breakdown. In addition, certain essential amino acids can be given which do not cause a rise in blood urea when they are synthesised to body proteins.

Parenteral fluids and nutrition.—If the patient is too ill to take any fluids by mouth he will have to be fed entirely intravenously and the great problem is to give sufficient calories without an excess of fluid.

20 per cent glucose will produce 800 cals/litre.

Examples of suitable parenteral regimes:

(a) Complete anuria.
    500 ml 40 per cent glucose (800 cals).
(b) Oliguria (500 ml urine in previous 24 hours).
    1000 ml 20 per cent or 40 per cent glucose (800 or 1600 cals).
(c) Oliguria (1000 ml urine in previous 24 hours) entering the diuretic phase.
    1500 ml 20 per cent or 40 per cent glucose (1200 or 2400 cals).

Because the parenteral solutions used are hypertonic they must be given into a large vein. In addition, heparin 1000 units per litre of fluid is usually given.

Anabolic steroids.—Protein breakdown can be reduced by giving anabolic steroids and it is customary to give norethandrolone 10 mg for the duration of the acute renal failure.

Hyperkalaemia.—This is the most dangerous complication of acute renal failure because it causes cardiac arrhythmias. The changes in the ECG which occur in hyperkalaemia are:

Tall T waves
Widening of the QRS complex
Prolongation of the PR interval
Disappearance of the P waves.

In an emergency the effects of potassium on the heart can be counteracted by intravenous calcium gluconate (20 ml of 10 per cent solution). The serum potassium can be temporarily lowered by giving insulin which promotes potassium transfer into the cells. 20 units of soluble insulin are given with 100 ml of 50 per cent glucose. Potassium can also be removed from the body by sodium ion exchange resin (Resonium-A). 40 g daily is given either by mouth or as a retention enema.

Other requirements.—(a) Vitamins should be given.

(b) Dry mouth can be prevented by sucking ice cubes, chewing gum or small pieces of lemon.

(c) *Severe* anaemia should be corrected with blood transfusion, but it must be noted that stored blood contains a large amount of potassium and protein.

Should these methods fail to control the metabolites before the patient begins to pass urine, then dialysis (either haemo or peritoneal) is considered. The main indications for dialysis are:

1. Hypercatabolic renal failure (rise in urea of more than 6·5 mmol/l per day)
2. Blood urea 30 mmol/l
3. Serum potassium above 6·0 mmol/l
4. Serum bicarbonate below 15 mmol/l (indicating acidosis)
5. Clinical deterioration and bleeding.

Peritoneal dialysis is usually the treatment of choice in the management of acute renal failure. It can be performed even if the patient has had a recent abdominal operation. It is particularly suitable for patients in whom it would be hazardous to perform haemodialysis, for example in those with a bleeding diathesis, poor cardiac output (e.g., after cardiac infarction), and in those patients who have uncommon blood groups for whom sufficient blood it not available for haemodialysis. Peritoneal dialysis is relatively simple to manage and requires the minimum of equipment and staff. Only two solutions are necessary, each contains the necessary concentration of electrolytes except potassium which has to be added. The solutions only differ in the amount of dextrose which they contain: one contains an excess of dextrose so that if the patient is overhydrated water will be absorbed into the fluid; the other solution used routinely is iso-osmolar with normal plasma (although, of course, not with plasma containing a high concentration of urea). The fluid is run into the peritoneum in hourly cycles, and is left in for 45 minutes before being siphoned out.

Potassium is added to the dialysis fluid if the patient is becoming hypokalaemic. The peritoneum exudes a certain amount of protein into the fluid and this can be replaced by allowing the patient to have some first-class protein in the diet, or by giving plasma. Each day, a sample of the dialysate is cultured after dialysis and if infection is present it is treated with the appropriate antibiotic. The incidence of infection is low and seems to be even less if the dialyses are kept down to 6–8 per day.

The main dangers of management to be avoided are:

Delay in starting dialysis until the patient has clinically deteriorated.

Inadequate care with catheterisation: technique should be irreproachable, and daily bladder washouts with antibiotic (neomycin usually) should be performed.

Over-enthusiasm once peritoneal dialysis is started: it is better to aim to dialyse for short periods and control the urea, potassium and hydration, than to aim for complete normality. After all, the aim of this treatment is only to tide the patient over; the number of dialyses should be kept to a minimum.

Stopping too soon. Once the diuretic phase has started, it is important to keep the dialysis tube in place until the blood urea and potassium are falling and the sodium and urea concentrations in the urine are rising.

Management of Chronic Renal Failure

It is worth emphasising two important functional differences between chronic and acute renal failure: in chronic renal failure the patient usually excretes too much water and too much sodium—the complete opposite to acute renal failure. *But* in the nephrotic syndrome, before chronic renal failure develops there is hypoproteinaemia which leads to fluid retention and sodium retention—this is why it is essential to grasp the difference between the nephrotic syndrome and chronic renal failure, and to appreciate that the nephrotic syndrome may terminate as chronic renal failure, necessitating alteration of treatment.

In other respects, acute and chronic renal failure cause similar functional disturbances, viz. rise in blood urea, rise in serum potassium, acidosis and anaemia. Hypertension may complicate chronic renal failure.

The important aspects of the management of chronic renal failure are:

1. Ensure adequate water intake. (Give the patient some idea by saying that he must fill a 2-litre container with urine each day.)
2. Ensure adequate sodium intake.
3. Control acidosis by prescribing oral sodium bicarbonate each day.
4. Prevent uraemic symptoms and protein breakdown by giving a modified Giovanetti diet which contains a known amount of first-class protein and essential amino acids. Restrict the intake of other proteins.
5. Control gently the blood pressure, urinary infections and anaemia if possible.
6. Treat osteodystrophy if present. Small doses of 1-α-cholecalciferol if the calcium is reduced, or possibly parathyroidectomy if the calcium becomes elevated as a result of tertiary hyperparathyroidism.
7. Consider haemodialysis and renal transplantation.

Before the stage of chronic renal failure in the nephrotic syndrome, the patient will usually require increased protein in the diet to compensate for excessive loss in the urine, but sodium intake should be restricted because the patient will have fluid retention due to hypoproteinaemia. If the blood urea begins to rise in the nephrotic syndrome or chronic renal failure develops, then protein intake will need to be restricted.

Fluid and Electrolyte Balance

It is possible to cope with any practical problem of fluid, electrolyte and acid-base imbalance if certain simple concepts and rules are applied (see p. 140 for discussion of Acid-Base Balance). The first of these is to remember the approximate volumes of the fluid compartments which are, in a 70 kg person:

Extracellular volume = 15 litres = 20 per cent of the body weight
(Plasma volume   = 3 litres = 4 per cent of the body weight)
Intracellular volume = 30 litres = 40 per cent of the body weight
Total body water   = 45 litres = 60 per cent of the body weight

Water is freely diffusible between extra- and intracellular compartments. Sodium is restricted to the extracellular compartment and potassium to the intracellular compartment; bicarbonate occurs in both.

Milliequivalents (Millimoles) and Available Solutions

One atom of hydrogen reacts with one atom of chloride which reacts with one atom of sodium. The weight of one atom of hydrogen is the unit, the weight of sodium is then 23 and of chloride is 35. Hence, 1 gram of hydrogen will react with 35 g of chloride, which reacts with 23 g of sodium. The weight of a substance which reacts with 1 g of hydrogen is known as the "gram equivalent weight". 23 g of sodium will combine with 35 g of chloride, but only one atom of chloride reacts with one atom of sodium, therefore, 35 g of chloride and 23 g of sodium each contain the same number of atoms (or "particles"). It is the number of "particles" present that determines the osmotic potential and the pH of solutions, and not the relative weight of the particles.

In chemical solutions which contain known weights of ions, we need to know, for physiological purposes, the number of "particles", in order to keep the pH and osmotic potential constant.

1 gram of hydrogen is equivalent to 35 g of chloride which is equivalent to 23 g of sodium.

1 gram equivalent (of hydrogen) is equivalent to 58 grams (23 + 35) of sodium chloride.

1 milligram equivalent of hydrogen is equivalent to 0·058 g or 58 milligrams of sodium chloride.

1 milligram equivalent is called a milliequivalent (mEq) or a millimole (mmol).

∴ 1 mEq or millimole = 58 milligrams of NaCl

∴ 1000 mEq or millimoles = 58 g of NaCl

∴ 1 gram NaCl contains 1000/58 mEq or millimoles = 17 mEq or millimoles.

We can, therefore, say that a gram of sodium chloride contains 17 milliequivalents of sodium and chloride. We need to know the number of milliequivalents in 1 gram of other salts, the most important of these are:

potassium chloride	13
sodium bicarbonate	12
calcium chloride	9

To summarise:

We need to bother with milliequivalents or millimoles for these reasons:

(i) All simple salts contain equal numbers of milliequivalents or millimoles of their constituent ions (but different weights of each ion).

(ii) To be at a neutral pH solutions must contain equal numbers of milliequivalents or millimoles of anions and cations, and not equal weights of each.

(iii) Solutions containing the same number of milliequivalents of different ions will be iso-osmotic with each other.

If we had to remember the number of milligrams of sodium which reacted with the number of milligrams of chloride or bicarbonate etc., it would be a monumental task to work out the amount of each ion that had to be given to combine with the other, and it would need separate calculations to work out the osmotic strength of the solution and whether its pH has changed.

Expressed simply, the pH and osmotic potential depend on the number of ionised "particles" present, and not on the weight of the "particles". Furthermore, simple salts consist of one "particle" of one ion joined to one "particle" of another ion, the relative weights of each "particle" do not matter.

In normal plasma, mmol/l of anions = mmol/l of cations = 150.

All parenteral solutions aim to be the same concentration (isotonic) as plasma. To achieve this, slightly different *concentrations* of each salt are necessary, for example, sodium chloride has to be a 0·9 per cent solution, and sodium bicarbonate a 1·4 per cent solution to be isotonic with plasma (i.e. 0·9 grams per 100 ml of NaCl and 1·4 grams per 100 ml of $NaHCO_3$).

It is convenient to consider all solutions in litres rather than in units of 100 ml, therefore a 0·9 per cent solution of sodium chloride will contain 9 grams per litre, and a 1·4 per cent solution of sodium bicarbonate, 14 grams per litre.

We already know that 1 gram of sodium chloride contains 17 mEq or mmol of sodium and chloride, therefore 9 grams will contain 153 mEq or mmol, i.e. a litre of isotonic (0·9 per cent) solution of NaCl will contain 153 mEq or mmol of sodium and chloride. Similarly, a litre of 1·4 per cent $NaHCO_3$ will contain 167 mEq or mmol of sodium and bicarbonate.

It is not recommended that complicated prepared intravenous solutions such as Ringer's, Hartmann's or Darrow's solutions be used, as the exact electrolyte content of each is not usually widely known.

Correction of Disturbed Electrolyte Balance

Sodium and Water

1. Depleted serum sodium.—This can be due either to (a) excessive water, or (b) a reduction in the amount of sodium (almost invariably accompanied by loss of water as well). Excess water is present if there is reduced excretion of water, for example acute renal failure, severe oedema or an excess of intake over excretion (for example, over-transfusion).

An excess of intake over excretion of pure water may result in *water intoxication*. The excess water is evenly distributed throughout both compartments. A small excess in circulating volume and extra-cellular fluid is not important but a small excess of intracellular water gives rise to water intoxication; it is the brain cells which are most sensitive to this increase in water, hence most of the symptoms are cerebral and the patient becomes stuporous and eventually comatose with convulsions.

Reduction of the serum sodium due to excessive loss of sodium is almost invariably accompanied by loss of water; when water is lost from the body (dehydration) it is first lost from the extracellular fluid in an attempt to conserve both the intracellular water and the circulating blood volume; if the loss continues water is removed from the intracellular compartment and finally from the circulating volume. The physical signs of dehydration reflect this sequence of salt and water loss.

Loss from extracellular compartment:
	dry tongue
	dry skin and loss of skin elasticity
	reduced intra-ocular pressure
Loss of intracellular fluid:	drowsiness
	pyrexia.
Loss of circulating fluid:	tachycardia
	reduced blood pressure
	constricted veins
Other signs of dehydration:	reduced flow of concentrated urine
	high packed-cell volume (increased haematocrit)
	increased blood urea.

Summary.—A low serum sodium with (a) signs of dehydration means loss of salt and water, (b) absence of signs of dehydration but with disturbance of cerebral function, means water intoxication.

2. Increased serum sodium.—In practice this means (a) excess loss of water over sodium or (b) over-transfusion with saline. Excess loss of water occurs in fistulae or excessive sweating and will be accompanied by the signs of dehydration. Over-transfusion with salt and water will result in an increase in volume of the extracellular and vascular compartments (not the intracellular, because sodium only occurs in the extracellular compartment). Excess fluid in the extracellular compartment affects mainly the lung, resulting in pulmonary oedema; later, oedema of the sacrum and finally the ankles may occur. Excess fluid in the vascular compartment results in elevation of the jugular venous pulse.

Summary.—An increased serum sodium (a) with signs of dehydration means excessive water loss; (b) without signs of dehydration but with elevation of the jugular venous pulse or pulmonary oedema means over-transfusion.

Treatment

A low serum sodium.—(a) With signs of dehydration (indicating loss of excessive salt and some water), give:
  (i) hypertonic saline (NaCl 5 per cent) which contains 855 mEq (mmol)/l of sodium and chloride;
  (ii) sodium bicarbonate (1·4 per cent) which contains 167 mEq (mmol)/l of Na and 167 mEq (mmol)/l of HCO_3.
(b) Without signs of dehydration but with disturbance of cerebral function (water intoxication). The aims of treatment are to reduce the cerebral oedema and promote the loss of water. This is best achieved by 20 per cent mannitol.

A high serum sodium.—(a) With signs of dehydration (indicating excess loss of water over sodium), give:
  (i) normal saline (0·9 per cent) NaCl which contains 154 mEq (mmol)/l of NaCl, that is, isotonic with plasma;
  (ii) dextrose/saline—NaCl (0·18 per cent) and 4·3 per cent dextrose (called "fifth normal saline"—note that 0·18 is $^1/_5$ of 0·9); this contains 31 mEq (mmol)/l of sodium and chloride;
  (iii) rarely, if water loss is truly excessive, dextrose 5 per cent. The sugar is metabolised leaving behind pure water.
(b) Without signs of dehydration usually means over-transfusion. The infusion should be stopped and a diuretic given (frusemide 40 mg intramuscularly).

How much of these solutions should be given?—The cardinal points to remember are the size of the compartments, the normal electrolyte content of plasma, and the fact that water is freely diffusible through both compartments but that sodium is found only in the extracellular compartment.

If the serum sodium is high it means that water has been drawn out from the cells to attempt to dilute the concentrated extracellular fluid; hence, sufficient water has to be given to dilute the serum so that the serum sodium returns to normal, and enough has to be given to replace that which has been drawn out from the cells. Hence, enough water has to be given to dilute the *total body water*—which is approximately 60 per cent of the body weight. Thus, if the observed serum sodium is 160 mmol/l it means that every litre of body water is concentrated to the same extent (although in the cells sodium will not be the ion which accounts for the concentration). Every litre, therefore, contains 20 mEq too much sodium.

∴ if the normal serum sodium is 140 mEq (mmol) every litre contains 20/140 more sodium than normal;

∴ to bring the serum sodium back to normal concentration each litre must be increased by 20/140 (that is, 1/7).

However, it has already been stated that every litre of body water has to be considered,

∴ the total amount of water required will be in litres 1/7×60 per cent of the body weight (kg);

that is, in hypernatraemia due to water and salt loss the amount of water required will be:

$$\frac{[\text{Na}]-140}{140} \times \frac{3}{5} \text{ body weight in litres.}$$

If the serum sodium is low in the presence of loss of sodium and water it means that water has been drawn into the cells so that the total body water is available for diluting any administered sodium.

Assuming the serum sodium is 120 mEq (mmol)/l, each litre will be 20 mEq (mmol) of sodium short. Hence, to increase the sodium content of the extracellular fluid to normal it must be assumed that the excess water in the cells is also available for diluting the administered sodium, that is, every litre of body water is 20 mEq (mmol) of sodium short, hence the amount of sodium which needs to be given is

20×60 per cent body water in mEq (mmol).

In practice in combined salt and water loss:

(a) if the serum sodium is 120–160 mEq (mmol)/l normal saline is given
(b) if the serum sodium is less than 120 mEq (mmol)/l, 1 litre hypertonic saline is given

(c) if the serum sodium is more than 160 mEq (mmol)/l, 3 litres 5 per cent dextrose is given.

Potassium

The serum level of potassium is a poor guide to potassium balance since potassium is found mainly inside the cells and the level in the serum will depend partly on the amount of water in the extracellular and vascular compartments. In addition potassium may leak out of cells in conditions causing an acidosis (for example, uraemia and diabetes) producing a high level in the serum due to depletion of normal intracellular potassium. Potassium depletion is best confirmed with an ECG (hypokalaemia causes lowering and inversion of T waves, prominent U waves and prolongation of the QT interval). Potassium depletion may cause:

cardiac arrhythmias
excessive sensitivity to digitalis
muscle weakness
renal damage.

Significant hypokalaemia is always accompanied by an alkalosis (hydrogen ion is lost by the kidney in an attempt to conserve potassium; hydrogen ion also passes into the cells to compensate for leakage of potassium leading to an intracellular acidosis). Accompanying water depletion may cause apparently normal serum levels of potassium due to haemoconcentration.

Hypokalaemia may only become obvious when the dehydration is treated. Similarly a metabolic acidosis may mask the accompanying alkalosis due to potassium depletion.

Potassium depletion occurs:

1. During loss of large volumes of intestinal contents (vomiting, diarrhoea, fistula)
2. During starvation (an adequate intake of glucose is essential for the functional integrity of cell membranes)
3. During hypercatabolic states when potassium is lost in the urine together with large amounts of endogenous protein
4. During diuretic therapy
5. In potassium-losing nephritis
6. In hyperaldosteronism (primary and secondary)
7. In severe salt and water depletion in which large amounts of aldosterone are produced causing sodium retention at the expense of potassium
8. In renal tubular disorders and certain rare potassium-losing tumours of the large intestine

9. In Cushing's syndrome
10. In familial periodic paralysis.

Correction of hypokalaemia.—If potassium deficiency is suspected, potassium should be administered in 5 per cent dextrose or 4·3 per cent dextrose/fifth normal saline. 1 g potassium chloride contains 13 mEq of potassium. It is seldom necessary to give more than 1–2 g per hour.

(For a discussion of acid-base disturbance, see p. 140)

Retroperitoneal Fibrosis

The most common presenting feature is hypertension, although weight loss, loin pain, urinary symptoms and low backache are also common symptoms. The condition is not confined to the retroperitoneal area: involvement of the pancreas may lead to diabetes, of the heart to heart block and conduction defects, of the liver to portal hypertension, of the mediastinum to vena caval and oesophageal obstruction, and of the lungs to pulmonary fibrosis. The sedimentation rate is usually elevated; the IVP shows narrowing of the mid-point of the ureters which are generally deviated medially. It is important that the whole of both ureters be seen on the IVP. Drugs which are reported to cause the condition are methysergide, dexamphetamine, ergotamine and hydralazine. Other sclerosing conditions such as sclerosing cholangitis, Riedel's thyroiditis and fibrotic contractures of the fingers are reported to have been associated. Retroperitoneal lymphomas can cause widespread fibrosis. Injection of sclerosing substances for haemorrhoids and varicose veins have been suggested as possible causes.

REFERENCES

ADDIS, T. (1949) *Glomerular Nephritis.* New York: Macmillan Co.
BRITISH MEDICAL JOURNAL (1979) Recommended terminology of urinary tract infection **2**, 717.
KASS, E. H. (1957) *Arch. intern. Med.,* **100**, 709.
KERR, D. N. S. (1978) *Progressive Clinical Medicine* 7th edit. Ed. HURLER, A. R. and FOSTER, J. B. Edinburgh: Churchill Livingstone.

GENERAL REFERENCE

BLACK, D. and JONES, N. F. (1979) *Renal Diseases,* 4th edit. Oxford: Blackwell Scientific Publications.

EPONYMS

1. PAUL ALBERT GRAWITZ (1850–1932)
Greifswald pathologist.

2. FRIEDRICH GUSTAV JAKOB HENLE (1809–1885)
Henle, a Jew, had liberal tendencies when young. He conceived two major conceptual advances: the first was that of epithelial surfaces, and the second was that micro-organisms are responsible for many diseases. Robert Koch, who was his pupil, later entirely vindicated Henle's novel views about the causes of infectious diseases.

3. GUIDO FANCONI (b. 1892)
Professor of Paediatrics at the University of Zürich (1929–1962).

4. SIR WILLIAM BOWMAN (1816–1892)
Bowman qualified at King's College Hospital, after which he travelled in Europe as mentor to Francis Galton. He was elected to the Royal Society at the age of 25, having been the first to note the difference between striated and involuntary smooth muscle; in the new specialty of ophthalmology he also made fundamental observations. He was first to use Helmholtz's ophthalmoscope and performed the first iridectomy for glaucoma in Britain.

5. THEODOR ESCHERICH (1857–1911)
Escherich was Professor of Paediatrics successively in Graz and Vienna.

9

SHOCK

Shock results from a complicated circulatory disorder affecting:

The pumping function of the heart
Blood distribution (arterioles)
Microcirculation (capillaries)
Capacitance vessels (veins)
Physical properties of the blood
The pulmonary circulation and lungs.

One of the simplest and most inclusive definitions of shock is *a clinical state in which the cardiac output is insufficient for tissue requirements*; the main tissue requirements are an adequate supply of oxygen and nutrients *and* adequate removal of the waste products of metabolism. Shock may be accompanied by or caused by acute heart failure; but all cases of heart failure are not necessarily shocked, because the dominant feature may be congestion behind the pump rather than forward failure of the pump and inadequate vascular compensation.

Shock results in reduced tissue perfusion, and therefore tissue hypoxia and accumulation of metabolites. The sympathetic and catecholamine activity cause cells to continue to metabolise at a normal or increased rate until hypoxia eventually causes reduced cell metabolism which soon becomes irreversible. The temporary continuation of cell metabolism is also encouraged by simultaneous increase in thyroid hormone and adrenal corticosteroids, while a reduction in insulin tends to impair cell utilisation of available glucose. Hypoxia tends to increase intracellular phosphorylation and accelerate the transfer of glucose across cell membranes, but glucose availability is further limited by reduced gluconeogenesis. Pyruvate accumulates locally because hypoxia damages cocarboxylase, the enzyme which allows pyruvate into the Krebs cycle.

Causes

A. Reduced venous return

Haemorrhage
Dehydration:
    Vomiting and diarrhoea   Addison's disease
    Diabetic ketosis   Heat stroke

Endotoxin shock
Anaphylaxis
Neurogenic shock (abdominal and testicular trauma, paracentesis)
Psychogenic shock
Acute peritonitis, pancreatitis and perforation
Burns.

B. **Reduced cardiac output (cardiogenic shock)**

Myocardial infarction
Pulmonary embolism
Myocarditis
Dysrhythmia
Cardiac tamponade
Ruptured valve cusp, papillary muscle, interventricular septum or chordae tendineae
Tight aortic or mitral stenosis.

Haemorrhage and loss of circulating fluid.—Following a sudden loss of blood or fluid from the intravascular compartment the cardiac output is maintained by an increase in the heart rate. Vasoconstriction of the arterioles occurs in such a way that perfusion of privileged tissues (brain and heart) is maintained while blood is diverted from less essential tissues. In the later stages of shock, due to fluid loss, there is a decrease in venous return, a fall in central venous pressure, a diminution in stroke volume and eventually a fall in blood pressure. The oxygen available to the tissues is very little reduced by a fall in haemoglobin of 30 per cent. The emphasis is swinging away from the rule "blood for blood lost". The most important factor is restoration of circulating volume. If dehydration has not reached the stage of causing a reduction in circulating volume electrolyte solutions can be used for rehydration. These will pass immediately into the dry extracellular space. If dehydration has progressed to the stage of diminished intravascular fluid volume as well as diminished extracellular fluid volume, early replacement is best made with solutions with a high oncotic pressure, i.e. the osmotic pressure is due to colloids (whole blood, plasma, albumin or dextrans). Later, electrolyte solutions can be used to rehydrate the extracellular compartment.

If electrolyte solutions are given to patients in whom dehydration has diminished the extracellular and vascular compartments most of the administered fluid passes straight into the extracellular compartment.

Endotoxin or Gram[1]-negative shock.—The endotoxin responsible for the peripheral circulatory failure in septicaemia due to Gram-negative organisms is a lipopolysaccharide within the cell wall of the organisms. The endotoxin has an intense sympathomimetic effect resulting in vasoconstriction of arterioles of the bowel, kidneys and lungs. The sympathomimetic effect is also partly due to release of endogenous catecholamines and the combination of the endotoxin with some substance in the blood producing an unknown sympathomimetic agent. The most usual organisms responsible are *E. coli, Str. faecalis, Bacteroides* and *Pseudomonas aeruginosa (pyocyanea)*. It is important to be aware that Gram-positive septicaemia can result in similar haemodynamic disturbances, although less commonly. The incidence of Gram-negative septicaemia is increasing due to increased use of intravenous infusions, corticosteroids, immunosuppressive drugs, and surgery in neonates and the elderly. Pulmonary oedema occurs more readily in septicaemia than other forms of shock even in the absence of left ventricular failure (shock lung).

Anaphylaxis.—Anaphylactic shock results from an antibody-antigen reaction occurring on the surface of the mast cells and releasing vasoactive substances such as histamine, 5-hydroxytryptamine, bradykinin and other kinins. These cause contraction of bronchial smooth muscle and airways narrowing, dilatation of the microcirculation and pooling of blood, increased capillary permeability, and loss of intravascular fluid. Sympathomimetic drugs are beneficial in the early stages of anaphylactic shock.

Neurogenic shock.—Sudden trauma to sensitive autonomic ganglia (e.g. a blow to the abdomen or testicles) can result in temporary dysfunction of the autonomic control of blood vessels. There is good evidence that some of the effects of shock due to pulmonary embolism and myocardial infarction are due to stimulation of local afferent nerve fibres and inappropriate response by peripheral blood vessels.

Psychogenic shock (vasovagal syncope).—Sudden emotional shock can cause widespread peripheral arteriolar dilatation and pooling of blood with a low cardiac output. Usually this is quickly reversible but occasionally it persists. Signs of disordered autonomic function, including disturbed vascular reflexes, are sometimes part of disordered emotional behaviour after sudden or sustained psychogenic shock (e.g. battle-fatigue). During the Second World War the use of immediate sedation after a harrowing experience reduced the incidence of subsequent hysterical behaviour. The situation is complicated if a patient has been physically injured *and* is suffering from psychogenic shock. This is seen in civilian practice when an injured driver sees his passenger mutilated in a road traffic accident. Severe pain and fear also gives rise to disordered vascular function through neurogenic or psychogenic mechanisms. For these reasons sedation and analgesia should be given to conscious casualties as soon as possible after injury. Morphia is given for its analgesic and sedative properties—if a casualty in an accident is not in pain, morphia is still indicated for its sedative properties. It should generally be given intravenously because of irregular absorption from intramuscular sites in states of shock.

Intra-abdominal emergencies and burns.—The causes of shock in these situations are due to several factors; fluid, protein and electrolyte loss, sudden pain, neurogenic factors and Gram-negative septicaemia.

Cardiogenic shock.—This is characterised by a sudden fall in cardiac output which brings into operation protective mechanisms similar to those in all other situations in which effective cardiac output is reduced. The response of the peripheral circulation to an inadequate cardiac output is the same whether it is due to Gram-negative septicaemia, anaphylaxis, haemorrhage and fluid loss, myocardial infarction, pulmonary embolism or dysrhythmia. In the case of cardiogenic shock two other adverse factors are in operation: one is the fact that the pump itself is damaged, and the other is the variable part played by neurogenic mechanisms in impairing peripheral circulatory function. It is thought that impulses from the injured myocardium or coronary arteries travel in afferent sympathetic pathways—probably via the vagus nerve—and disturb peripheral vascular responses. In acute cardiac failure there is often a simultaneous reduction in venous return, so that pulmonary congestion does not always occur.

Pathophysiology of Shock

All blood vessels contain both types of adrenergic receptors—α and β. In general, stimulation of the α receptors results in constriction of arterioles, capillaries and veins, while stimulation of the β receptors results in vasodilatation. The relative numbers of α and β receptors varies in different blood vessels, hence the exact response to adrenergic receptor stimulation varies in different parts of the body. Stimulation of β receptors of the heart results in an increase in myocardial contractility (inotropic action); β receptors predominate in the heart. Alpha receptors predominate in the gut, skin and kidney. In the muscles, α and β receptors are present in roughly equal amounts. In the heart and brain there are very few receptors. In general α receptors are innervated by the sympathetic system, whereas β receptors are not innervated and respond to circulating catecholamines. A further factor to be taken into account is the variable responsiveness of local blood vessels to accumulation of metabolites; the coronary circulation for example is very responsive to local metabolites.

The capillaries are freely permeable to water and electrolytes. Flow through capillaries is controlled by sphincter mechanisms at both ends—the pre- and postcapillary sphincters. The precapillary sphincters tend to open in response to accumulation of local metabolites. The postcapillary sphincters respond to catecholamines both directly and via the sympathetic nervous system. A rise in catecholamines results in constriction of postcapillary sphincters. Control of capillaries is such that only one-third of all the capillaries is open at any one time. If all the capillaries in the body opened at the same time the capillary circulation could contain two to three times the circulating blood volume.

All types of shock are associated with a high level of circulating catecholamines. In the early stages this is beneficial and is responsible for maintaining the central blood pressure and allowing perfusion of privileged tissues, particularly the brain and heart. This is possible because the arterioles of muscle, skin and splanchnic beds are richly innervated with α receptors—the vessels of the brain and heart are poorly innervated with α receptors. As a result of sustained catecholamines production the peripheral resistance increases. The pressure of fluid in a closed system is equal to the flow times the resistance ($P = F \times R$). If the blood pressure is kept constant and the peripheral resistance is increased by catecholamines or sympathomimetic drugs, then it follows that flow must decrease. Decreased flow of blood in the microcirculation is responsible for the invariably fatal outcome of severe shock. Modern forms of therapy aim at preventing prolonged reduction of flow to the microcirculation particularly in the splanchnic organs. It is convenient to consider the pathophysiology of shock in two stages. Stage I is that in which increased catecholamines production is a temporary necessity, beneficial if not prolonged. Stage II is that in which catecholamine production is prolonged and harmful, resulting in irreversible damage within the microcirculation.

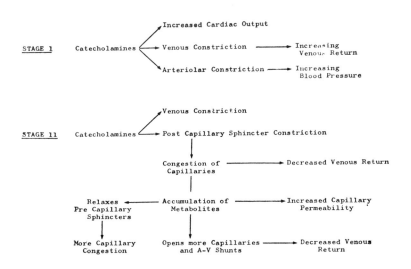

Stage I: Catecholamines result in an increase in cardiac output due to direct stimulation of the heart. This is offset later because the increased work of the heart must be carried on by anaerobic metabolism, leading to local acidosis which reduces contractility. Catecholamines cause constriction of the capacitance vessels (veins) which contain 80 per cent of the circulating blood volume and so they temporarily increase venous return. Catecholamines also cause differential arteriolar constriction, causing preferential perfusion of privileged tissues.

Stage II: Sustained catecholamine production causes further vein constriction which now acts as an *obstruction* to further venous return. Catecholamines also constrict the postcapillary sphincters, leading to capillary congestion and a further fall in venous return. Capillary congestion allows the local metabolites of anaerobic metabolism to accumulate, leading to:

1. Precapillary sphincter *relaxation* and more capillary congestion.
2. Opening of some of the two-thirds of capillaries which are normally closed at any one time, causing further pooling of blood, direct shunting from the arterial to venous side and bypassing of the microcirculation. These changes further decrease venous return and tissue perfusion.
3. Increased capillary permeability and loss of intravascular fluid into the extracellular compartment.
4. Further cell damage, causing release of vasoactive substances (histamine, 5-hydroxytryptamine and other kinins) and resulting in further pooling in the microcirculation.

In cardiogenic shock, death usually occurs because of irretrievable damage to the pump; infarction of more than 40 per cent of the myocardium is inevitably fatal. Strenuous therapeutic attempts to sustain patients with cardiogenic shock are based on:

1. The fact that peripheral circulatory compensatory mechanisms may be inadequate in the presence of recoverable pump failure.
2. The possibility of recovery of some myocardium which is only temporarily impaired in the vicinity of an infarct.
3. The fact that cardiac dysrhythmias may result from a small infarct and that it is the dysrhythmia which is often responsible for the reduced cardiac output.

Physiological and Metabolic Disturbances of Shock

Coronary blood flow.—The diastolic pressure in the ventricle is normally zero, but in heart failure and shock it is always raised. The coronary arteries are perfused during diastole and elevation of the intraventricular diastolic pressure must decrease the coronary blood flow.

Lung function.—Hyperventilation occurs in the early stages of shock and heart failure because of hypoxic stimulation of the respiratory centre. Because of the raised pulmonary venous pressure there are profound disturbances of V/Q ratios within the lungs. In the normal lung the bases are relatively over-perfused and in shock this effect is increased, resulting in arteriovenous shunting and hypoxaemia. Reduced systemic blood flow causes increased oxygen removal from the available blood so that any shunting results in disproportionately severe hypoxaemia. All these disadvantages are compounded by local areas of collapse, alveolar-wall oedema and reduction in surfactant.

Catecholamines.—The concentration of endogenous catecholamines in the plasma increases proportionately with the degree of hypotension, leading to vasoconstriction, particularly in the splanchnic, renal and cutaneous vessels. Catecholamines are produced both from the adrenal medulla and from local sympathetic nerve endings. In the later stages of shock and heart failure the synthesis of noradrenaline is markedly reduced, a process accelerated by metabolic acidosis. The reason for the reduced noradrenaline synthesis is that it is dependent on tyrosine hydroxylase, which becomes depleted.

Blood volume.—The blood volume has been monitored during the bleeding of animals. At the stage of maximum blood loss, the volume of blood remaining in the circulation is greater than the amount calculated from the original blood volume and the amount in the reservoir. This is due to fluid passing from extracellular compartments into the circulation. Towards the end of the critical stage of four and a half hours and the beginning of the stage of irreversible shock, the blood volume falls sharply as fluid is removed from the effective circulation by pooling in the splanchnic bed. Normally only one-third of the capillary bed is open, in man. Acidosis or anoxia causes the remaining two-thirds to open, leading to a 10 to 15 per cent loss of effective circulating blood. As stagnant anoxia within the microcirculation continues, ulceration causes intravascular fluid to be lost into the gut.

Blood flow.—Measurements of the blood flow in the superior mesenteric artery indicate that during hypotension the flow is reduced to 10 per cent of normal. If the superior mesenteric artery is perfused with blood at a normal pressure in a hypotensive dog, the state of irreversible shock does not occur, nor do the other metabolic and physiological disturbances. It was suggested that the hypotension of irreversible shock is due to endotoxins from Gram-negative organisms in the blood as a result of loss of gut-wall resistance. However, the hypotension still occurs when the gut is sterilised with antibiotics and the animals kept in a germ-free atmosphere.

Protein metabolism.—In the early stages of hypotension, the blood urea rises, due to catabolism of muscle proteins. Later, in the stage of irreversible shock, the urea falls, due to diminished formation by the anoxic liver. Because of the liver anoxia there is loss of the ability to deaminate the amino acids which accumulate in the plasma. The blood ammonia also rises, but never to toxic levels in clinical shock.

Carbohydrate metabolism.—The blood sugar is generally elevated in clinical shock, probably because of the increase in catecholamines. In the stage of irreversible shock, hypoglycaemia occurs, due partly to reduced gluconeogenesis in the anoxic liver, and partly to increased tissue uptake of glucose.

Renal function.—Following an episode of hypotension, oliguria may occur when the renal blood flow is again normal. Although total renal blood flow may be normal, the blood is shunted through the juxtamedullary glomeruli and the renal cortex becomes ischaemic. The volume of glomerular filtrate may be normal but there is often widespread necrosis and destruction of the renal tubules. This allows fluid to leak into the interstitial tissue of the kidneys. There is usually metabolic acidosis in shock, but occasionally in endotoxin shock there is respiratory alkalosis, probably the result of stimulation of the respiratory centre by endotoxins.

Viscosity of blood.—The flow properties of blood are such that at slow rates the viscosity is 10 times that at normal flow rates. This is due to the formation of aggregates between red cells and the plasma proteins, particularly fibrogen and globulins, which may be increased in shock. This increase in viscosity in the slow-moving blood will tend to increase the stagnation in the congested capillaries.

MANAGEMENT

The treatment of shock must aim at increasing effective blood flow through the microcirculation. To this end the fundamental considerations are the ability of the heart to pump, of the arterioles to distribute to the microcirculation and of the microcirculation to distribute to the cells. Other important considerations are the flow properties of the blood, the function of the lungs and the kidneys, acid-base balance, and correction of the *cause* of the shock.

Physical Examination and Observations

1. *Assessment of pump function:*

    (i) Ability to pump blood forward (state of the peripheral circulation).

(ii) Ability to prevent blood draining back behind the pump (central venous pressure and evidence of pulmonary oedema).

(iii) Evidence of impaired function from examination of the pump itself:
    (a) Gallop rhythm.
    (b) Reversed splitting of the second sound due to left ventricular dysfunction.
    (c) Papillary muscle or valve dysfunction.
    (d) Pericardial friction rub or tamponade.

2. *Assessment of peripheral circulation:*

(i) Pulse volume and blood pressure. (It is important to note that as the arterioles are the main resistance vessels the pulse may appear of good volume in the proximal arteries without necessarily indicating adequate forward flow and tissue perfusion.)

(ii) Skin colour and temperature.

(iii) Speed of filling of superficial veins on the dorsum of the hands and feet. As a rule filling of veins within 5 seconds of emptying them indicates adequate tissue perfusion *of the part examined*.

(iv) Skin capillary circulation. Blanching the skin should be followed by return of colour 3 seconds later if tissue perfusion is adequate.

3. *Central venous pressure.*—This is a most useful method of monitoring the venous return. It is *not* a substitute for careful clinical observation of the jugular venous pulse. Its value lies in the fact that it can be measured by the nurses at frequent intervals, and that it can be measured when the patient is flat or on a respirator. It cannot be emphasised strongly enough that the central venous pressure measures not one parameter but three, viz:

(i) The ability of the pump to prevent fluid damming back.

(ii) The blood volume.

(iii) The tone of the veins and size of the microcirculation.

These three have to be assessed independently and by other means before the significance of changes in the central venous pressure is known. In general two of these factors do not change at the same time, *but they may*.

4. *Urine output:*

(i) Volume. An output of 50 ml/hour usually indicates adequate renal function.

(ii) Colour. Dark-coloured urine is not always a concentrated urine. Urochrome pigments may be excreted in severe oliguria.

(iii) Concentration. Specific gravity above 1015 *usually* indicates an ability to concentrate the urine and, if associated with a low urine output, indicates prerenal uraemia; however, again there are exceptions. Occasional cases of cortical necrosis and acute glomerular nephritis are associated with a urine concentration above 1015.

(iv) Urine urea. A urine urea concentration above 1·0 g/l indicates that renal function is adequate.

(v) Urine sodium. This can be misleading: complete inability to concentrate the urine is associated with a near-absence of sodium from the urine, whereas severe cortical necrosis causes leakage of plasma through the kidneys and hence a urine sodium of 140 mEq (mmol)/l. As a rule a urine sodium concentration between 30 and 80 mEq (mmol)/l indicates adequate renal function.

(vi) Urine and plasma osmolality. Urine osmolality twice that of the plasma, or over 500 osmoles per litre, indicates adequate renal function.

5. *Blood cultures* are mandatory in *all* forms of shock.

6. *Blood gases and acid-base balance.*—Most cases of shock are accompanied by a metabolic acidosis. Some cases of septicaemic shock have a respiratory alkalosis, presumed to be due to stimulation of the respiratory centre by endotoxin.

7. *ECG monitoring.*

8. *Daily chest x-rays.*—It is important to note that the appearances of pulmonary oedema on the chest x-ray can be misleading. It is occasionally seen in the absence of a raised end diastolic left ventricular pressure (i.e. left ventricular failure). It may take 24 hours to disappear after left ventricular failure has been reversed and it may take 24 hours to appear after left ventricular failure. Nevertheless, frequent chest x-rays are essential because in some instances radiological signs are the only evidence of left ventricular or left atrial failure. Portable chest x-rays may be misleading with regard to pleural fluid—large effusions can be missed if the portable is taken with the patient lying flat or nearly flat. Dilated upper-lobe veins, even in a portable film, may be valuable pointers to pulmonary venous hypertension. Blurring of the outline of hilar vessels may be the only sign of pulmonary oedema.

9. *Cardiac output and other measurements.*—It is relatively easy to measure cardiac output using a Swan-Ganz catheter and a thermodilution technique; with the same catheter pulmonary capillary pressure can be measured. The catheters are easy to insert, but familiarity with

the necessary equipment is essential for meaningful and reproducible results. The mixed venous oxygen saturation has been found to be a useful measurement, and correlates with cardiac output, arterial hypoxia and excess tissue extraction of oxygen. Thus, clinical assessment, central venous pressure, diastolic blood pressure, mixed venous oxygen saturation and pulmonary capillary wedge pressure are among the most useful parameters (Robinson, 1977).

MANAGEMENT OF SHOCK

The main therapeutic aims are:

Increasing or decreasing ventricular preload, whichever is necessary, so that among other things the most effective portion of the Starling curve relating ventricular stroke volume to filling pressure is utilised
Improving myocardial function
Reducing ventricular afterload
Other useful manoeuvres:
(i) correction of acidosis
(ii) increasing inspired oxygen concentration
(iii) correction of dysrhythmias
(iv) prevention of intravascular coagulation
(v) prevention of secondary septicaemia.

Altering Ventricular Preload

The amount of ventricular preload is assessed clinically by measuring the central venous pressure, and if possible by the pulmonary capillary pressure, using a Swan-Ganz catheter. If the ventricular preload is too high, the main therapeutic aims are improvement in myocardial function and positive-pressure assisted ventilation, which reduces preload by increasing the intrathoracic pressure, so reducing the venous return. If the ventricular preload is too low, which is often the case, judicious fluid infusion together with attempts to improve myocardial function are indicated. It is not usually appreciated that the loop diuretics have an initial vascular action of decreasing venous tone and so increasing the pooling in the capacitance vessels; later they induce a natriuresis and diuresis. All these effects are useful in reducing preload. Loop diuretics need not be given in large doses initially although large doses may be required later in order to combat acute renal failure.

Intravenous fluids.—Blood is the best fluid for shock due to haemorrhage. Saline or plasma are better if the haematocrit is over 55 per cent and if fluid has been lost from extensive burns or dehydration. As a rule saline is indicated if there is depletion of salt and water from extracellular fluid; solutions with a high oncotic pressure are indicated for expansion of the vascular compartment. It is important to note that in dehydration the vascular compartment is affected after the extracellular *but* when saline is given, most of it passes into the extracellular compartment before the vascular compartment is expanded.

Dextrans.—Low-molecular-weight dextrans (Rheomacrodex, average molecular weight 40 000) are of special value in cardiogenic shock and in situations where the flow properties of the flood are impaired, e.g. severe dehydration, polycythaemia and slow flow rate. Rheomacrodex improves the flow properties of blood by:

> Preventing aggregations of red cells
> Expanding the circulating plasma volume
> Reducing intravascular clotting

For these reasons dextrans have a place in the management of acute arterial insufficiency, and Rheomacrodex is of proven value in the prophylaxis of deep vein thrombosis and pulmonary embolism (Lambie et al., 1970). Because the average molecular weight of Rheomacrodex is 40 000 and the renal threshold for dextrans is around 50 000, Rheomacrodex is excreted into the urine, most of it within 6 hours; it therefore has some value as an osmotic diuretic.

Mannitol (25 per cent) should be given as early as possible in cardiogenic and septicaemic shock, because of its known beneficial effect in delaying the acute renal failure to which patients with septicaemia are particularly prone. Not more than 200 ml should be given if the patient does not appear dehydrated and does not pass 50 ml urine in the first hour after the infusion.

Improving Myocardial Function

Most of the drugs which affect the heart also affect the peripheral circulation. Some manoeuvres aimed at improving myocardial function are concerned with reducing the likelihood of dysrhythmias.

Glucagon.—Glucagon has a positive inotropic effect on the heart and also a small effect in reducing peripheral vascular resistance. It has a variable effect on heart rate. It is not used when other drugs are controlling the heart failure, but occasionally it has a remarkably beneficial effect in severe low cardiac output states (Diamond et al., 1971). The usual dose is about 5 mg per hour by infusion. It is available in 1 mg ampoules.

Glucose, potassium and insulin.—The transport of glucose into myocardial cells depends on insulin and insulin levels are usually low in severe heart failure. Increasing the concentration of insulin in the blood has been shown to improve ventricular function in severe heart failure (Majid *et al.*, 1972 and Bukesfield *et al.*, 1973). Furthermore, loss of potassium from injured myocardial cells causes dysrhythmias. Glucose partially prevents the loss of potassium from injured cells and infusions of potassium will tend to maintain the intracellular concentration of potassium.

Following myocardial damage there is rise in plasma and local concentrations of free fatty acids and it is known that these are harmful in that they promote electrical instability and also reduce the contractility of myocardial cells. The concentration of free fatty acids are reduced by insulin, beta blockers and heparin. They may exert their harmful effects by binding with magnesium potassium or calcium and lowering the local concentration of these ions. Nicotinic acid has a possible therapeutic role in that it prevents mobilisation of free fatty acid from adipose tissue (Oliver 1975).

Dobutamine.—Dobutamine is a synthetic analogue of isoprenaline with few of the peripheral effects of dopamine. Its inotropic effects on the heart are similar to those of isoprenaline except that it does not increase heart rate to the same extent. Dobutamine is available as Dobutrex in vials of 250 mg, which are diluted with 250 ml dextrose, giving a concentration of 1000 μg/ml. The average requirement is 150–500 μg/minute.

Isoprenaline.—Isoprenaline has beta 1 and beta 2 (vascular and cardiac) adrenergic agonist activity. It also causes increase in volume of capacitance vessels and therefore reduces preload and afterload. It may however cause dysrhythmias and increased myocardial oxygen consumption, although clinical experience suggests that the advantages may outweigh the disadvantages in cardiogenic shock. (Mueller *et al.*, 1972). Isoprenaline is infused in doses up to 10 μg/minute, the usual requirement being 2–5 μg/minute. It is available as Saventrine I.V. in 2 ml ampoules containing 2 mg. One ampoule should be diluted with 500 ml dextrose giving a solution containing 4 μg/ml.

Reducing Ventricular Afterload

Drugs acting mainly on the peripheral circulation reducing afterload and preload.—Most drugs which dilate peripheral arteries also cause dilatation of veins. Unfortunately some drugs preferentially cause vasodilatation in non-essential tissues, resulting in lack of perfusion of essential organs. Isoprenaline is an example of a drug which reduces peripheral resistance in some patients in this way. It is crucial to appreciate that these drugs can only be used if the circulating blood volume is adequate. They should never be used if the central venous pressure is below 10 cm.

Phentolamine.—Phentolamine is an alpha adrenergic blocking drug which also has some direct action on smooth muscle and is a mild beta

2 agonist. Phentolamine is available as Rogitine 1 ml ampoules containing 10 mg phentolamine. The dose in shock is 1–2 mg/minute.

Sodium nitroprusside.—Sodium nitroprusside is a direct-acting vasodilator with a short duration of action. Once prepared the solution should be protected from light by wrapping in aluminium foil. It is metabolised to thiocynanate and cyanide, and this limits its usefulness. The dose in shock is 20–120 μg/minute starting with 20 μg and increasing by 10 μg every 10 minutes. Nitroprusside is available as Nipride in ampoules which contain 50 mg sodium nitroprusside, which is diluted in 500 ml of 5 per cent dextrose, giving a solution containing 10 μg per ml.

Nitrates (nitroglycerine and isosorbide dinitrate).—Nitrates have a greater direct effect on the capacitance vessels than on the arterioles. Their role in the clinical management of shock is still being evaluated.

Salbutamol.—Salbutamol is a relatively specific beta 2 adrenergic receptor agonist and has little effect on the heart (beta 1 adrenergic receptors). It has little effect on backward failure but is useful in improving peripheral perfusion without increasing myocardial oxygen consumption. Sulbutamol is administered in doses up to 40 μg/minute. It is available as Ventolin solution for intravenous infusion, 5 ml ampoules containing 5 mg. One ampoule should be diluted in 500 ml of dextrose/saline to produce a solution containing 10 μg per ml.

Corticosteroids.—Corticosteroids have a number of known actions which theoretically could be of benefit to damaged cells in severe shock. They have a stabilising effect on cell membranes which could reduce the liability to dysrhythmias and further metabolic cell damage. They may also have a positive inotropic action on contracting myocardial cells and a peripheral alpha-blocking effect on blood vessels. Their role in the management of cardiac shock is still controversial but it is generally agreed that in septicaemic shock they do have a beneficial role in reducing the toxicity of endotoxin. Hydrocortisone is available in vials containing 500 and 1000 mg. The usual dose in shock is 500 mg every 2–6 hours. Increased physiological amounts of corticosteroids have three important functions:

1. They have a direct inotropic action on the myocardium probably by facilitating the transfer of ions across cell membranes.
2. They enable the mineralocorticoids to exert their effect on the distal renal tubules and are therefore important in regulating fluid losses.
3. In physiological doses they potentiate and revive the effects of circulating catecholamines on the blood vessels. In the *early* stages of shock this has an important beneficial action.

In pharmacological doses of the order of 50 mg/kg hydrocortisone, corticosteroids have different, definite, but often poorly explained effects.

In pharmacological doses they:

Cause a fall in peripheral resistance (mild alpha-blocking effect)
Influence the tone of veins
Increase splanchnic blood flow
Protect against the effects of bacterial endotoxin
Protect against the effects of excess catecholamines
Increase gluconeogenesis
Increase utilisation of lactate.

Dopamine.—Dopamine is the immediate precursor of noradrenaline but it has the additional property of stimulating specific dopamine receptors in the splanchnic and renal vascular beds resulting in vasodilatation and improved perfusion (Goldberg *et al.*, 1977). It also has a beta agonist effect on the heart without increasing heart rate and therefore myocardial oxygen demand. The effects of dopamine are critically dependent on dose; in higher doses its actions are similar to those of noradrenaline and therefore may be harmful; in lower doses (up to 250 μg per minute) its effects are likely to be beneficial. Dopamine (Intropin) is available in 5 ml ampoules containing 200 mg. It should not be diluted with sodium bicarbonate but can be diluted with 5 per cent dextrose or normal saline. The main side-effect is cardiac dysrhythmia.

Management of Cardiogenic Shock

A reasonable therapeutic procedure for cardiogenic shock is:

Digoxin, corticosteroid plus dopamine
If the heart rate is below 60 per minute, isoprenaline; if cardiac output and peripheral perfusion improve, continue with isoprenaline
If heart rate is rapid, dobutamine
If pheripheral perfusion remains low consider phentolamine and/or salbutamol
If cardiac output remains low consider boluses of glucagon

This regime may be supplemented with:

High concentrations of inspired oxygen
Transfusion if necessary
Glucose, potassium and insulin if indicated
Correction of acidosis and dysrhythmias
Consideration of balloon aortic pulsation, if the shock is due to ruptured papillary muscle or interventricular septum, and surgery is contemplated.

TABLE XXI

SHOCK: DRUGS AND PROCEDURES ACTING ON THE
CARDIOVASCULAR SYSTEM.

Alteration of Ventricular Preload

To *Decrease* preload	Positive-pressure ventilation
	Diuretics
	Expansion of capacitance vessels
	nitrates
	hydralazine
To *Increase* preload	Transfusion

Improvement in Myocardial Function
  Digoxin
  Glucose, potassium and insulin
  Glucagon
  Dobutamine
  Isoprenaline
  Dopamine
  Steroids
  Reduction in FFA

Alteration of Ventricular Afterload

Alpha blockers	phentolamine
Direct acting	nitroprusside
	nitrates
Beta 1 agonists	salbutamol
	isoprenaline
Dopaminergic	dopamine

Oxygen and Positive-Pressure Ventilation

Positive-pressure ventilation is important in the management of shock. Hypoxia is virtually always present in clinical shock. Positive-pressure respiration is the most suitable means of increasing blood Po_2 if hypoxia persists after the patient breathes 100 per cent oxygen through a properly fitted Ventimask. Pulmonary oedema is common in all types of shock. Pulmonary oedema increases the stiffness of the lungs; most positive-pressure respirators deliver gas at a predetermined pressure. The volume of gas (the tidal volume) delivered at this pressure is usually 500–600 ml per cycle. If the machine creates a constant pressure, any increase in stiffness of the lungs will mean that a smaller volume of gas is delivered. A check on the tidal volume should be made and recorded every 30 minutes: at a fixed pressure a fall in the tidal volume means increased resistance to flow of air into the lungs, of which the commonest cause is pulmonary oedema. The fall in tidal volume is often the earliest evidence of pulmonary oedema.

Positive-pressure ventilation can play an important part in treating pulmonary oedema once it has developed by:

Increasing intra-alveolar pressure, preventing interstitial fluid entering the alveoli.

Reducing venous return (by increasing the amount of air in the chest and so diminishing the amount of blood which can enter).

Allowing fluid to be sucked out of the airways through the endotracheal tube or tracheostomy.

When positive end-expiratory pressure is used, the lung closing volume may be reduced so that compliance is increased and ventilation is improved as a result of small airways remaining open, so allowing ventilation of distal alveoli. If shock lung is present, however, there may be such profound V/Q disturbance that increasing ventilation cannot overcome the venous admixture effect.

Hyperbaric oxygen.—Oxygen at a high pressure causes an increased solution of molecular oxygen in a physically dissolved form in the blood so that relatively more oxygen is delivered to the tissues. Hyperbaric oxgen has been used in the treatment of dogs with experimental shock. In one series, improvement only occurred if it was given early, in the less severe stage of shock. Other workers showed a reduction in mortality in dogs with shock exposed to oxygen at two atmospheres pressure. However, only 50 per cent of the extra oxygen was utilised.

Depression of cardiac output has been shown to occur at increased tensions of inspired oxygen; vasoconstriction is also seen. These effects offset the improvement in oxygenation of the tissues and hyperbaric oxygen probably is not indicated in the treatment of shock in man.

Correction of Acidosis

The administration of 8·4 per cent sodium bicarbonate, which contains 1 mEq (mmol)/ml is a convenient way of combating excess metabolic acidosis in shock. Correction of acidosis is usually not possible until shock has been reversed by other methods, and indeed, complete correction of acidosis may not be desirable, since acidosis shifts the oxygen dissociation curve of haemoglobin to the right which means that at the tissues haemoglobin gives up its oxygen more readily—clearly an advantage if cellular oxygen supply is compromised for other reasons.

Gram-negative Shock

Gram-negative septicaemia (endotoxin) shock should be suspected if there is a history of recent operation or urological instrumentation.

Other suspicious findings are leucocytosis, fever, petechiae, jaundice and cyanosis. Endotoxin shock should always be considered if there is no other obvious cause for the shock. Urine and blood cultures should be taken before treatment is started.

Other features which should alert to the possibility of septicaemic shock are:

Cold, sweating skin
Tachypnoea
Leucopenia and thrombocytopenia as evidence of diffuse intravascular coagulation

The extreme toxicity of endotoxin is due to the presence of "Lipid A", a fatty acid which interferes with cell and mitochondrial membranes. "Lipid A" may give rise to specific antibodies and can be detected by the Limulus assay

Endotoxins act as:

Direct pyrogens
Indirect pyrogens by promoting release of pyrogens from leucocytes
Activators of coagulation and fibrinolysis
Necrotic agents on blood vessels
Releasers of complement, prostaglandins and kinins
Glucocorticoid antagonists
Depressors of cellular respiration
Direct damaging agents to cell surface phospholipids, especially in the alveoli of the lungs.

Choice of antibiotics in endotoxin shock.—Gentamicin and clindamycin (to counteract possible *Bacteroides*). Chloramphenicol is sometimes still indicated; metronidazole may also be effective against *Bacteroides*. Polymyxin is believed to have additional endotoxin neutralising properties but is rather toxic. Carbenicillin is indicated if Pseudomonas is the responsible infecting organism.

Disseminated Intravascular Coagulation (DIC)

Tissue thromboplastins will activate the coagulation cascade; intravascular coagulation occurs if there is extensive tissue damage or activation by proteolytic lysosomal enzymes released from leucocytes as a result of endotoxins. The effects of intravascular coagulation are a combination of organ damage due to platelet aggregation, fibrin deposition and thrombosis, and severe hypocoagulability due to consumption of clotting factors and platelets. There is also a disturbance in the release and function of prostaglandins. Prostacyclin

(PGI$_2$) is released from vascular endothelium, resulting in non-opposed platelet aggregation to vessel walls. Platelet destruction leads to release of thromboxane (TxA$_2$), which promotes further platelet aggregation and PGE$_2$, which increases vascular permeability. Heparin is usually recommended in shock to reduce the possibility of severe DIC.

REFERENCES

BUKESFIELD, R. P., LANKIECH, P. G. and BOLTE, H. D. (1973) *Brit. med. J.*, **2**, 365.

DIAMOND, G., FORRESTER, J., DANZIG, R., PARMLEY, W. W. and SWAN, H. J. C. (1971) *Brit. Heart J.*, **33**, 290.

GOLDBERG, L. I., HSIEH, Y. and RESNEKOV, L. (1977) *Progr. in Cardiovascular Dis.*, **19**, 327.

LAMBE, J. M., BARBER, D. C., HALL, D. P. and MATHESON, M. A. (1970) *Brit. med. J.*, **3**, 144.

MAJID, P. A., SHARMA, B., MEERAN, M. K. and TAYLOR, S. H. (1972) *Lancet*, **2**, 719.

MUELLER, H., AYRES, S. M., GIANELLI, S., CONKLIN, E. F., MAZZARA, J. T. and GRACE, W. J. (1972) *Circulation*, **45**, 335.

OLIVER, M. (1975) *Modern Trends in Cardiology—3*, London: Butterworth.

ROBINSON, B. F. (1977) Advanced medicine. *Topics in Therapeutics—3* (Royal College of Physicians). London: Pitman Medical.

EPONYM

1. HANS CHRISTIAN JOACHIM GRAM (1853–1938)
Christian Gram was a physician with a large private practice in Copenhagen. While working with Friedländer in Berlin, Gram was experimenting with staining bacteria with modifications of some of Ehrlich's dyes when he accidentally tipped some Lugol's iodine on to one of the slides. When he attempted to remove the iodine with absolute alcohol, some organisms retained the stain while others did not.

10

DISORDERS OF MINERAL METABOLISM

Introduction

Mineral metabolism abounds with accounts which so intertwine the experimental data with the workaday clinical account that for most people the subject holds terrors which are quite unfounded.

You can be extremely competent at interpreting electrocardiograms and know almost nothing about muscle action potentials or intracellular metabolism, but you won't be much good at cardiograms if you don't know which are the PQRST waves on the electrocardiogram. Similarly in considering disorders of mineral metabolism certain facts must be remembered to make the thing intelligible.

1. Parathyroid hormone (PTH)
   (*a*) Causes hypercalcaemia by mobilising calcium from bone
   (*b*) Increases calcium and phosphorus reabsorption by the renal tubules
   (*c*) Variably increases serum calcium by increasing absorption of calcium from the gut.

2. Vitamin D is absorbed from the diet (ergocalciferol) and formed in the skin (cholecalciferol). These substances are converted in the liver to 25-hydroxycholecalciferol and this is converted in the kidney to the metabolically active 1, 25-dihydroxycholecalciferol and/or the inactive metabolite 25, 26-dihydroxycholecalciferol.

3. The actions of 1, 25-dihydroxycholecalciferol are:
   (*a*) Increased intestinal absorption of calcium
   (*b*) Promotion of mineralisation of bone if mineralisation is deficient
   (*c*) Promotion of resorption if bone mineralisation is already normal.

4. Vitamin D deficiency
   (*a*) Causes reduced tubular reabsorption of phosphorus which returns to normal when normal doses of vitamin D are given *but* overdose with vitamin D does not cause excessive tubular reabsorption of phosphorus.
   (*b*) Causes a myopathy
   (*c*) Prevents the action of PTH on bone and gut.

5. Deficiency of PTH causes the effects of vitamin D deficiency because PTH is necessary for the conversion of vitamin D into its active metabolite 1, 25-dihydroxycholecalciferol.

Clinically the two commonest disorders of mineral metabolism encountered in adult general medicine are firstly an accidental finding of hypercalcaemia and secondly bone disease due to renal failure.

HYPERCALCAEMIA

The total serum calcium consists of three components: ionised calcium, protein-bound calcium and citrated calcium. It is the ionised calcium which is altered by Vitamin D and PTH. If the sources of error in estimating and interpreting levels of serum calcium are borne in mind, the normal range of serum calcium is 8·9–10·3 mg/100 ml (2·2–2·6 mol/l). A number of factors influence the serum calcium other than changes due to bone disease.

Factors causing an increase in serum calcium:

Recent meal
Upright posture and exercise
Venous occlusion
Increase in plasma proteins particularly the serum albumin.

Factors causing a decrease in serum calcium:

Recumbency
Precipitation of the proteins in the blood sample (e.g. by delay in performing the calcium estimations). For practical purposes, therefore, *if* the sample reaches the laboratory reasonably quickly and the serum calcium is reported as being in the normal range (particularly if it is at the lower end), one can be pretty certain that hypercalcaemia is not present.

So far as the serum phosphorus is concerned, the levels are high in childhood, in renal failure and sometimes when bone is being rapidly destroyed. The symptoms and signs of hypercalcaemia are not often the presenting feature—it is no truism to say that the commonest presenting sign of hypercalcaemia is a raised serum calcium. The serum levels of phosphorus are otherwise of remarkably little value in adults except in rare instances of hypophosphataemic osteomalacia (see p. 532).

The only true physical sign of hypercalcaemia is corneal calcification, which usually needs to be looked for very carefully and is often difficult to distinguish from arcus senilis; it is usually a thin band, best seen on the medial side, and is separated from the conjunctiva by a clear band of cornea. However, if arcus is also present this clear band of normal cornea may not be seen. The symptoms of hypercalcaemia are non-specific but certain of the symptoms are caused by the complications of hypercalcaemia, e.g. hypertension, peptic ulceration, pancreatitis and renal calculi. Hypercalcaemia itself may cause poly-uria, constipation, skin itching, headache, depression, generalised muscle weakness and almost any psychiatric disturbance.

The causes of hypercalcaemia are:

Osteolytic bone metastases
Non-metastatic bone resorption
(a) due to tumours producing a PTH-like polypeptide
(b) due to production of vitamin D-like sterol by tumours
Hyperparathyroidism
Vitamin D ingestion
Paget's disease
Sarcoidosis
Thyrotoxicosis
Immobility
Addison's disease
Thiazide diuretics.

Sorting out the Cause of Hypercalcaemia

The first step is to confirm that hypercalcaemia is in fact present by repeating the blood sample, taking all the correct precautions and using the correction factors for plasma protein levels and blood specific gravity.

A raised alkaline phosphatase will generally confirm that hypercalcaemia is probably present and that the hypercalcaemia is arising from bone destruction (thus usually excluding sarcoidosis, excess vitamin D ingestion, Addison's disease and diuretic ingestion). The level of alkaline phosphatase tends to be higher in hyperparathyroidism with predominantly bone involvement, and less high with renal involvement.

Estimation of the serum phosphorus contributes almost nothing. If persistently low it favours (but does not indicate) the diagnosis of hyperparathyroidism.

Skeletal radiology should come next. The purist will start only with the x-ray of the hands and skull. If subperiosteal erosions of the distal phalanges and/or fragmentation of the cortices and a "pepperpot" skull are present, the diagnosis of hyperparathyroidism is definite. In hyperparathyroidism more extensive skeletal radiology may reveal single or multiple lesions of osteitis fibrosa cystica or subperiosteal erosions affecting the outer third of the clavicles, inner side of the neck of the femur or inner aspect of the upper tibia.

If hyperparathyroidism is not the cause of the hypercalcaemia, skeletal radiology may reveal osteolytic bone secondaries, myeloma, reticulosis or leukaemia. If none of these is present radiologically and no other cause of hypercalcaemia is found, a radioisotope bone scan may reveal metastatic bone lesions not seen on the skeletal x-rays.

If sarcoidosis is present the gamma globulins should be raised and routine chest x-rays may show hilar adenopathy or parenchymal lung lesions. In sarcoidosis, bone lesions may be seen in the x-rays of the hands. If by this time sarcoidosis is seriously possible as the cause of hypercalcaemia a Kveim test should be performed.

By this stage the majority of cases of hypercalcaemia will have an established cause—however some will not. So at this point go back and take the history again, particularly for ingestion of any tablets or tonics containing any form of vitamin D, and also check the thyroid function and adrenal function.

If you are still struggling by this time, the problem is almost invariably:

(a) Is it hyperparathyroidism? or
(b) Is it a primary carcinoma with non-metastatic hypercalcaemia?

The next step is the *standard* hydrocortisone test. Hydrocortisone in a dose of 40 mg t.d.s. for 10 days will not affect the serum calcium levels in hyperparathyroidism, but will reduce the serum calcium levels in other causes of hypercalcaemia. The *only exceptions* to this rule have been patients with hyperparathyroidism or metastatic bone lesions in whom the bony lesions have been diagnostic on the x-rays.

Estimation of the serum parathyroid hormone is available but should not usually be necessary to establish the cause of the hypercalcaemia. In a really difficult case it will be helpful, but it is important to realise that PTH is measured by radioimmunoassay and that the immunologically active part of the polypeptide is not the same as the biologically active part. Further, some tumours produce a PTH-like hormone which, if present, will not distinguish between hyperparathyroidism and hypercalcaemia due to non-metastatic malignant disease which is producing an immunologically similar although not biologically identical polypeptide.

The main use of assaying the PTH level is to locate the site and side of the presumed parathyroid adenoma, having established that the cause of the hypercalcaemia is hyperparathyroidism.

HYPERPARATHYROIDISM

Primary hyperparathyroidism refers to excessive output of parathyroid hormone arising from spontaneously occurring parathyroid adenoma or hyperplasia. Secondary hyperparathyroidism refers also to an excessive output of parathyroid hormone, but the increased output is stimulated by a low level of serum calcium. Tertiary hyperparathyroidism refers to those cases of secondary hyperparathyroidism which go on to adenoma formation and uncontrolled and autonomous release of parathyroid hormone.

The majority of cases of primary hyperparathyroidism are due to a single adenoma, although in about 5 per cent of cases there are two adenomas and in about the same number the affected parathyroid gland is situated in the mediastinum. For this reason it is sensible before exploring the neck to obtain venous samples by means of selective venous catheterisation of the innominate and jugular veins draining different parts of the lower neck, to measure the parathyroid hormone levels, so that the site of excess hormone production can be found. Selective venous catheterisation and sampling may not be necessary for first explorations of the neck, but in re-explorations it is mandatory. Re-exploration may be necessary if the hypercalcaemia is not cured by removal of an adenoma or if hypercalcaemia recurs.

Occasionally hyperparathyroidism is of familial origin or associated with multiple endocrine-gland neoplasia. There are two types of multiple-gland neoplasia:

Type 1 consists of adenomas of parathyroid, pituitary and pancreas glands

Type 2 consists of parathyroid adenoma, phaeochromocytoma, medullary thyroid carcinoma and Cushing's disease. This type is sometimes inherited as an autosomal dominant.

Patients with hyperparathyroidism are more likely to have renal stones than they are to have osteitis fibrosa, but it is extremely unusual for the two to occur together in the same patient. The reason for this is quite unknown. Paradoxically, patients who have osteitis fibrosa are likely to have a greater impairment of renal function than those with renal calculi because they often have nephrocalcinosis (but not renal stones).

Hyperparathyroidism accounts for about 5 per cent of renal calculi and about 15 per cent of recurrent calculi.

There are a few additional points which on occasions may be useful in the diagnosis of hyperparathyroidism.

(a) Phosphorus deprivation (with aluminium hydroxide) *sometimes* causes a rise in serum calcium in hyperparathyroidism especially if the routine calcium levels have been only equivocally raised.

(b) Patients with hyperparathyroidism have an aminoaciduria and sometimes a myopathy.

(c) Hydroxyproline excretion is increased but usually only if there is obvious bone involvement.

(d) Hyperparathyroidism causes a hyperchloraemic acidosis by decreasing the ability of the renal tubules to excrete hydrogen ion. The plasma chloride is therefore often marginally raised.

(e) The requirement for vitamin D is increased in hyperparathyroidism. Vitamin D given in the presence of hyperparathyroidism may re-mineralise the bones. Excessive rise in serum calcium can be prevented with a low-calcium diet and high phosphorus intake. It is usually worth doing this only if there is extensive pre-operative bone disease. This relative vitamin D deficiency is probably responsible for the occasional x-ray and histological appearance of osteomalacia in hyperparathyroidism.

Following parathyroidectomy the following points should be borne in mind (Dent, 1962):

1. The patient should be warned that symptoms of hypocalcaemia may occur and particularly that depression may occur after the operation.
2. Hypocalcaemia is worse when there is severe bone involvement pre-operatively.
3. The lowest calcium levels occur 4–10 days after operation. Tetany may precede hypocalcaemia.
4. The presence of hypocalcaemia should always be confirmed before treatment is started.
5. If hypocalcaemia occurs, and provided that renal function is normal, 20 ml of 20 per cent calcium gluconate should be given by *slow* intravenous injection daily.
6. If bone disease is severe pre-operatively vitamin D (2·0 mg/day) should be given for 2 months and then stopped. Vitamin D is not necessary if the hypocalcaemia is not causing symptoms.
7. The serum calcium and phosphorus levels should be followed twice weekly for the first 6 weeks. A return of serum calcium to pre-operative levels suggests that some tumour has been left behind. A rise in serum phosphorus means either hypoparathyroidism or the development of renal failure.
8. Alkaline phosphatase levels should also be monitored. A return to normal levels means that vitamin D can be stopped.
9. If tetany occurs and the serum calcium is normal the tetany is probably due to hypomagnesaemia. This is particularly likely if there is extensive bone disease.

Management of Severe Hypercalcaemia

A rise in serum calcium has a potentially reversible deleterious effect on renal function. Glomerular filtration is reduced because of vasoconstriction, and tubular reabsorption of water and salt is diminished, so that hypercalcaemia is accompanied by salt and water depletion. If the situation is not corrected quickly, irreversible renal failure will occur. The following points should be considered:

1. Infusion of saline (often large amounts are required).
2. Increasing calcium excretion by using a loop diuretic such as frusemide.
3. Corticosteroids. These are usually only effective in hypercalcaemia due to sarcoidosis or vitamin D intoxication; their beneficial effect may take a week to be seen.
4. Mithramycin is probably the most effective way of lowering the calcium. Once the calcium has started to fall it may go on falling after the drug is stopped; bone marrow suppression may occur.
5. Calcitonin. This usually produces a small fall in serum calcium but in about 20 per cent of patients it is ineffective.
6. Peritoneal dialysis or haemodialysis
7. Inorganic phosphates are generally too dangerous because they lower the calcium by promoting calcium phosphate deposition in the tissues (including the kidneys).

URAEMIC BONE DISEASE (URAEMIC OSTEODYSTROPHY)

There are four principal manifestations of bone disease in chronic glomerular failure:

1. Osteomalacia, or rickets in children (bone pain and myopathy)
2. Osteitis fibrosa
3. Soft-tissue calcification and osteosclerosis
4. Osteoporosis.

Table XXII shows the main mechanisms involved in the pathogenesis of these manifestations.

With progressive renal damage there is failure of the kidneys to convert circulating 25-hydroxycholecalciferol into the more active 1, 25-dihydroxycholecalciferol, leading effectively to a deficiency of vitamin D and osteomalacia which can only be corrected by giving very large doses of vitamin D, hence the term "vitamin D resistance". Phosphorus retention in glomerular failure leads to hyperphosphataemia and hypocalcaemia and hence secondary hyperparathyroidism. The hyperphosphataemia may encourage excessive precipitation of calcium phosphate in soft tissues (leading to ectopic calcification) or in the bones (leading to osteosclerosis). Secondary hyperparathyroidism will lead to osteitis fibrosa and an autonomous adenoma may develop, leading to tertiary hyperparathyroidism. The acidosis of renal failure also contributes to osteomalacia.

Following regular haemodialysis some patients develop osteoporosis. The incidence of this varies considerably; it was particularly high in Newcastle and is sometimes known as Newcastle bone disease.

TABLE XXII

MECHANISMS CAUSING THE CLINICAL MANIFESTATIONS OF
CHRONIC RENAL FAILURE

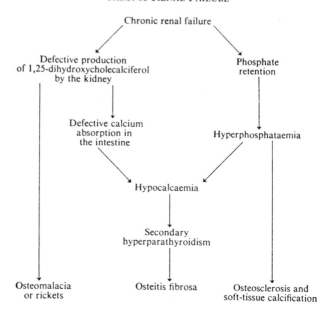

Chronic renal failure

Defective production
of 1,25-dihydroxycholecalciferol
by the kidney

Phosphate
retention

Defective calcium
absorption in
the intestine

Hyperphosphataemia

Hypocalcaemia

Secondary
hyperparathyroidism

Osteomalacia
or rickets

Osteitis fibrosa

Osteosclerosis and
soft-tissue calcification

(*By courtesy of Dr C. R. Patterson*)

Management

Osteomalacia.—The main features are severe bone pain and muscle weakness (myopathy). Most patients with renal failure have hyperphosphataemia as well as malabsorption of calcium; the hyperphosphataemia is controlled with oral aluminium hydroxide (up to 20 g/day) and the malabsorption of calcium, the bone lesions and myopathy are treated with large doses of vitamin D. The two main problems with the administration of vitamin D are firstly that the effective dose may be variable even in the same patient, and secondly that ectopic calcification may occur. It is therefore necessary to monitor the serum calcium and alkaline phosphatase levels frequently as well as the bone x-rays. Treatment is not necessary once the bone lesions and myopathy have healed. Vitamin D should be stopped if the serum calcium level rises to within the normal range. The serum alkaline phosphatase level should fall on treatment but the treatment should stop before the alkaline phosphatase reaches the normal range otherwise overdosage with vitamin D will occur—this may lead to renal calcification (nephrocalcinosis), which will worsen the renal failure and may also lead to ectopic soft-tissue calcification. It is customary to start treatment with 1·25 mg vitamin D_2 daily. Improvement in the myopathy and appetite occur early, the relief of bone pain and healing of osteomalacia take several weeks. The bone changes of any secondary hyperparathyroidism take several months to heal even on adequate doses of vitamin D. Vitamin D therapy should be *stopped immediately* if the serum calcium rises above 10·8 mg per cent, if anorexia, nausea or vomiting occur or if there is an unexplained rise in the blood urea. Once the myopathy and osteomalacia have healed it is customary to leave patients on a small dose of vitamin D (0·5 mg daily). It should be noted that the half-life of administered vitamin D in renal failure may be as much as six months. Shorter-acting metabolites of vitamin D obviously have advantages over vitamin D itself.

Opinion is divided on the value of calcium supplements. Calcium absorption can be increased with oral calcium supplements and also a rise in serum phosphate may be prevented. However, metastatic calcification can occur if the serum calcium phosphorus product is over 70.

Uraemic hyperparathyroidism is less common than osteomalacia and more difficult to treat. The secondary hyperparathyroidism may respond slowly to aluminium hydroxide, vitamin D therapy and if necessary haemodialysis, with an adequate calcium concentration in the dialysate. However if osteitis fibrosa cystica and the radiological features of hyperparathyroidism in the fingers are severe or persistent or if metastatic calcification is increasing, parathyroidectomy is indicated. Occasionally tertiary (autonomous secondary) hyperparathyroidism develops and this too should be treated with parathyroidectomy. Following parathyroidectomy in renal failure, large doses of vitamin D are usually required.

Osteomalacia and Rickets

Osteomalacia (adults) and rickets (children) occur when there is effectively a deficiency of vitamin D. Vitamin D is essential for the calcification of bone osteoid and the calcification of cartilage in growing bones. The causes of vitamin D deficiency are:

Inadequate dietary content
Inadequate sunlight
Malabsorption:
   Partial gastrectomy
   Pancreatic disease
   Biliary obstruction
   Intestinal malabsorption

Defective production of active metabolites of vitamin D:
Renal failure
Liver disease
Anticonvulsant therapy
"Resistance" to vitamin D due to renal tubular disorders:
Generalised tubular damage (Fanconi syndrome)
Isolated tubular defects
Renal tubular acidosis

Biochemically, osteomalacia and rickets are characterised by a low serum calcium and usually, in adults, a low phosphorus and a raised alkaline phosphatase. Urine calcium and phosphorus excretion are also correspondingly low. Radiologically the effects of rickets are seen on the growing parts of the long bones, i.e. the epiphyses; these are widened, the ends of the long bones are irregular (tufted) and also widened (splayed). These changes are due to the growing cartilage failing to become calcified. The increased cartilage at the epiphyses causes the swellings which may be seen at the ends of the ribs (rickety rosary). The skull may also be affected, being softer than normal and therefore misshapen. The associated vitamin D deficient myopathy may prevent the child moving its head so that one particular part of the skull becomes flattened. The persistence of rickets during childhood causes the weight-bearing bones to become deformed, causing either knock or bowed knees. Occasionally patients with rickets and osteomalacia get tetany, but this is not common.

The radiological features of osteomalacia are the pathognomonic pseudo-fractures and Looser's zones which are usually seen in characteristic sites, e.g. neck of femur, upper ends of tibia, pubic ramus or clavicles. In the spine osteomalacia causes all the vertebrae to soften and hence the intervertebral discs can push into the vertebrae, especially at their centres, causing the "codfish" spine. Osteoporosis tends to be patchy and causes individual vertebrae to collapse or become wedge-shaped. Sometimes osteomalacia is superimposed on osteoporosis, e.g. in malabsorption or in liver disease.

Nutritional Rickets and Osteomalacia

There has to be both a deficiency of vitamin D in the diet and inadequate synthesis of vitamin D in the skin for nutritional rickets to occur. The condition is probably more frequent in Britain than is generally appreciated. It occurs particularly in immigrants, in whom skin pigmentation or seclusion may prevent adequate exposure to what little sun there is. This is aggravated by the fact that many immigrants habitually eat food which is deficient in the vitamin. Nutritional vitamin D deficiency is also seen in the elderly in whom the skin becomes less effective in synthesising vitamin D. It may well be that subclinical osteomalacia is an important factor in the pathogenesis of fractures in the elderly.

Malabsorption of Vitamin D

Most vitamin D is absorbed in the duodenum, so malabsorption is particularly likely if the duodenum has been by-passed. Bile salts are necessary for vitamin D absorption, so malabsorption of vitamin D is likely after prolonged biliary stasis or in the stagnant loop situation where bile salts are excessively deconjugated.

Defective Production of the Metabolites of Vitamin D (see p. 523)

Vitamin D Resistance (see p. 532)

OSTEOPOROSIS

Osteoporosis refers to the condition in which the collagen matrix of bone is reduced while the size of the bone remains normal. Along with a reduction in collagen there is also a reduction in the amount of bone salt. The biochemical structure of the bone matrix collagen and polysaccharides in osteoporosis are probably normal.

There are three principal types of osteoporosis:

1. Senile
2. Idiopathic juvenile
3. Secondary.

With increasing age there is generalised reduction in bone collagen and hence an increased incidence of osteoporosis. However, there is a group of patients who appear to have an accelerated and even localised form of the disease. In both forms the main symptoms are bone fractures, bone pain and loss of height. In the absence of these symptoms, which occur relatively late in the progression of the disease, the real problem lies in detecting the disorder before it has caused symptoms, particularly because at least 50 per cent of the bone mass must be lost before there is any demonstrable change in the density of the bones on x-ray.

There are available methods of refining the detection of osteoporosis in a preclinical stage, although there is yet no convincing evidence that any useful purpose is served by large-scale screening programmes to detect the asymptomatic disease.

Methods of detecting preclinical osteoporosis:

1. Presence of unsuspected crush fractures of vertebrae (these are not always painful).

2. Thinning and reduction in trabecular pattern of bones—usually the vertebrae and femoral necks are the most common sites.

3. Sophisticated bone densitometry using known standards of bone density.

4. Cortical thickness indices; there is always a reduction in the cortical thickness of the bones in osteoporosis but this is not always easy to measure and is complicated by the fact that the cortical thickness depends on the height of the patient (and therefore the length of the long bones). Nevertheless there are available percentile charts for indices of cortical thickness related to the length of the bone which indicate whether at a given age the cortical thickness index falls within the normal range. The two commonest sites for measuring the cortical thickness are the right second metacarpal and the midpoint of the femur. There are other indices which measure the biconcavity of the vertebrae by comparing the height of the outside of the lumbar vertebrae with the height of the centre of the bone.

5. Bone biopsy.

It is usually part of the definition of osteoporosis that there are no detectable biochemical abnormalities such as abnormal serum calcium, phosphorus or alkaline phosphatase levels, or urinary levels of calcium or hydroxyproline. By and large this is true, but it is most important to remember that a recent fracture (even an asymptomatic crush fracture) may cause a rise in serum alkaline phosphatase which may remain elevated until the fracture heals; also immobilisation (such as may occur with severe pain or fracture) may cause a negative calcium balance, so that 24-hour urinary calcium excretion may appear to be abnormally high. Calcium absorption may be reduced in juvenile idiopathic osteoporosis and there is a statistical tendency in a series of women for the serum calcium and the 24-hour urinary calcium to be higher after the menopause compared with premenopausal levels. There is now convincing evidence that in women, senile osteoporosis begins at around the age of the menopause. Administered oestrogens can reduce the serum levels and urinary calcium excretion and delay the onset of osteoporosis. In tissue culture oestrogens block the action of parathyroid hormone on bone, and also postmenopausal osteoporosis is rare in hypoparathyroidism. These pieces of evidence suggest that postmenopausal osteoporosis is at least partially due to the increased action of parathyroid hormone on bone due to the absence of the protective effect of gonadal hormones. Nordin (1973) suggests that after the menopause most of the bone resorption occurs at night, because calcium levels tend to fall at night and so slightly stimulate the parathyroids. It is also suggested that in the elderly, minor and undetectable states of subclinical vitamin D deficiency are common, and that conversion of vitamin D to its active metabolites may also be impaired in old age.

Other factors in the pathogenesis of osteoporosis may be fluoride deficiency, and a high-protein diet which produces a mild acidosis that is partly buffered by bone minerals, which are thereby depleted.

Management of Osteoporosis

One important rule in the management of osteoporosis is to avoid immobilisation and bed rest even if pain is quite severe. In the acute juvenile form of osteoporosis the symptoms and probably the whole disease process are episodic. Careful and continuous follow-up of cases of osteoporosis are necessary to detect the exacerbations.

All cases of symptomatic osteoporosis should have a series of 24-hour urinary calcium levels done and if there is evidence of excessive calcium excretion it is reasonable to try to reduce calcium excretion with a thiazide diuretic and phosphorus supplement. If urine calcium excretion is low it is reasonable to try to increase calcium absorption from the gut by giving a calcium supplement and small dose of vitamin D (0·25 mg/day, i.e. 10 000 iu). Once the urine calcium excretion has either risen to or fallen to the normal range it is probably wise to stop any calcium or phosphorus supplements and any vitamin D after about 3 months. There is now good evidence that vitamin D or 1 alpha OH D_3 with ethinyloestradiol (or norethisterone if oestrogens are contra-indicated) will prevent the bone loss in postmenopausal women (Nordin et al, 1980).

Secondary Osteoporosis

It should not be forgotten that like hypertension the secondary causes of osteoporosis must be looked for because, although rare, most of them are treatable.
Causes of secondary osteoporosis:

Partial gastrectomy	Hyperthyroidism
Malabsorption	Liver disease
Cushing's disease	Scurvy
Hypogonadism	Mast cell disease (urticaria pig-
Acromegaly	mentosa).

HYPOCALCAEMIA

The main symptom of hypocalcaemia is tetany. The level of total calcium at which tetany occurs is extremely variable—some individuals can tolerate only a small fall in serum calcium; in others a much larger fall occurs before tetany develops. The development of tetany depends on the level of ionised calcium.

Hypocalcaemia may produce a wide variety of clinical features, which include papilloedema and benign intracranial hypertension, epilepsy, "asthma" (due to laryngeal stridor), dementia, depression, dry skin, psoriasis, "pins and needles", constipation and moniliasis. The main causes of hypocalcaemia are:

Hypoparathyroidism
Vitamin D deficiency (nutritional or malabsorption)
Uraemic bone disease
Acute pancreatitis
Alkalosis
Renal tubular disorders and relative resistance to vitamin D
Hypomagnesaemia
Anticonvulsant therapy
Obstructive jaundice
Medullary carcinoma of the thyroid.

HYPOPARATHYROIDISM

In hypoparathyroidism there is deficient secretion of parathyroid hormone which leads to hypocalcaemia and a raised serum phosphorus. Idiopathic hypoparathyroidism may be associated with pernicious anaemia, Addison's disease and malabsorption. Moniliasis appears most frequently in this variety of hypoparathyroidism.

A proportion of patients with idiopathic hypoparathyroidism have skeletal abnormalities which are not related to the hypocalcaemia, e.g. irregular length of the fingers, soft-tissue calcification, short stature and tooth defects. These patients also have the biochemical abnormalities of hypoparathyroidism which, however, do not respond to injected parathyroid hormone; there is considered to be "end-organ resistance" to parathyroid hormone. This condition is called pseudo-hypoparathyroidism. A small number of patients have the same skeletal abnormalities without the biochemical disturbances—these patients are said to have pseudo pseudohypoparathyroidism. These conditions associated with skeletal abnormalities are much more frequently inherited than is idiopathic hypoparathyroidism.

The incidence of secondary hypoparathyroidism following thyroid surgery is low, but the reported incidences vary very much and several reputable authors have quoted incidences of up to 50 per cent—to some extent the incidence will depend on the criteria for hypoparathyroidism and the methods of assessment. Hypoparathyroidism has also been described following radioactive iodine therapy for hyperthyroidism. The treatment of hypoparathyroidism should be with dihydrotachysterol (DHT), which is an analogue of vitamin D and requires hydroxylation in the liver, but not in the kidney. It is suggested that calcium supplements may also increase the serum calcium in some patients with hypoparathyroidism and they are worth trying in an individual patient. DHT has the great advantage over vitamin D that it is much shorter acting, so that when it is stopped the toxic effects wear off much sooner.

RENAL TUBULAR DISORDERS

Disordered function of the renal tubules is commoner than is generally appreciated. Nearly all forms of acute or chronic renal damage produce impairment of tubular functions, the most familiar being failure of water reabsorption in pyelitis and failure of sodium and chloride reabsorption in chronic renal failure. The functional defects associated with damage to the tubules will obviously relate to the normal functions of the tubules, which are:

Reabsorption of calcium and phosphorus
Reabsorption of glucose
Reabsorption of some amino acids
Excretion of potassium
Excretion of hydrogen ion as ammonia, carbonic acid and dihydrogen sodium phosphate.

It follows therefore that the features of renal tubular disorders will be related to any of the following:

Hypocalcaemia and hypophosphataemia
Glycosuria
Aminoaciduria
Hypokalaemia
Retention of hydrogen ion (acidosis).

Some of the tubular disorders are due to widespread damage from a toxic substance, either endogenous or exogenous. When tubular damage is due to a toxin, all tubular functions are likely to be impaired, although often to a varying degree. Isolated or single disorders of tubular function occur usually as a hereditary disorder which affects only one or only a few of the enzymes involved in the transporting of a substance normally reabsorbed or excreted. The name "Fanconi syndrome" is applied to the *generalised* disorders of tubular function; in the Fanconi syndrome there is a generalised aminoaciduria because most or all the transport enzymes will be affected. Other forms of aminoaciduria occur either because there is an overproduction and hence high blood levels of an amino acid, e.g. phenylalanine, or because there is an isolated defect of one enzyme system responsible for reabsorption of one amino acid (e.g. cystinuria).

Causes of Fanconi Syndrome

Cystinosis
Wilson's disease
Myelomatosis
Cadmium poisoning
Ingestion of degraded tetracycline
Glycogen storage disease
Lead poisoning
Neurofibromatosis and other benign fibromas of mesenchymal origin.

Besides the generalised tubular disorders there are a number of important disorders producing isolated tubular defects. The most important are:

Hypophosphataemic osteomalacia (excess loss of phosphorus)
Cystinuria (failure to reabsorb cystine and certain related amino acids)
Renal tubular acidosis (failure to excrete hydrogen ion).

Hypophosphataemic Osteomalacia

This condition occurs in two forms—one presents in childhood and is inherited, the other occurs in adult life and is sporadic. The inheritance of the childhood type is unusual in that it is inherited as an X-linked dominant, which means that a female carrier may pass the disease to half her sons and half her daughters and that a male carrier may pass the disease to all his daughters but none of his sons. Males tend to have the disease more severely than females. A male patient must have inherited the condition from his mother. A female patient is theoretically twice as likely to have inherited from her father as from her mother. The childhood form of the disease may remit spontaneously and re-occur later in life; however when this happens the stigmata of childhood rickets are always present. There are other differences between the sporadic adult type and the inherited childhood type (Dent and Stamp, 1971); for example, in the adult type the vertebrae appear to be much more severely affected by the osteomalacia, the myopathy is much more severe, and frequently there is glycinuria. It is an important distinction because the adult type requires large doses of phosphate in addition to vitamin D, whereas the childhood type does not require phosphate supplements.

The relative phosphaturia and hypophosphataemia result in rickets or osteomalacia. Unlike nutritional rickets, in which there is nearly always radiological evidence of healing followed by relapses, the rickets of hypophosphataemia is constant. The disease usually remits in the teens although hypophosphataemia remains. Other members of the family may have hypophosphataemia or mildly raised alkaline phosphatase without having any other stigmata of the disease.

Cystinuria (see section on Renal Calculi, p. 537)

RENAL TUBULAR ACIDOSIS (RTA)

RTA is a cause of osteomalacia as well as renal calculi and nephrocalcinosis. The basic defect is an inability to excrete hydrogen ion. There is a tendency to excrete potassium instead of hydrogen ion, which leads to hypokalaemia and muscle weakness. The rickets and osteomalacia are probably due to a combination of hypophosphataemia, acidosis and hypercalciuria, which leads to hypocalcaemia and secondary hyperparathyroidism. This tends to cause phosphaturia in addition to the inherent tubular defect of phosphorus reabsorption.

Diagnosis of RTA

The condition should be considered in all cases of acidosis, nephrocalcinosis, renal calculi, hypokalaemia and osteomalacia. In the severe form there will be acidosis in the presence of alkaline urine; however the commonest variety ("incomplete RTA") does not have an acidosis unless the patient is given an acid load. This form can be detected by the short acid load test of Wrong and Davies (1959).

Varieties of RTA

The body, as a result of metabolism, produces about 2000 mEq per day of hydrogen ion. Most of this is excreted by forming carbonic acid which then forms CO_2 and water and is eliminated by the lungs. However about 70 mEq/day of hydrogen is excreted by the kidneys. This happens in three ways:

1. Formation of NaH_2PO_4 from Na_2HPO_4
2. Formation of HCO_3 some of which is excreted and some reabsorbed
3. Formation of ammonia (NH_3).

The formation of ammonia is relatively fixed and is small at a urine pH around 7·4; it is higher at a lower urine pH. Around pH 6·5–7·4 hydrogen is predominantly excreted as phosphate; above 7·4 hydrogen ion is excreted mainly as bicarbonate. At lower urine pH there is little or no bicarbonate in the urine.

There are three ways in which the body may fail to eliminate hydrogen ion and in which the urine will be inappropriately alkaline when it should be acid.

1. Hydrogen ion release by tubular cells may be limited by the relative concentration of hydrogen ion in the cells and tubular lumen ("gradient failure").
2. Hydrogen ion release from tubular cells may be too slow ("rate failure").
3. Ammonia production may be reduced (in this type the urine may be acid but ammonia production at lower urine pH is reduced. Normally at low urine pH ammonia production is high). This type is diagnosed by finding a low urine ammonia.

Hydrogen ion *gradient* failure is known as Type I RTA; this disorder affects mainly the distal renal tubule. In this type the urine pH is fixed (because of the failure of hydrogen ion excretion), there is acidosis and hence a low plasma bicarbonate. However, if the plasma bicarbonate is raised by infusion of bicarbonate the pH of the urine will rise, i.e. become more alkaline as more bicarbonate passes into the urine.

Hydrogen ion *rate* failure affects mainly the proximal tubule and the rate of hydrogen ion production is so slow that bicarbonate in the tubule is not neutralised and consequently is "wasted" and lost from the body. The urine pH is therefore high (alkaline) because it contains an excess of bicarbonate. However if the body is made very acidotic so that plasma bicarbonate falls and production of bicarbonate by the proximal tubule also falls, no excess bicarbonate appears in the urine; thus at very low plasma pH levels the urine can be acidified in the Proximal type of RTA whereas in the Distal type of RTA the urine cannot be acidified no matter how severe the acidosis. Also in the Proximal type of RTA more bicarbonate than normal appears in the urine at all levels of plasma bicarbonate, i.e. hydrogen ion *rate* failure RTA is synonymous with "bicarbonate wastage".

Congenital RTA is generally Type I. It is commoner in women and presents in childhood with rickets, nephrocalcinosis, renal calculi, hypokalaemia and muscle weakness.

Acquired RTA is generally a mixture of Types I and II, although occasionally it is Type II only. The causes of acquired RTA are:

Renal calculi	Heavy-metal poisoning
Pyelonephritis	Outdated tetracycline
Myeloma	Amphotericin B nephropathy.
Hypergammaglobulinaemia	

The main complications of RTA are:

Osteomalacia (due to phosphaturia and hypophosphataemia, secondary hyperparathyroidism and acidosis).

Nephrocalcinosis or renal calculi (due to hypercalciuria, hyper-phosphaturia and alkaline urine). There is a predisposition to urinary infection which may of course make the RTA worse. The renal stones which form may be triple phosphate stones (due to the urinary infection), calcium phosphate stones, or a mixture of these. In all cases of renal stone formation or nephrocalcinosis it is always worth looking for a complete or incomplete acidification defect of the urine. One of the main pitfalls in the diagnosis of incomplete RTA is the presence of urinary infection with urea-splitting organisms, which produce ammonia and so may keep the urine alkaline despite adequate acidification by the tubules. It is therefore important to eliminate urinary tract infection before testing for RTA. It is also important to check plasma bicarbonate levels during the ammonium chloride acid load test to ensure that the plasma bicarbonate levels have been lowered sufficiently.

Treatment of RTA

The main treatment is with alkalis (sodium and potassium bicar-bonate); this may heal the osteomalacia, but usually vitamin D is required as well. The main danger of alkaline treatment is that the urine will be made more alkaline and so encourage renal infection and stone formation. The hypokalaemia and sodium depletion (if any) can be corrected with supplements.

RENAL CALCULI

Renal calculi consist either of relatively pure substances or mixtures of salts. Pure stones are generally due to a specific and recognisable disorder—unfortunately pure stones are the exception and the main problem with renal stones is to decide whether they are metabolic stones or whether they are due to infection or obstruction. The pure or metabolic stones with a rough indication of their percentage frequency of all stones are:

Calcium oxalate	(12 per cent)
Cystine	(3 per cent)
Uric acid	(3 per cent).

Stones which contain magnesium ammonium phosphate are almost always due to infection and most of these also contain varying amounts of calcium phosphate and calcium oxalate (triple phosphate stones). This group accounts for about 25 per cent of renal stones in this country.

The largest single group of stones (roughly a half) are those which contain a mixture of calcium phosphate and calcium oxalate. From a diagnostic point of view it is this group which provides the real problems because infection may be present coincidentally even though the stones are "metabolic" in origin. Hyperparathyroidism characteristically causes calcium phosphate (and calcium oxalate) stones although hyperparathyroidism in fact accounts for only about 5 per cent of renal calculi (about 15 per cent of recurrent calculi). A small proportion of stones consist of calcium oxalate but pure calcium phosphate stones are rare. Calcium phosphate is nearly always present either with calcium oxalate or magnesium ammonium phosphate.

Causes of Renal Calculi

Pure stones   (i) Uric acid
                  (ii) Hyperoxaluria
                  (iii) Cystinuria

Mixed stones   (i) Infection
(non-metabolic) (ii) Obstruction

Mixed stones   (i) Hypercalciuria due to hypercalcaemia
(metabolic)   hyperparathyroidism
                    vitamin D excess
                    sarcoidosis
                    immobilisation
                    milk alkali syndrome
                    carcinoma
                    hyperthyroidism
              (ii) Idiopathic hypercalciuria (largest single group)
            (iii) Renal tubular acidosis
           (iv) Medullary sponge kidney
            (v) Bowel disease (ulcerative colitis, ileostomies).

Some Factors in the Pathogenesis of Mixed Metabolic Stones

Calcium oxalate excretion in the urine is very nearly enough to cause a saturated solution, so it is not surprising that any tendency to dehydration and low urine volume will produce stones consisting mainly of calcium oxalate. Calcium phosphate tends to precipitate in an alkaline solution, hence calcium phosphate stones (with some calcium oxalate) will tend to occur in an alkaline urine (infection, RTA and other tubular disorders). In the absence of any obvious metabolic cause there must be other factors predisposing to renal stone formation; after all, the majority of renal stones occur in the absence of any infective or metabolic cause. Other proposed mechanisms are:

Excess of nucleating substances. All stones contain a matrix consisting of mucoproteins—mucopolysaccharides which *in vitro* encourage precipitation of calcium salts.

Lack of an inhibitor to stone formation. Known inhibitors of crystal aggregation and accretion are pyrophosphate, cations (magnesium, zinc, etc) and polysaccharide inhibitor.

Uric Acid Stones

The most important factor in the formation of urate stones is an acid urine. Not all uric acid stone formers have hyperuricosuria. There appears to be a deficiency of ammonia production in many uric acid stone formers. Uric acid stones also occur in patients with leukaemia and polycythaemia, particularly if there is a rapid response to antimitotic drugs. The treatment of uric acid stones is high fluid intake combined with alkalis (sodium bicarbonate 10g/day). At pH 7·0 uric acid is nearly 20 times as soluble as at pH 5.

Xanthine stones occasionally occur, particularly in the rare inborn error of metabolism called xanthinuria. It is theoretically possible that the drug allopurinol, which is a xanthine oxidase inhibitor, could lead to xanthine stones by causing an accumulation of xanthine.

Pure Oxalate Stones

These usually occur in primary hyperoxaluria, which is a rare and serious inborn error of metabolism associated with oxalate deposition in all the tissues of the body. It is usually fatal in childhood but more adult cases are being discovered.

Cystine Stones

Cystinuria is a tubular disorder in which there is a defect in reabsorption of cystine and the other related amino acids (lysine, arginine and ornithine). Cystine precipitates in an acid and concentrated urine. The treatment therefore consists of giving enough fluid (particularly at night) to keep the urine volume high. This will then prevent cystine stones forming and also dissolve any which are present. Cystine stones are not so radio-opaque as calcium-containing stones but if they are over 1 cm in diameter they can normally be seen on abdominal x-ray. The disease shows two forms of inheritance—recessive and incompletely recessive. In both forms the homozygotes have a high urinary cystine excretion whereas in the completely recessive form the heterozygotes have a normal cystine excretion and in the incompletely recessive form the heterozygotes have intermediate levels of cystine excretion. The same enzyme defect is present in the gut as in the renal tubule, so there is also a failure to absorb these amino acids from the gut.

Idiopathic Hypercalciuria

This is probably the most common single cause of metabolic renal stones and of nephrocalcinosis. Most normal people only absorb as much calcium from the diet as they need. Patients with idiopathic hypercalciuria absorb much more calcium from the diet than they need and the excess is excreted in the urine. When testing for the condition it is important to ensure that the patient is on a diet which contains enough calcium. If the dietary calcium is low even patients with idiopathic hypercalciuria may not excrete more than 300 mg calcium per 24 hours. Peaks of calcium oxalate excretion during the 24 hours are probably the initiating factors in stone formation in idiopathic hypercalciuria. The condition is much commoner in men and appears to become less frequent with increasing age. Treatment is with a low-calcium diet together with cellulose phosphate.

Renal Stones in Gut Disorders

Urate stones are liable to occur in patients with ileostomies and ulcerative colitis. All the reasons are not known, but dehydration and low urine sodium excretion are partly responsible. Some patients with ileal dysfunction may form oxalate stones; this is probably because bile salts are not reabsorbed in the terminal ileum and, together with the glycine to which they are conjugated, they pass into the large gut where bacterial action removes the glycine which is then absorbed and excreted as oxalate. Normally bile salts are conjugated to taurine and not glycine, but because of failure to reabsorb bile salts most taurine is lost from the body and the liver only has a limited ability to produce taurine. Change in pH of the intestines also promotes glycine rather than taurine conjugation.

Management of Renal Stones

It is obviously essential that any stone or gravel passed should be examined—preferably by x-ray defraction crystallography. It may be necessary for stone formers always to pass urine through a net filter in order to have a specimen of the stone for examination. Any stone which contains triple phosphate is related to infection, but whether this is primary or secondary will have to be determined. It is obviously important to measure 24-hour urine excretion of uric acid, calcium oxalate and cystine as well as amino-acid chromatography of the urine. All the causes of hypercalcaemia and hypercalciuria should be excluded. Measuring the pH of the urine is important and if the urine is persistently alkaline in the absence of infection, RTA should be excluded. It may also be necessary to test for other tubular disorders or evidence of tubular dysfunction; still the best screening test for tubular dysfunction is the urine concentration and dilution test.

Treatment of Mixed Metabolic Stones

Encourage high fluid intake.

Low calcium intake particularly in idiopathic hypercalciuria. It may be necessary for the patient to have a water softener. Cellulose phosphate will reduce calcium absorption and also increase urinary phosphate excretion.

If the stones contain a high proportion of calcium phosphate a reduced phosphate intake may be indicated. This can be achieved by giving aluminium hydroxide (Aludrox), which binds phosphorus in the gut.

If the stones contain a high proportion of oxalate a low-oxalate diet may be indicated.

Alkalis will obviously be indicated for the treatment of renal tubular acidosis and urate stones although in RTA care should be taken not to make the urine too alkaline.

Magnesium salts (magnesium oxide) have been found to be effective in some series.

Thiazide diuretics reduce urinary calcium excretion.

Nephrocalcinosis

This tends to be either cortical or medullary. Cortical calcium deposition occurs following renal cortical necrosis and sometimes after glomerulonephritis. Medullary calcium deposition occurs with any of the known causes of hypercalciuria. The medullary nephrocalcinosis of medullary sponge kidney tends to be localised.

MISCELLANEOUS DISORDERS

Magnesium Metabolism

Disturbances of magnesium metabolism play a small but occasionally significant part in disturbances of mineral metabolism. This is not particularly surprising because magnesium is the most abundant intracellular cation after potassium. About half the body magnesium is in the bone, where it is involved in bone crystal architecture, although it is not part of the molecular crystal structure.

Hypomagnesaemia causes tetany, muscular weakness, depression and epilepsy, all of which may also occur with hypocalcaemia. The two sometimes co-exist, particularly in malabsorption syndromes and in the presence of intestinal fistulae. The hypocalcaemia may not respond to vitamin D treatment until the hypomagnesaemia has been corrected. Hypomagnesaemia is fairly common in cirrhosis, particularly alcoholic cirrhosis; all the causative factors are not known, but the secondary aldosteronism and high gut ammonia probably play a part. The excess ammonia in the gut precipitates magnesium as insoluble magnesium ammonium phosphate, preventing its absorption. The same phenomenon is seen in cattle fed on grass that has been fertilised with ammonium fertilisers; the resulting tetany is referred to as "grass staggers".

Serum magnesium may also be reduced in renal tubular disorders, although in glomerular failure hypermagnesaemia occurs. There are now several reports of low magnesium excretion in some recurrent stone formers as well as reports of beneficial results in reducing stone formation by increasing magnesium intake. Magnesium excess produces muscle weakness, leading eventually to peripheral and central nervous system depression and anaesthesia. Vasodilatation also occurs.

The Significance of Calcitonin

Calcitonin is a calcium-lowering hormone produced by the C cells of the thyroid gland. It is, however, doubtful whether calcitonin plays a major part in normal calcium homeostasis. The only known disorder of calcitonin production is excess output due to medullary carcinoma of the thyroid, but even in this condition, when calcitonin levels may be several hundred times the normal range, no disorder of serum or urinary calcium occurs. Medullary carcinoma of the thyroid may be a familial disorder and is sometimes associated with phaeochromocytoma and parathyroid adenoma.

The main use of calcitonin is in the treatment of Paget's disease. The indications for treatment are: bone pain, hypercalcaemia, rapidly increasing bone deformity and increasing neurological compression due to the disease. Treatment has to be given by injection and has to be continued for at least six months. It is important to monitor the effects of treatment by sequential measurements of urinary hydroxyproline, serum alkaline phosphatase and serum calcium, particularly if this was elevated originally.

Diphosphonates

Diphosphonates are compounds which resemble pyrophosphate except that they are not susceptible to the action of the phosphatase enzymes in the body. They have many of the other properties of pyrophosphate and they can become bound to bone hydroxyapatite crystals; if they do, the crystals cannot be dissolved by normal phosphatase enzymes. Diphosphonates may thus inhibit bone resorption and in higher doses they also inhibit bone mineralisation. They have therefore been used in a variety of conditions, including Paget's disease, in which prevention of mineralisation is likely to be beneficial. As diphosphonates become generally available they are likely to find a definite role in some disorders of mineral metabolism, including Paget's disease; they are effective when given by mouth.

REFERENCES

DENT, C. E. (1962). *Brit. med. J.*, **3**, 1419 and 1495.
DENT, C. E. and STAMP, T. C. (1971). *Quart. J. Med.*, **40**, 303.
NORDIN, B. E. (1973). *Metabolic Bone & Stone Disease*. Edinburgh: Churchill Livingstone.
NORDIN, B. E., HORSMAN, A., CRILLY, R. G., MARSHALL, D. H. and SIMPSON, M. (1980). *Brit. med. J.*, **1**, 451.
PATTERSON, C. R. (1974). *Metabolic Disorders of Bone*, Oxford: Blackwell Scientific Publications.
WRONG, O. W. and DAVIES, H. E. (1959). *Quart. J. Med.*, **28**, 259.

INDEX OF EPONYMS

(Figures refer to Chapter and Note number.)

INDEX